BOTANICAL MEDICINE

FROM BENCH TO BEDSIDE

BOTANICAL MEDICINE

FROM BENCH TO BEDSIDE

Editors: Raymond Cooper, Ph.D. and Fredi Kronenberg, Ph.D.

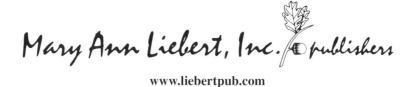

Mary Ann Liebert, Inc. publishers

www.liebertpub.com

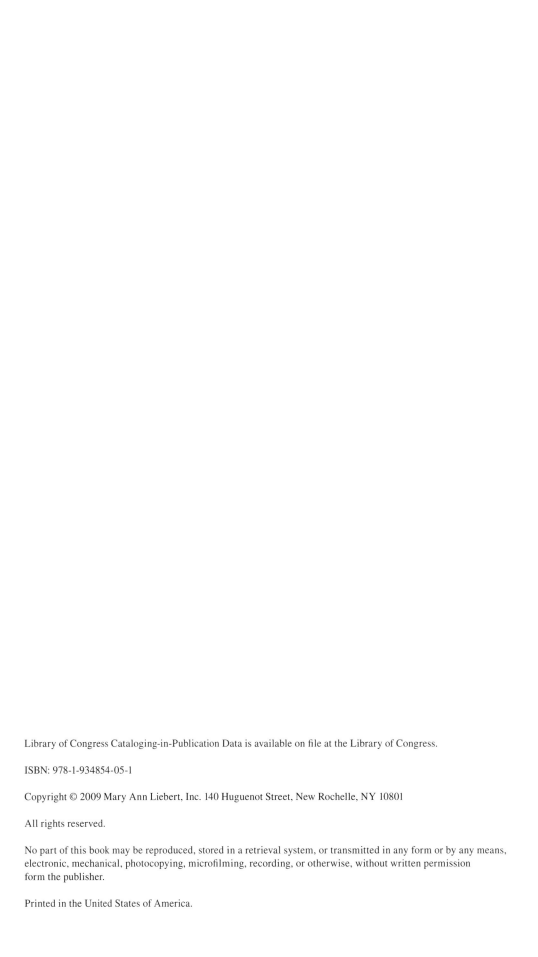

Library of Congress Cataloging-in-Publication Data is available on file at the Library of Congress.

ISBN: 978-1-934854-05-1

Copyright © 2009 Mary Ann Liebert, Inc. 140 Huguenot Street, New Rochelle, NY 10801

Printed in the United States of America.

CONTENTS

FOREWORD

The editors have produced a valuable book that will serve the broad community of researchers who seek to conduct scientifically sound research on botanicals used for medicinal purposes. The content evolved from an American Society of Pharmacognosy workshop titled "Clinical Pharmacognosy: Contribution of Pharmacognosy to Clinical Trials of Botanicals and Dietary Supplements" and highlights some of the best quality research, the complexities of studying botanical extracts, and potential pitfalls and challenges of searching for active compounds.

The book contains authoritative chapters, ranging from how to ensure quality products through to clinical aspects of widely used and emerging botanical medicines. The topics and particular botanicals chosen are illustrative of the detailed examination and knowledge needed to take an herb from the field to the phytochemistry laboratory, to a clinically useful product. It is important, given significant marketing spin in product advertising, labels, and Internet sites, that the book as a compilation, enables the reader to see the links between the extracting methods, the design of basic scientific studies, and the questions asked in a clinical trial, based on scientific rationale, as well as documented use.

Data are succinctly presented and include multicomponent interactions; detailed pharmacology; mechanisms of action, safety and toxicology; and exemplify issues to take into consideration when conducting research or reading scientific papers on botanicals.

Organized into three sections—selection and quality of botanical preparations, preclinical and clinical approaches, and a practitioner's view of the challenges for those interested in exploring botanical preparations—this book is, to the best of my knowledge, the first to address all three of these subject areas under the same cover. This book enables clinical researchers to appreciate the unique challenges of researching herbal products, and basic scientists and developers of the final products to be cognizant of what is relevant to clinicians who seek to guide patients on the choice and use of herbal products. It is important to understand the biological activity for a particular indication, which would lead to more informed and productive clinical trials. This approach will facilitate the development of effective dosing and should reduce the ambiguity created by multiple clinical trials of the "same" product with different intended outcomes. This book is valuable for anyone seeking to understand the intricacies of researching botanical medicines.

More than twenty scientific contributors have prepared chapters based on their own expertise and experience, or from detailed analyses of the literature. The editors, Drs. Ray Cooper and Fredi Kronenberg, should be congratulated for bringing together such a diverse group of contributors with such high expertise with the goal of facilitating high-quality botanical research.

NORMAN R. FARNSWORTH, PH.D.

CONTRIBUTORS

Vladimir Badmaev, M.D., Ph.D.
Sabinsa Corporation
Piscataway, New Jersey

Marilyn Barrett, Ph.D.
Pharmacognosy Consulting
Mill Valley, California

Gina B. Benson, B.S.
Nature's Sunshine Products
Spanish Fork, Utah

Veronika Butterweck, Ph.D.
College of Pharmacy
Department of Pharmaceutics
University of Florida
Gainesville, Florida

Raymond Cooper, Ph.D.
Novus International Inc.
St. Charles, Missouri

Steven Dentali, Ph.D.
American Herbal Products Association
Silver Spring, Maryland

Joseph L. Evans, Ph.D.
JERIKA Research Foundation
Redwood City, California

Norman R. Farnsworth, Ph.D.
College of Pharmacy
University of Illinois at Chicago
Chicago, Illinois

James W. Forsythe, M.D.
Cancer Screening and Treatment Center of
    Nevada
Reno, Nevada

Amy B. Howell, Ph.D.
Marucci Center for Blueberry Cranberry
    Research
Rutgers University
Chatsworth, New Jersey

Uwe Koetter, Ph.D.
Dr. Koetter Consulting
Uttwil, Switzerland

Fredi Kronenberg, Ph.D.
New York Botanical Garden
Bronx, New York

Arizona Center for Integrative Medicine
College of Medicine
University of Arizona
Tucson, Arizona

Tieraona Low Dog, M.D.
Arizona Center for Integrative Medicine
University of Arizona Health Sciences Center
Tucson, Arizona

Jerry L. McLaughlin, Ph.D.
Department of Medicinal Chemistry and
    Molecular Pharmacology
School of Pharmacy and Pharmaceutical
    Sciences
Purdue University
West Lafayette, Indiana

Irmgard Merfort, Ph.D.
Institute of Pharmaceutical Sciences
University of Freiburg
Freiburg, Germany

Christina L. Nance, Ph.D.
Department of Pediatrics
Baylor College of Medicine
Houston, Texas

Jess D. Reed, Ph.D.
Department of Animal Sciences
University of Wisconsin
Madison, Wisconsin

Juliane Reuter, M.D.
Competence Center Skintegral
Department of Dermatology
University Medical Center Freiburg
Freiburg, Germany

Christoph M. Schempp, M.D., Ph.D.
Competence Center Skintegral
Department of Dermatology
University Medical Center Freiburg
Freiburg, Germany

Günter Seelinger, Ph.D.
Medical and Pharmaceutical Services
Berlin, Germany

William T. Shearer, M.D.
Department of Pediatrics
Baylor College of Medicine
Houston, Texas

Michael S. Tempesta, Ph.D.
Phenolics LLC
El Granada, California

Tad A. Turgeon, B.S.
Nature's Sunshine Products
Spanish Fork, Utah

Bettina Vinson, Ph.D.
Department of Clinical Research
Steigerwald Arzneimittelwerk GmbH
Darmstadt, Germany

Ute Wölfle, Ph.D.
Competence Center Skintegral
Department of Dermatology
University Medical Center Freiburg
Freiburg, Germany

INTRODUCTION

Plants have been used for medicinal purposes across history and cultures and even across species. Over the past several decades, scientific literature, popular media articles on adverse drug effects, and an increased interest in natural products by the general public have helped fuel a greater scientific awareness of botanical medicine.

A majority of the world still relies heavily on herbal remedies for their primary health care. With the increasing movement of people across countries, there is an accompanying movement of their respective traditional medicines. While globalization of medicine has typically been thought of as being the movement of Western medicine to developing countries, there is now, in China, for example, significant discussion of the "globalization of traditional Chinese medicine" and discussion of how to improve the quality of Chinese medicinal products and interest in developing a body of research evidence for their effectiveness. This is particularly relevant given the establishment of traditional Chinese medicine programs and practitioners around the world. The interest in traditional herbal medicines has also contributed to a resurgence of interest in Western herbal medicine (natural products), particularly in the United States and Europe, and a desire for information about its safety and efficacy.

Further, as societies have improved methods for treating acute medical problems and have improved public health measures, there is now greater attention on the chronic illnesses that are beginning to consume a significant portion of health care budgets, particularly in the face of an aging world population. Some chronic illnesses may be ameliorated, and the search for natural means of optimizing the health of aging populations may be facilitated through the use of botanical remedies. Yet, some of the top-selling dietary supplements, although popular with the consumer, do not possess sufficient scientific data to support their intended use.

Botanical Medicine: From Bench to Bedside is based loosely on the workshop "Clinical Pharmacognosy: Contribution of Pharmacognosy to Clinical Trials of Botanicals and Dietary Supplements" held at the American Society of Pharmacognosy (ASP) Meeting in Portland, Maine. The book offers chapters by leaders in the field from academe and industry that address critical issues facing the field of botanical medicine. These include the challenges of conducting sound scientific studies of botanicals: from the sourcing of appropriate products to details on the preparation of the products and understanding the types of scientific inquiry that will advance this field. This discussion also includes challenges to the dietary supplement industry to continue to improve the quality of botanical products and to increase the industry's commitment to facilitating the collection of data that will provide the evidence base for the safety and effectiveness of the products being produced. This will reassure current consumers and health care providers and bring into the user group clinicians and a wider public who all seek treatments that are safe and effective and that have the fewest side effects possible.

Pharmacognosy, commonly referred to as the pharmacology of natural products, derives from two Greek words, *pharmakon*, or drug, and *gnosis*, or knowledge. Its scope includes the study of the physical, chemical, biochemical, and biological properties of drugs, drug substances, or potential drugs or drug substances of natural origin as well as the search for new drugs from natural sources. Research in pharmacognosy often includes studies in the areas of phytochemistry, microbial chemistry, biosynthesis, biotransformation, chemotaxonomy, and other biological and chemical sciences.

The role of pharmacognosy in furthering the quality of botanical preparations and the quality of clinical research is evident throughout. Examples are provided of high-quality scientific research required to achieve higher-quality preclinical and clinical studies of herbal preparations and better-quality herbal products. Topics in the book were chosen to illustrate many of the issues and a variety of scientific approaches that address the challenges in botanical research.

As the number of studies increases, there is increased concern over the quality and specific composition of botanical preparations that are tested in clinical trials, because the manufacture of poor-quality product may contribute to ambiguous, incorrect, or nonreproducible results. The quality of the outcome is only as good as the quality of the product used. This is true for preclinical and clinical research alike.

For example, several preparations of St. John's wort used in earlier research studies were based on levels of hypericin; valerian extracts were based on valerenic acids; and the popular echinacea extracts are standardized to echinacosides, alkylamides, or phenolic acids. These compounds may be considered as the plants' respective biomarkers but may not necessarily be the components that are key to any therapeutic effect (1, 2). For many botanical medicines, there is little information, or maybe controversy, about which constituents are the "actives" for particular medical indications. Inconclusive or negative results may be due to the use of extracts with less-than-optimal composition. In the absence of an identified bioactive constituent, at a minimum the extract requires identification of a biomarker for the plant. Dosing also is often insufficiently examined prior to initiating a large-scale clinical trial. Optimally, dose-ranging studies should be conducted on the population to be studied before large clinical trials are undertaken.

The methods used in extraction of the plant material can influence the chemical composition of the resulting extracts and potentially, the biological activity. The more information on the product that is provided in research publications, the greater will be the ability to compare among studies and understand differences in results that may emerge.

This book addresses the characterization of phyto- equivalence/generic herbal issues facing the supplement industry. The preparations must be qualified at all stages of research, and the chapters deal with the following stages: preclinical and clinical studies on botanicals and the safety, efficacy, and dose of botanical preparations. We have chosen as topics either popular botanical preparations—for example, valerian, St. John's wort, and cranberry—or subjects that highlight issues germane to broader questions—for example, Iberogast to highlight analysis of multicomponent mixtures, and chaste tree to highlight challenges facing the health practitioner.

The book is organized into three parts: selection and quality of botanical preparations, preclinical and clinical approaches to botanical preparations, and a practitioner's view of the challenges for those interested in exploring botanical preparations.

Part I addresses how high-quality scientific research, and thus clinically relevant outcomes, depend on a well-characterized product including the accurate identification of the plant and its constituents. Chapter 1 addresses product quality issues, botanical standards, and approaches to characterizing product consistency and stresses the importance of including chemical and biological profiling. Accurate identification of plant content requires a careful analysis (by the company making a product or by another laboratory) of the chosen botanical preparations (intermediate extracts and the end product). Companies providing botanical products for research (or making any product for sale) should be able to provide the researcher with detailed documentation including the plant's Latin botanical name; an authentic voucher specimen; the plant part uscd, collection dates, and geographical collection location; a detailed description of extraction, drying methods, and preparation; a Certificate of Analysis, the extract "fingerprint" and method of analysis; and the manufacturing protocol following the guidelines of the Food and Drug Administration's (FDA) Good Manufacturing Procedures (GMPs). Chapter 1 reviews the information with which everyone conducting botanical research should at least be conversant. It is with high-quality, reproducible research in mind that the National Institutes of Health's (NIH) National Center for Complementary and Alternative Medicine (NCCAM) has issued guidelines for botanical products used in clinical research.

Chapter 2 offers a review and a critical commentary on botanicals chosen for research on controlling blood glucose levels. With diabetes a growing cause of morbidity and mortality for an already large and rapidly growing number of adults and obese children, botanical therapies to control blood glucose levels are gaining attention. While there are antidiabetic pharmaceutical medications that are well studied for lowering blood glucose levels (3), there are traditional herbal remedies for diabetes used in the United States and elsewhere, and some intriguing basic and clinical research is evolving. Chapter 2 describes the extent of the research to date while pointing out the challenges for future research.

Topical botanical preparations are also emerging as more natural approaches for treating various skin ailments. Studies of these products also exemplify how information on traditional use and some knowledge of the mechanism of action of plant constituents guide current research and product development. This research includes products for skin conditions as well as products to meet a growing demand of a large aging population seeking to remain youthful looking. Chapter 3 is a comprehensive review of botanical preparations used for various skin ailments and safety issues regarding the use of these products.

In Part II, we selected botanicals that exemplify ways to address the issue of whole extract versus particular constituents and to study the complexity of herb-drug interactions (St. John's wort) and the painstaking preclinical work necessary to develop a multicomponent herbal mixture (Iberogast). We also present valerian and hops as examples of herbs studied both individually and in combination for the additive properties conferred by different mechanisms of action.

The chapters in Part II offer examples of the rigorous attention to detail that is necessary at the preclinical stage to achieve botanically relevant and appropriately targeted clinical studies. This is not meant to be an exhaustive discussion of well-researched botanicals. Such a list might include, for example, ginkgo and black cohosh, which have been substantively reviewed elsewhere. Rather, we chose to present botanicals perhaps not as often reviewed, such as St. John's wort, paw paw, and cranberry; Iberogast; a standardized curcuminoid extract from the rhizomes of turmeric; and green tea as a therapeutic intervention in HIV-1 infection.

Cranberry, with a long traditional use in folk medicine, was until recent times manufactured as extracts based on the organic acid content. Although it is well known that cranberries contain up to 25–30% organic acids, there was no serious consideration to link the bioactivity related to urinary tract infections to the presence of the proanthocyanidins in cranberries. Chapters 10 and 11 lay out the preclinical and clinical evidence linking these tannin-like compounds with bioactivity, as well as discuss evidence for broader use for cardiovascular and other medical indications.

Even if the active compounds or mode of action is not yet clear for many herbal products, nutraceuticals, and dietary supplements, there is a need to enforce quality standards for these products. Product standards define the consistency of the content, using a chemical constituent or a class of compounds (e.g., a phytochemical marker, using the active principal[s] when known), and offer some quality control over potency and efficacy. It should be noted that standardization to one constituent does not guarantee the levels of other components, does not represent any synergistic effects, does not describe unidentified actives, and is not a description of the plant, its part, or the extraction process.

Information about biological activity, using in vivo studies, ideally will provide information to answer the following questions:

- Is there significant evidence for the intended biological activity or improvement of the condition?
- Does the herbal preparation (active compound if known) reach the biological target within the body in a bioavailable form?
- What are the pharmacokinetics of the product?
- What is the required daily dose for achieving the desired effect or a maximum effect (as this may not be derived only from in vivo studies in animals)?
- How does the efficacy profile of the product change over time (i.e., what are the shelf life attributes of the product)?

Questions related to safety can be addressed in a variety of ways, including animal testing (LD50) and evaluating human safety via clinical trials, establishing postmarketing surveillance, and creating an adverse event reporting (AER) system (see Chapter 6 on Iberogast).

In designing clinical studies on botanicals, it also may be helpful to consider knowledge of prior human experience and traditional use to choose the end point most relevant to the plant's use. This will increase the likelihood of obtaining a reproducible and desired clinical end point. Ancient and traditional ethnomedicines are now often modified from "tea-style" consumption (i.e., a diluted form) to concentrates (powders and tablets) by the modern industry. Accompanying claims of safety based on a long history of use are presumptive, given the new formulations and concentrations not seen in traditional use, and rarely sufficiently studied before marketing.

Finally, in Part III, a perspective from a health practitioner is offered. Currently, many products on store shelves raise significant concerns because of insufficient information and misleading label claims. When independently tested, identification and concentration of the labels' ingredients are often found to not match the claim or reveal inconsistencies from batch to batch. These and other concerns relevant to clinical recommendations are discussed in Chapter 12 on the use of chaste tree extract.

In conclusion, our intent is to present information on the science required to achieve (a) better-quality botanical products; (b) research well designed to match the product to its intended use, to ensure adequate quality control, and to take into consideration the complexities of activities of biological products on biological systems, with the product described adequately to enable reproducibility; and (c) setting clinical end points based on results from historical use or preclinical studies. If we can make a small contribution to this important discussion that will increase the quality of botanical preparations, and thus the quality of research, we may help consumers and manufacturers create safe, effective, and clinically proven botanical medicines.

RAYMOND COOPER, PH.D.
FREDI KRONENBERG, PH.D.

REFERENCES

[1]Mitscher L, Cooper R. Echinacea and immunostimulation: a critical review. In: L Packer, CN Ong, B Halliwell, eds. *Herbal and Traditional Medicine: Molecular Basis of Health.* New York, NY: Marcel Dekker; 2004: 634–664.

[2]Pillai S, Pillai C, Mitscher LA, Cooper R. Use of quantitative flow cytometry to measure ex vivo immunostimulant activity of echinacea: the case for polysaccharides. *J Altern Complement Med.* 2007;13(6): 625–634.

[3]Inzucchi SE. Oral antihyperglycemic therapy for type 2 diabetes. *JAMA.* 2002;287:360–372.

PART I

Botanical Preparations: Selection and Quality Issues

Botanical Medicine: From Bench to Bedside
Edited by R. Cooper and F. Kronenberg
© Mary Ann Liebert, Inc.

Chapter 1

Botanical Preparations: Achieving Quality Products

Steven Dentali

The scientific study of botanical materials for their medicinal properties, squarely in the domain of natural product chemists and ethnobotanists, is once again receiving greater attention from investigators with expertise in clinical and preclinical applied research. However, these latter researchers are not often sufficiently acquainted with botanical preparations to make good choices when choosing them for scientific investigations. They generally have little to no exposure either to botanical research standards or to basic requirements for qualifying botanical study materials. Research on botanical products for therapeutic or dietary supplement applications requires specific knowledge in order to ensure that the materials chosen for scientific study have met appropriate identity and quality specifications. The determination of these specifications (and ensuring that they are met) requires expertise not generally found within the ranks of biomedical researchers.

Historically, herbs have always played a significant role in treating illness or preventing disease. Accepting the effectiveness of well-established traditional botanical use helps explain the wide use of medicinal plants prior to the development of more modern pharmaceutical agents. The challenge now is to understand and employ botanical preparations in the context of our modern medical system in which practitioners are largely uninformed about their use and effective applications (1). Mass manufacturing, distribution, and acceptance of botanical drug standards for safety and efficacy may require clinical trials, for which high-quality, standardized materials must be employed (2). It is also desirable to demonstrate some mode of action in vitro and in vivo in order to identify efficacious and safe dosages and establish consistent results through clinical studies.

Creating an appropriate research team for the study of botanical medicines requires familiarity with issues specific to botanicals. While individual researchers are themselves not likely to produce the materials they will be studying, they should be familiar with these issues so that they will know which questions to ask and whom to consult, in order to obtain the products most appropriate for their research. This chapter reviews ways to choose and qualify botanical products successfully as materials suitable for scientific study. It also presents basic concepts of plant identity, characterization, reasonable chemical consistency,

American Herbal Products Association, Silver Spring, Maryland; sdentali@ahpa.org

"fit-for-purpose" standardization, and standardized reporting of results from clinical trials employing botanical materials.

QUALITY

Quality botanical preparations are achieved through the development of procedures and practices designed to ensure conformity to specifications—the conditions and circumstances under which a consistent, high-quality product is produced. The activities necessary to implement such procedures and practices, including the determination of appropriate specifications, fall within the purview of several disciplines: botany, chemistry, pharmacology, and the one that encompasses all of these, that of pharmacognosy (3).

VOUCHER SPECIMENS

Correctly identifying plant materials may require the acquisition of a reference standard known as a voucher specimen. A *voucher specimen* "is a sample of collected or studied material that serves as permanent documentation of that specific material, and that can be re-examined to confirm the identity and nature of the material from which research results were derived. The essential character of a voucher for medical research is not its form or quality, but that it is material preserved from the same batch as the test material, collected in the same place at the same time. It is essential that the location of vouchers be specified in print" (4). Voucher specimens can be obtained at any stage of processing, such as an initial small amount of bulk material, the dried herb before it is ground to powder, ground material, or a sample of commercial extract, and then stored for possible future re-examination in order to confirm the identity of material from which the study results were derived.

For research that solely focuses on identifying the chemical constituents of a particular botanical through phytochemical analysis, the collection and deposition of a voucher plant specimen into an herbarium are essential. No further identification may be required because the voucher specimen can be reviewed at a later date if there is any question regarding its identity. Standard reference materials, certified reference materials, and other commercially available botanical reference materials have distinct uses, including standards for chemical analysis both as markers of identity and as references from which the analytical method's performance may be evaluated.

REASONABLE CHEMICAL CONSISTENCY

Genetic and environmental factors influence the chemical composition of plants, leaving the possibility that botanical preparations may not be absolutely uniform from batch to batch. With single chemical compounds it is possible to create products that are exactly uniform, with no variations in detail, as is the case for most prescription drugs. Botanical preparations, however, are complex, containing scores of chemical constituents. Expecting the type of uniformity possible with single active ingredients is not a realistic goal when dealing with whole-plant products. The goal, therefore, is to work with material that agrees with or conforms to appropriate specifications within an acceptable range of variation. This approach usually includes conforming to chemical specifications that can help establish minimum quality; however, chemical measurement is not always an absolute requirement for achieving reasonable product consistency and therefore acceptable quality.

The type of product uniformity desired for clinical research depends on the type of study material and its origins. For example, reasonable chemical consistency of an exotic fruit beverage used in clinical research may be ensured by securing juice that is obtained from fruit from the same farms from year to year. A properly stored sample from material of the same harvest as that of the test material may be reasonable enough to achieve future product consistency. If specific biological activities of individual chemicals or chemical classes are to be evaluated, then standardization must include specifications for the chemicals of interest and any other information that helps ensure reasonable chemical consistency of the study material.

Accurate identification of bioactive compounds in this case may begin with a combination of phytochemical, in vitro, and in vivo studies; screening and identifying the highest-yielding species; and selecting the correct plant parts during the optimal growing season in order to obtain the compounds identified as having biological activity in the assays or systems of interest. This is followed by extraction using appropriate solvents and drying methods to ensure safety and stability. The final extract can then be examined for chemical consistency and adjusted to achieve the desired concentration and efficacy of biologically active compounds, if they are known.

One way to ensure a minimum defined quality is to ensure that the botanical materials conform to pharmacopoeial monograph standards. However, while monographs can establish minimum quality parameters, they do not always provide adequate assurance that all materials that conform to their standards will always give the same research results, because only certain specified standards are measured and activity may also reside elsewhere. Nevertheless, pharmacopoeial quality standards are important quality references if properly developed and observed.

"FIT-FOR-PURPOSE" STANDARDIZATION

"Fit-for-purpose" standardization is an approach that is appropriate to the question being asked and condition being studied, as was discussed for the exotic fruit juice example previously.

In a different example, for example, the evaluation of coffee or tea ingested for the purpose of increasing alertness, a good measure for standardizing the potency of a preparation is the caffeine concentration of a cup of the beverage because the activity of caffeine accounts for the increase of alertness from the consumption of that beverage. In a similar way the sennosides in senna (*Senna alexandrina*) account for the laxative effect of a tea made from senna. Caffeine and sennosides have very similar, if not the same, potencies when delivered in a non-purified tea form or as single purified compounds. The action of most botanicals is not simplistically determined by the identification of single compounds. Often classes of compounds such as catechins in tea are identified, with each individual compound contributing to the activity of the extract and with no single compound able to account for the whole of the extract's biological activity. The different situations regarding identification of single active compounds, or groups of compounds, and their relationship to the activity of the whole plant or extract can be defined, but before doing so here, it is important to understand how quantitative standards, such as the relationship of starting material to finished product, are properly described. One place to start is with a brief discussion of the term "standardization."

A common misconception is that standardization of botanical products is achieved by simply controlling a small percent of chemical constituents. For example, a ginger extract "standardized" to 5% gingerols says nothing about the content of individual gingerols (there are more than one) or the composition of the other 95% of the extract. The 5% designation is a statement of strength but not of the *biological effect*: that is, the potency of the extract. Two different extracts meeting the same 5% gingerol strength claim could vary significantly in their biological activity because of the composition of that 5% and bioactivity that might be contributed by some compound in the other 95% of the extract. Thus, standardization requires a thorough description of the starting plant material and of the whole extraction process because factors such as good agricultural and collection practices (GACP) and good manufacturing practice (GMP) affect the outcome of the final product. Standardization is not accomplished simply through the assay of an active principle or marker. "Standardization signifies the body of information and controls that are necessary to guarantee constancy of composition" (5).

Standardizing a fruit juice by obtaining cultivated material from a single farm's harvest may be appropriate for research involving the dietary intake of that food. The juice studied would be a reasonable representation of material found in the marketplace and yet would have a known production history. Additional material of reasonable consistency for similar studies could be secured. Another example, previously mentioned, is the standard of botanical identity assured through proper taxonomic identification and a deposited voucher specimen. This taxonomic standard may adequately define botanical identity for wild harvested materials intended for phytochemical exploration. Other materials for other studies may require much greater characterization.

Some finished products, including well-characterized, registered, European phytomedicines, have well-defined specifications and processes in place to ensure consistent and well-characterized products. Such processes and procedures include generating crude herbs produced according to GACP, manufacturing ingredients according to GMP, and matching products characterized to bioactive compounds or bioactive fractions to rigorous specifications throughout the shelf life of the product. Other products may have reasonable standards for their raw material but cannot be adjusted to a concentration of an active chemical compound because no such entity has been identified.

FDA GUIDELINES ON LABELING AND IDENTIFICATION OF STANDARDS USED FOR FINISHED PRODUCTS

The Food and Drug Administration (FDA) specifies certain labeling requirements for foods, supplements, and drugs. For example, the federal regulations that specify how an herbal tincture may be labeled include the following statement: "Information may be included on the concentration of the dietary ingredient and the solvent used, e.g., 'fresh dandelion root extract, x (y:z) in 70% ethanol,' where x is the number of milliliters (mL) or mg of the entire extract, y is the weight of the starting material and z is the volume (mL) of solvent.

Where the solvent has been partially removed (not to dryness), the final concentration, when indicated, shall be stated (e.g., if the original extract was 1:5 and 50 percent of the solvent was removed, then the final concentration shall be stated as 1:2.5)" (6). This spells out useful information necessary to express and understand how much plant material was used in the creation of the finished product and the ratio of starting plant material to the volume of finished tincture in a standardized fashion.

The FDA also regulates how solid extracts are to be defined. "For a dietary ingredient that is an extract from which the solvent has been removed, the weight of the ingredient shall be the weight of the dried extract" (7). Because the FDA provided no information to guide labeling of solid extracts, the American Herbal Products Association (AHPA) has further defined solid extracts similarly to liquid extracts, and in both cases fresh material should be identified as such if used in processing. Solid (dry) extracts can be labeled with the portion of the preparation that originates from the extraction of the plant without any added fillers, excipients, binders, or other ingredients.

This portion of an extract that derives from the plant alone is expressed as *percent native extract*: the extract that is "native" to the plant. For example, using AHPA's definition of an extract, one kilogram of dried valerian root would be required to yield 250 g of a valerian root extract identified as 4:1 (80% native). The 80% native designation would indicate that of the 250 g of extract, the amount of actual material that was native to the dried root would have been 200 g. Added carriers and excipients, etc., amounting to 50 g would give a total extract weight of 250 g. This 250 g represents one part finished extract derived from four parts (by weight) of dried valerian root (8). Other representations, such as basing the ratio on the amount of material used to the amount of native extract yield without added carriers, are also possible. In fact, this is the convention in Europe. In this example, the same valerian extract would be represented as 200 g of dried valerian root extract 5:1 with the carriers, etc., disclosed separately. In addition to defining the amount of extract as the native extract, the European Union (EU) also has standard ways to describe products relating descriptions to standards of activity.

EU EXTRACT DEFINITIONS

The European Union differentiates extracts depending on the ability to attribute bioactivity of the extract to its known chemistry. When the activity of the botanical material can be attributed wholly to its known chemistry, such as in the earlier examples of caffeine in coffee or tea, and sennosides in senna, then the term *standardized* may be used. If the activity of the botanical material can be partly, but not wholly, attributed to specific known chemical constituents, then the term *quantified* is employed. In cases where the bioactivity of the botanical material cannot be explained by its known chemistry, as is often the case, materials are referred to as *other*. These definitions are applied equally to herbal substances (the starting material of a preparation), to herbal preparations that contain only milled or powdered herbs, and to herbal extracts. They are used to help define the quality of an ingredient or the product containing the ingredient in relation to what is known about the connection to its chemistry and biological activity (9). Each example is explained in a bit more detail below. It is important to keep in mind that such terms can serve to identify crude dried plant material, intermediate preparations, and the presence of either of these classes of substances in a finished product.

The EU Definition of "Standardized"

In the European Union, standardized herbal substances are adjusted within an acceptable tolerance to a given content of constituents with known therapeutic activity. This is a way to standardize the therapeutic effect and can be achieved only with materials for which the identified active compounds completely account for the activity of the substance. In this case standardization may be achieved by adding excipients in order to adjust the potency of the herbal substance or by blending different batches of the herbal substance with higher or lower concentrations of the target active(s) as needed. In describing such herbal substances, the name and quantitative content of the constituent(s) with known therapeutic activity should be stated. The equivalent quantity of the genuine herbal substance should be also given, which, if applicable, can also be represented as a range of values.

The EU Definition of "Quantified"

In the European Union, a quantified herbal substance is one that is adjusted to a defined range of constituents where those constituents are known to be partially responsible for the activity of the herbal substance. Adjustments are made by blending different batches of herbal substances used in the manufacturing process. As in the standardized example above, different strengths of batches can be combined to achieve the desired concentration of the specified compound. Unlike the situation for standardized materials, the addition of inert excipients to dilute material too high in the compounds to be quantified is not permitted. For quantified herbal substances, the name of the active compounds (those constituents that contribute to but do not fully account for the biological activity of the material) should be stated and their quantitative content should be given as a range. The equivalent quantity of the genuine herbal substance should also be given.

The EU Definition of "Other" Herbal Substances

When neither constituents with known therapeutic activity nor marker compounds contributing partial activity have been identified in an herbal substance, it is essentially defined by its production process and specifications. For such "other" herbal substances, the quantity of the herbal substance itself should be specified. In the EU model, the names and quantitative content of analytical markers, the known chemical constituents that do not contribute to the activity of the herbal substance, should not be stated in finished product labeling as they provide no useful information with regard to the potency of the material. Table 1.1 provides examples of each of these three definitions for herbal substances and preparations and how their presence in the product containing them should be described.

DEFINING PRODUCTS BEFORE AND AFTER CLINICAL TRIALS

The National Center for Complementary and Alternative Medicine (NCCAM) at the National Institutes of Health (NIH) instituted a procedure for ensuring the integrity of ma-

Table 1.1. EU Guidelines for Herbal Substances and Preparations

Standardized herb example: cut senna leaf

Constituents with known therapeutic activity are identified and quantified.	2.55% hydroxyanthracene glycosides, calculated as sennoside B
Quantity of the genuine herbal substance is presented as a range.	85–96%
Quantity of excipients for adjustment is disclosed.	4–15%
Declaration of the quantity of the standardized herbal substance (herbal substance and excipients for adjustment) in the product is given.	1.3 g per sachet or tea bag

Quantified herb example: cut willow bark

Co-active compounds are identified and quantified.	1.5–1.7% of total salicylic derivatives calculated as salicin
Quantity of the herbal substance in the herbal medicinal product is identified.	3.0 g per sachet or tea bag
Declaration of the quantity of the ingredient in the finished product is given.	One tea sachet/bag contains 3.0 g willow bark, corresponding to 45–51 mg of total salicylic derivatives, calculated as salicin.

Other substance example: dried valerian root extract

Quantity of the genuine extract is stated.	80% genuine extract Herb extract ratio = 3–6 : 1
Quantity of other excipients is stated.	20%
Extraction solvent is identified.	Ethanol 70% v/v
Quantity of the dry extract (genuine herbal preparation with excipients) in the herbal medicinal product is given.	200 mg/capsule
Declaration of the quantity of the extract in the finished product is provided with either the extract ratio or the equivalent amount of raw herb stated. Extraction solvent is identified.	One capsule contains 160 mg of extract from valerian root [(3–6:1) OR (equivalent to 480 mg – 960 mg of valerian root)]. Extraction solvent: ethanol 70% v/v

terials to be studied in grants that it funds. Researchers with successful grant applications have been responsive to the botanical guidance that details the type of information needed on the raw material and finished preparations that form the test materials (10). This is a requirement for reproducible scientific work. For this reason a researcher must not only properly qualify the material used but also include sufficient detail in reporting the study so that the reader may know what was used and be able to compare studies that employed equivalent test materials. Fortunately, standard reporting recommendations for studies that employ botanical materials are available.

CONSORT GUIDELINES

The Consolidated Standards of Reporting (Randomized Controlled) Trials (CONSORT) recommendations were designed as guidelines for the minimum of information that should be provided in reports of clinical trials. Those guidelines have been modified to include descriptions of trials that employ herbal interventions (11, 12). For botanicals, this information includes the Latin binominal of the plant used, its family and common names, the herbal product name, the brand or extract and manufacturer names, and whether the product is licensed or registered. Characteristics of the herbal product that should be reported include the plant part(s) used to make the product or ingredient and the type of product it is, that is, fresh, dry, raw, extract, or some identified other. The type and concentration of solvent used in the extraction and the ratio of herbal raw material used to finished extract are also important herbal product characteristics to report. For example, an extract should be described as to the solvents needed to prepare it and the ratio of starting material to native extract reported, or to the amount of total extract with the percent native revealed. The method of authentication of raw material, who authenticated it, the manufacture lot number, the voucher specimen number, and where the voucher is retained also need to be noted. Knowing these guidelines in advance makes it possible for researchers to be sure up front that they will be able to get the desired information from the manufacturer.

Additional reported information should include product dosage, the duration of the product's administration, and how this information was determined. The content, by weight and percent of quantified constituents, and added materials such as excipients should be reported. In trials in which standardized products (according to the EU definition) (9) are employed, the quantity of active and/or marker constituents per unit dosage should be identified. Where quantified and "other" types of extracts are used as the bioactive test agent in clinical trials, the reporting of qualitative analytical testing may be important. This information may include a chemical fingerprint and the methods used to obtain it and by whom. The location of any retained voucher samples of the test material should be identified. Other important descriptors for the quality of an herbal intervention in the reporting of clinical trials are descriptions of any special testing, including purity tests. These tests may represent the standardization information employed and how the material was measured (for example, as active or marker compounds) for quality to be assured. The placebo or control should be described as well as the rationale for the appropriateness of its choice.

ACCEPTABLE IDENTITY OF BOTANICAL STUDY MATERIALS

Sometimes it helps to understand what to do by understanding what not to do. For example, it is unacceptable to specify "ginseng" as the test material for a clinical trial without determining the exact source: American ginseng (*Panax quinquefolius*), Asian ginseng (*P. ginseng*), the misnamed "Siberian ginseng" correctly termed eleuthero (*Eleutherococcus senticosus*), or some other plant. Describing only where a product was purchased and identifying the manufacturer of the botanical ingredient by the company name on the label and not the supplier of the active material are likewise insufficient for describing the product. When investigators deal with botanical study materials, these types of shortfalls invariably occur because investigators are unaware of the field of pharmacognosy and fail to secure the cooperation of a pharmacognosist or other qualified expert during the early stages of planning investigations that are to involve herbal study materials.

TRADITIONAL COMBINATION PRODUCTS

Securing botanical study material for single-plant products where adequate information is available to ensure reasonable chemical or biological consistency and appropriate standardization for the study at hand can be daunting even for an expert. Additional care and attention are required to characterize formulas made from several crude herbs that are combined prior to extraction. In most general cases, using marker compounds and fingerprinting is inadequate for determining adequate characterization standards for combination products. One possible solution may begin with the evaluation of the individual raw herbs that comprise each of the ingredients of the final formula. This approach requires a voucher sample for each ingredient prior to combination and subsequent extraction. Adequate quality specifications and analytical evaluations for each ingredient would have to be obtained, such as documentation of conformance to pharmacopoeial monograph quality specifications. An example of a multicomponent mixture is presented in Chapter 9.

COMMERCIAL FOODS AS A STUDY MATERIAL

Commercial foods do not come with specifications of levels of active ingredients and are often not highly processed. As botanical materials, commercial foods can also represent quality botanicals suitable for study materials in a clinical trial as long as appropriate specifications are created and met. It is essential that the agricultural source of the material be identified even if purchased at a farmer's market or grocery. The particular variety of the botanical material must be identified and some idea of annual product consistency should be ascertained. It could also be useful to obtain some chemical characterization of the food product test item.

CONCLUSIONS

A study of product quality guidelines (10) can be very helpful in understanding the scope and depth of information essential to adequately describing botanical study materials both prior to initiating research and when reporting the results of scientific investigations. The quality of herbal study materials requires interdisciplinary research teams when the research design is still at the stage of inception. It should be clear that to conduct clinical trials using botanical materials, researchers should take pains to avail themselves of appropriate expertise such as botanical and natural product experts, phytochemists, pharmacognosists, or other similarly qualified individuals very early in the design of a scientific investigation.

The specific product quality requirements for every possible research study cannot be specified and cannot be elucidated by a simple checklist. Different research aims and different types of botanical products require customized approaches in order to match the requirements of the investigation with the attributes of the desired study material. As an increasing number of investigators enter this field, it is hoped that the growing body of information and available guidelines will result in more well-designed studies reported accurately and completely in order to provide information desired by clinicians and the public alike.

REFERENCES

[1]Ashar BH, Rice TN, Sisson SD. Medical residents' knowledge of dietary supplements. *South Med J.* 2008 Oct;101(10):996–1000.

[2]Chen ST, Dou J, Temple R, Agarwal R, Wu KM, Walker S. New therapies from old medicines. *Nat Biotechnol.* 2008 Oct;26(10):1077-1083. Available for free download from www.nature.com/nbt/journal/v26/n10/pdf/nbt1008-1077.pdf.

[3]Malone MH. The pharmacological evaluation of natural products: general and specific approaches to screening ethnopharmaceuticals. *J Ethnopharmacol.* 1983;8(2):127–147.

[4]Applequist W, Miller J. Personal communications.

[5]Bonati A. How and why should we standardize phytopharmaceutical drugs for clinical validation? *J Ethnopharmacol.* 1991;32:195–197.

[6]Title 21Code of Federal Regulations §101.36(b)(3)(ii)(B).

[7]Title 21Code of Federal Regulations §101.36(b)(3)(ii)(C).

[8]*Guidance for the Retail Labeling of Dietary Supplements Containing Soft or Powdered Botanical Extracts.* American Herbal Products Association; 2003.

[9]Guideline on Declaration of Herbal Substances and Herbal Preparations in Herbal Medicinal Products/ Traditional Herbal Medicinal Products in the Summary of Product Characteristics. Available at www.emea. europa.eu/pdfs/human/hmpc/28753905en2.pdf. Accessed May 23, 2008.

[10]NCCAM Interim Applicant Guidance: Product Quality: Biologically Active Agents Used in Complementary and Alternative Medicine (CAM) and Placebo Materials. Available at http://grants.nih.gov/grants/guide/notice-files/NOT-AT-05-004.html. Accessed June 3, 2008.

[11]Gagnier JJ, Boon H, Rochon P, Moher D, Barnes J, Bombardier C; CONSORT Group. Recommendations for reporting randomized controlled trials of herbal interventions: explanation and elaboration. *J Clin Epidemiol.* 2006;59(11):1134–1149.

[12]Gagnier JJ, Boon H, Rochon P, Moher D, Barnes J, Bombardier C; CONSORT Group. Reporting randomized, controlled trials of herbal interventions: an elaborated CONSORT statement. *Ann Intern Med.* 2006 Mar 7;144(5):364–367. Available at www.annals.org/cgi/reprint/144/5/364. Accessed May 23, 2008.

Botanical Medicine: From Bench to Bedside
Edited by R. Cooper and F. Kronenberg
© Mary Ann Liebert, Inc.

Chapter 2

Preclinical and Clinical Evidence for Botanical Interventions for Type 2 Diabetes

Joseph L. Evans

Diabetes mellitus has reached epidemic proportions in the United States and worldwide (20.8 million and 171 million individuals, respectively) and is projected to increase dramatically (1, 2). In the United States, 7% of the population suffer from diabetes, including 14.6 million diagnosed cases and 6.2 million undiagnosed cases. The epidemic of diabetes is not restricted to affluent, westernized countries but is also affecting developing countries such as Brazil, China, India, and Russia (Table 2.1). In less than 25 years, diabetes in these countries will account for nearly 38% of the worldwide burden. Globally, the direct health care cost of diabetes for people in the 20–79 age group is estimated to be at least $153 billion annually (3).

Type 2 diabetes accounts for about 90% to 95% of all diagnosed cases of diabetes. It usually begins as insulin resistance, a disorder in which the cells do not respond to insulin adequately. As the need for insulin rises, the pancreas gradually loses its ability to produce it. Type 2 diabetes is associated with older age, obesity, a family history of diabetes, a history of gestational diabetes, impaired glucose metabolism, physical inactivity, and race or ethnicity. Furthermore, the prevalence of insulin resistance, an independent risk factor for cardiovascular disease and the metabolic syndrome X, is even more widespread (4–6). This situation is exacerbated by obesity, a major risk for developing type 2 diabetes. The number of adults overweight or obese is 125 million in the United States (65% of the population) and 1.3 billion worldwide (20% of the population) (7). Since dietary modification and increased physical activity provide insufficient glucose control over the long-term course of the disease, the vast majority of patients require some type of pharmacological intervention (8).

Although pharmacological options for the management of type 2 diabetes have been increasing and will continue to do so (9–14), not all patients benefit from them. In addition, the cost of prescription medications may exceed the financial capacity of an increasing number of older citizens, those without adequate health insurance, and those living in poverty (15,

JERIKA Research Foundation, Redwood City, California 94061; jevansphd@earthlink.net

Table 2.1. Global Prevalence of Diabetes

Country	2000	2030
India	31,705,000	79,441,000
China	20,757,000	42,321,000
Brazil	4,553,000	11,305,000
Russia	4,576,000	5,320,000
BRIC Total	61,591,000	138,387,000
World Total	171,000,000	366,000,000
BRIC, as % of World Total	36.0	37.8

Source: World Health Organization
BRIC=Brazil, Russia, India, China; CAGR=Current Annual Growth Rate

16). Furthermore, certain ethnic groups who are at increased risk for developing diabetes (e.g., Asians, Hispanics, and Native Americans) come from cultures with a long history of use of traditional medicines and are likely to employ one or more traditional (botanical) treatments rather than prescription medications (17–26). Though a majority of diabetic patients are being treated, many are unable to achieve the current American Diabetes Association–recommended goal of $HbA_{1C} < 7\%$ (Hemoglobin A_{1C}, the gold-standard surrogate marker for long-term glycemic control). Thus, in patients with poorly controlled type 2 diabetes, especially those who are obese, there is a need to identify and evaluate adjunctive therapies that are safe, efficacious, and cost-effective.

Botanical extracts represent a rich, potential source of affordable therapies for type 2 diabetes and insulin resistance for the impoverished in developed countries and throughout much of the developing world. Several recent comprehensive reviews have focused on the use of botanicals for diabetes (21, 23, 27–32). The overall objective of this chapter therefore is to provide a concise, comparative overview of those botanicals that have received the most scientific attention and hold the most promise for qualifying as clinically validated "alternate therapies," defined here as significantly lowering HbA_{1C} in multiple, randomized, double-blind, placebo-controlled clinical trials.

BOTANICAL INTERVENTIONS

Botanicals have been used for medicinal purposes since the dawn of civilization (33). It is well documented (26) that many pharmaceuticals commonly used today are structurally derived from natural compounds found in traditional medicinal plants. The development of the antihyperglycemic drug metformin (dimethlybiguanide) can be traced to the traditional use of *Galega officinalis* to treat diabetes and the subsequent search to identify active compounds with reduced toxicity (34–36). *G. officinalis* is far from the only botanical to have been used as a treatment for diabetes. Chinese medical books written as early as 3000 B.C. spoke of diabetes and described therapies for this disease (37, 38). These historical accounts reveal that type 2 diabetes existed long ago, and medicinal plants have been used for many millennia to treat this disease. To date, the antidiabetic activities of well over 1,200 traditional plants have been reported, although scant few have been subjected to rigorous scientific evaluation for safety and efficacy in humans (37, 39–43). This section will provide an overview of those botanicals used for diabetes that have received the most scientific attention, have been evaluated for their antidiabetic effects in individuals with diabetes, and deserve additional research. The botanicals are presented in the order of their relative (highest-to-lowest) ranking for safety and efficacy and are summarized in Table 2.2.

Ipomoea batatas (Caiapo)

Caiapo is derived from the skin of a variety of white sweet potato of South American origin, *Ipomoea batatas*, which is cultivated in a mountainous region in Kagawa Prefecture, Japan. It has been eaten raw for centuries in the belief that it is effective for anemia, hypertension, and diabetes. Caiapo is commercially available throughout Japan without prescription and used for the prevention and treatment of type 2 diabetes. In rodents, caiapo exhibits antidiabetic activity, and the active component is thought to be a high-molecular-weight acid glycoprotein (44, 45).

A beneficial effect of caiapo on glycemic control, including the reduction of HbA_{1C}, has been reported and confirmed in several clinical studies. In a pilot study, a total of 18 male patients with type 2 diabetes (age: 58 ± 8 years; weight: 88 ± 3 kg; BMI [body mass index]: 27.7 ± 2.7 kg/m^2; means $\pm$ SEM [standard error of the mean]) treated by diet alone were randomized to receive placebo (n=6) or 2 g (low dose; n=6) or 4 g (high dose; n=6) caiapo (four tablets each containing 168 or 336 mg powdered white-skinned sweet potato, respectively) before breakfast, lunch, and dinner for six weeks (46). At the end of treatment, no statistically significant changes in fasting glucose, insulin, or lipids occurred in either the low-dose caiapo or placebo groups. In the group treated with the high-dose caiapo, fasting plasma glucose (−13%) as well as cholesterol (total [−10.5%] and LDL [−13%] cholesterol) were significantly decreased ($P < 0.05$, compared to baseline). Body weight and blood pressure remained unchanged in all three groups. In patients receiving low-dose caiapo, insulin sensitivity (S_I) increased by 37% (2.02 ± 0.70 vs. 2.76 ± 0.89 10^4 min$^{-1} \cdot \mu U^{-1} \cdot ml^{-1}$, $P < 0.05$); in those on high-dose caiapo, the FSIGT (frequently sampled intravenous glucose tolerance test) demonstrated an increase of S_I by 42% (1.21 ± 0.32 vs. 1.73 ± 0.40 10^4 min$^{-1} \cdot \mu U^{-1} \cdot ml^{-1}$, $P < 0.03$). No changes were seen for S_I in patients receiving placebo (1.52 ± 0.28 vs. 1.35 ± 0.21 10^4 min$^{-1} \cdot \mu U^{-1} \cdot ml^{-1}$). Glucose tolerance was significantly increased (~72%; $P < 0.02$) in the high-dose group (47). No adverse events were reported.

The results of this pilot study have been confirmed in a randomized, double-blind, placebo-controlled trial (48). A total of 61 patients with type 2 diabetes treated by diet were given 4 g caiapo (n=30; mean age 55.2 ± 2.1 years; BMI 28.0 ± 0.4 kg/m^2) or placebo (n=31; mean age 55.6 ± 1.5 years; BMI 27.6 ± 0.3 kg/m^2) once daily for 12 weeks. Each subject underwent a 75 g oral glucose tolerance test (OGTT) at baseline and after one, two, and three months to assess two-hour glucose levels. Additionally, fasting blood glucose, HbA_{1C}, total cholesterol, and triglyceride levels were measured. Fasting blood glucose levels decreased in the caiapo group (143.7 ± 1.9 vs. 128.5 ± 1.7 mg/dl; $P < 0.001$) and remained unchanged in the placebo group (144.3 ± 1.9 vs. 138.2 ± 2.1 mg/dl; $P = 0.052$). In the caiapo group, HbA_{1C} decreased significantly (−0.53%; $P < 0.001$) from 7.21 ± 0.15 to 6.68 ± 0.14% and remained unchanged in the placebo group (7.04 ± 0.17 vs. 7.10 ± 0.19%; $P = 0.23$). Two-hour glucose levels were significantly ($P < 0.001$) decreased in the caiapo group (193.3 ± 10.4 vs. 162.8 ± 8.2 mg/dl) compared with the placebo group (191.7 ± 9.2 vs. 181.0 ± 7.1 mg/dl). Mean cholesterol at the end of the treatment was significantly lower in the caiapo group

Table 2.2. Most Promising Botanicals for Type 2 Diabetes

Botanical	Putative Bioactives	Antidiabetic Activity	Mode of Action	Typical Daily Dose	Potential Side Effects	Relative Rating
I. batas (caiapo)	High-molecular-weight acid glycoprotein	Glucose control; reduces HbA$_{1c}$	Not well characterized; possibly increases insulin sensitivity	4 g of white-skin sweet potato (capsule)	None reported	5
C. indica	Not yet characterized	Glucose control; reduces HbA$_{1c}$	Not characterized; possibly insulin mimetic	1 g (alcoholic extract); 1.8 g (powdered leaves)	None reported (limited data)	5
T. foenum-graecum (fenugreek)	Fiber, 4-hydroxyisoleucine, saponins, coumarins, alkaloids, glycosides	Glucose control; anti-hyperlipidemic	Delays gastric emptying; inhibits glucose absorption in gut; enhances insulin secretion	2.5–15 g (defatted seeds)	Hypoglycemia; additive with other glucose-lowering agents and insulin; GI irritation; anti-coagulant	4
O. streptacantha (nopal; prickly pear)	Fiber, pectin	Glucose control; anti hyperlipidemic	Delays gastric emptying; inhibits glucose absorption in gut	2.4 g	None reported (limited data)	3+
M. charantia (bitter melon)	Charantin, vicine, morrordicine (alkaloid), polypeptide P	Glucose control	Inhibits glucose absorption in gut; enhances insulin secretion; increases glucose transport and glycogen synthesis	300–600 mg (juice extract); 1.8 g (capsule)	Hypoglycemia; additive with other glucose-lowering agents and insulin; GI irritation	3

A. sativum (garlic)	Allicin, allyl methyl thiosulfonate, 1-propenyl allyl thiosulfonate, γ-L-glutamyl-S-alkyl-L- cysteine	Anti-hyperlipidemic; anti-hypertensive	Anti-inflammatory (antioxidant)	600–1000 mg	GI irritation; anti-coagulant; heartburn; garlic odor	2+
G. sylvestre (gurmar)	Gymnemic acids, gymnemosides	Glucose control	Inhibits glucose absorption in gut; enhances insulin secretion	200–600 mg	Hypoglycemia; additive with other glucose-lowering agents and insulin; GI irritation	2
P. quinquefolius (American ginseng)	Ginsenosides (saponins), polysaccharides, peptides, fatty acids	Glucose control	Delays gastric emptying; inhibits glucose absorption in gut; hormonal and CNS activity	100–200 mg	Estrogenic effects; ginseng abuse syndrome; interacts with many drugs	2
A. vera (aloe)	Fiber (glucomannan), aloins, anthra quinones, barbaloin, polysaccharides, salicylic acids	Glucose control	Not characterized; possibly delays gastric emptying and inhibits glucose absorption in gut	1.2 g (capsule)	None reported (limited data)	2
C. cassia (cinnamon)	Methyl hydroxyl chalcone polymer (MHCP)	Glucose control	Possibly insulin mimetic	3–6 g (capsule)	None reported	1+

Ranking scale: 5, most promising; 1, least promising

(214.6 ± 11.2 mg/dl) than in the placebo group (248.7 ± 11.2 mg/dl; $P < 0.05$). A decrease in body weight was observed in both the placebo group ($P = 0.0027$) and the caiapo group ($P < 0.0001$); in the caiapo group, body weight was related to the improvement in glucose control ($r = 0.618$; $P < 0.0002$). No significant changes in triglyceride levels or blood pressure were observed. Unfortunately, possible effects on fasting insulin, C-peptide, or insulin sensitivity were not reported in this study. Caiapo was well tolerated without significant adverse effects. This study confirms the results of the pilot with regard to the beneficial effects of caiapo on short-term glycemic control (as well as cholesterol levels) and documents the efficacy of caiapo on long-term glycemic control in patients with type 2 diabetes. The magnitude of the effect of caiapo at reducing HbA_{1c} (-0.53% absolute decrease) is comparable with that of acarbose, an approved oral antihyperglycemic medication (10), although it falls short of what has been suggested as the minimal acceptable level for a new antihyperglycemic medication (-0.7% absolute decrease) (49).

A five-month follow-up of this study (48) was conducted to further evaluate the mode of action of caiapo on insulin sensitivity over an extended period of time as well as its effects on fibrinogen and other clinical markers of low-grade inflammation (50). In the group receiving caiapo (4 g/day), insulin sensitivity and adiponectin both increased significantly, while fibrinogen decreased. This was associated with an improvement in HbA_{1C} (decreased from $6.46\% \pm 0.12\%$ to $6.25\% \pm 0.11\%$; $P = 0.008$), fasting glucose, and triglycerides. Body weight, lipid levels, and C-reactive protein were not altered. No changes were observed in the placebo group except for HbA_{1C}, which significantly increased from $6.25\% \pm 0.10\%$ to $6.50\% \pm 0.12\%$; ($P = 0.0001$). This study confirms the beneficial effects of caiapo on glucose and HbA_{1C} control in patients with type 2 diabetes after five months' follow-up. Improvement of insulin sensitivity was accompanied by increased levels of adiponectin and a decrease in fibrinogen. Thus, caiapo can be considered a natural insulin sensitizer with potential antiatherogenic properties. It will be of interest and important to see if the results of these very exciting outcomes with caiapo can be confirmed in other well-designed clinical trials by other groups and to establish that caiapo does not exhibit any adverse interaction with existing antihyperglycemic medication.

Coccinia indica

Coccinia indica is a creeper plant (one that spreads by means of stems that creep) that grows wildly in Bangladesh and in many other parts of the Indian subcontinent. Although *C. indica* has a long history of use as an antidiabetic treatment in Ayurvedic medicine (a holistic system of healing that originated among the Brahmin, the Hindu priestly caste) (25), it has not been subjected to the number of clinical trials that have evaluated *M. charantia*, fenugreek, or *G. sylvestre* (based on published reports). Neither the bioactive compounds nor mode of action of *C. indica* has been well characterized, but there is some suggestion that a component or components of the plant possess insulin-mimetic activity (30).

In a double-blind, placebo-controlled trial, a preparation from the leaves of the plant was administered to patients with uncontrolled type 2 diabetes for six weeks (51). Of the 16 patients who received the experimental preparations, 10 showed significant improvement in their glucose tolerance ($P < 0.001$), while none out of the 16 patients in the placebo group showed improvement. Several other studies also offered supporting evidence of the beneficial effect of this treatment (reviewed in [30]). No adverse effects were reported.

Convincing evidence for the clinical utility of this extract has recently been provided (52). The design of this study was a double-blind, placebo-controlled, randomized trial employing subjects with type 2 diabetes. Sixty newly diagnosed patients with type 2 diabetes (aged 35 to 60 years) needing only dietary or lifestyle modifications with fasting blood glucose in the range of 110 to 180 mg/dl were recruited into the study. The subjects were randomly assigned into the placebo (n = 30) or treatment (n = 29) group and were provided with 1 g alcoholic extract of *C. indica* for 90 days. In the treatment group, there was a significant decrease in both the fasting (−16%) and postprandial blood glucose (−18%) of the experimental group compared with placebo. Most importantly, there was a significant reduction in HbA_{1c} of the experimental group at day 90 (6.1 ± 1.1%) compared with baseline (6.7 ± 1.2%), while there was no change in the placebo group (baseline HbA_{1c} = 6.4 ± 0.9%). The magnitude of the effect of *C. indica* at reducing HbA_{1c} (−0.6% absolute decrease) is comparable with that of acarbose, an approved oral antihyperglycemic medication (10), and it approximates what has been suggested as the minimal acceptable level for a new antihyperglycemic medication (−0.7% absolute decrease) (49). No significant changes were observed in the serum lipid levels or daily energy intake. No serious adverse events were reported. In the experimental group, 17 (59%) experienced mild hypoglycemic symptoms such as perspiration, excessive hunger, and slight dizziness once or twice during the study period. The other observed adverse events were minor and limited to mild symptoms of the gastrointestinal tract such as abdominal distention, flatulence, constipation, and gastritis. Seven (24%) of the subjects from the experimental group and eight (27%) of the subjects from the placebo group experienced these minor adverse effects. These symptoms were present in both groups of subjects and subsided within a week. This study indicates that *C. indica* extract has an antihyperglycemic action in patients with mild type 2 diabetes. However, further studies clearly are warranted to confirm this activity, to assess its potential efficacy in patients with more severe diabetes and in combination with other antidiabetic medications, and to elucidate the mechanism(s) of action.

Trigonella foenum-graecum (Fenugreek)

Trigonella foenum-graecum, also known as fenugreek, is an herb native to southeastern Europe, northern Africa, and western Asia but is also widely cultivated in other parts of the world (53). Fenugreek has a long history of traditional use among Ayurvedic sages of ancient India and Nepal (approximately 3000–5000 years ago) and Chinese medicine (54) and has been widely used for the treatment of diabetes (41). The defatted seeds of the fenugreek plant contain ~ 50% fiber (similar to guar gum), along with a variety of bioactive saponins, alkaloids, coumarins, and 4-hydroxyisoleucine, the principal bioactive compound (40, 41). This last compound exhibits insulinotropic activity (55–57); following a six-day subchronic administration, 4-hydroxyisoleucine (50 mg/kg/day) reduced fasting hyperglycemia and insulinemia and improved glucose tolerance in diabetic rats (57). In addition, an aqueous extract of fenugreek seeds contains insulin-like activity, including the stimulation of hepatic glucokinase and hexokinase activities, suggesting an extrapancreatic mode of action (58).

The clinical studies that have evaluated the efficacy of fenugreek in individuals with both type 1 and type 2 diabetes have been reviewed (23). In one study, 17 of 21 patients with type 2 diabetes showed a reduction in two-hour postprandial glucose averaging 30 mg/dl following administration of 15 g of ground fenugreek seed (59). In a crossover, placebo-controlled trial with 60 individuals with type 2 diabetes, the treatment group received 12.5 mg defatted fenugreek at lunch and dinner with isocaloric diets for 24 weeks (60). Fasting blood glucose was 151 mg/dl at baseline and decreased to 112 mg/dl after 24 weeks ($P<0.05$). Fenugreek also caused a significant decrease in the area under the glucose curve by approximately 40%.

In a small study, the effects of fenugreek seeds on glycemic control and insulin resistance in mild to moderate type 2 diabetes was performed using a double-blind, placebo-controlled design (61). Twenty-five newly diagnosed patients with type 2 diabetes (fasting glucose <200 mg/dl) were randomly divided into two groups. Group I ($n=12$) received 1 g per day of fenugreek seeds, and group II ($n=13$) received standard care (dietary control, exercise) plus placebo capsules for two months. After two months, fasting blood glucose and two-hour postglucose load-levels were not significantly different. However, following an oral glucose challenge, the area under the curve (AUC) for blood glucose (2375 ± 574 vs. 27597 ± 274) and insulin (2492 ± 2536 vs. 5631 ± 2428) was significantly lower ($P<0.001$), as was the HOMA-IR index (112.9 ± 67 vs. 92.2 ± 57; $P<0.05$) in the treatment group compared to control. Serum triglycerides decreased and HDL cholesterol increased significantly (both $P<0.05$) following fenugreek treatment. Significant reductions in total cholesterol and triglycerides have also been reported in other studies following fenugreek treatment (23).

In an open-label pilot study, fenugreek seeds were evaluated in combination with *M. charantia* and jamun seeds (*Syzigium cumini*) for effects on glycemic control in patients with type 2 diabetes (62). The patients were divided into two groups of 30 each. The patients of group I were given the raw powdered mixture in the form of capsules; the patients of group II were given this mixture in the form of salty biscuits. Daily supplementation of 1 g of this powdered mixture for a 1.5-month period and increased to 2 g for another 1.5 months significantly reduced the fasting as well as the postprandial glucose level of the diabetic patients. A significant decrease in oral hypoglycemic drug intake and decline in percentage of the subjects who were on hypoglycemic drugs were found after the three-month feeding trial. The authors concluded that 2 g of this powdered mixture of traditional medicinal plants in either raw or cooked form can be used successfully for lowering blood glucose in diabetics.

The doses of fenugreek used in clinical studies have ranged from 2.5 g to 15 g daily of the crushed and defatted seeds. Crushing is important to release the viscous gel fiber, which presumably contributes to the efficacy of fenugreek. Typical doses of seeds are in the range of 1 to 3 g mixed with food and taken at mealtime. The most common side effects are gastrointestinal upset (diarrhea and flatulence), which often can be alleviated by dose titration. Since the fenugreek fiber might absorb other oral medications, fenugreek should be taken independently (e.g., one to two hours) of other medications. Because of the ability of fenugreek to lower blood glucose, individuals should monitor their glucose levels carefully when they use fenugreek in combination with insulin or other glucose-lowering agents. Fenugreek can exhibit anticoagulant activity; it should not be used with other anticoagulating agents because of the increased risk for bleeding.

The potential genotoxicity of a fenugreek seed extract (THL) containing a minimum of 40% 4-hydroxyisoleucine was evaluated using the panel of assays recommended by the U.S. Food and Drug Administration for food ingredients (i.e., reverse mutation assay, mouse lymphoma forward mutation assay, and mouse micronucleus assay). THL was determined not to be genotoxic under the conditions of the tested genetic toxicity battery (63).

Opuntia (*fuliginosa, streptacantha*) (Prickly Pear Cactus; Nopal)

Nopal, a member of the *Opuntia* genus, is widely used in Mexico as a treatment for glucose control (64). It grows in arid regions throughout the Western Hemisphere and is known in the United States as prickly pear cactus. This plant produces a vegetable called nopal and a red egg-shaped fruit called tuna. Nopal is a common component of everyday foods including soups, salads, and sandwiches and is blended in drinks. When used for glucose control, nopal is prepared as a food and is available in bulk, as dried powder, or in capsules. The glucose-lowering activity of nopal is likely due to its very high soluble fiber and pectin content (40, 41, 65), although its ability to reduce fasting glucose is suggestive of additional modes of action (64).

The results of most human studies of this plant have been reported in Spanish-language journals (30, 64); two studies evaluating the acute effects of nopal have been published in English by Frati et al. (66, 67). Both studies used *Opuntia streptacantha Lemaire* and reported improved glycemic control (decreased serum glucose) and improved insulin sensitivity (decreased serum insulin) following a single dose (500 g of broiled or grilled nopal stems) in patients with type 2 diabetes (n = 14 and n = 22). No effect was observed in healthy individuals (66), nor were any adverse effects reported.

A more recent study has reported that the addition of nopales (prickly pear cactus pads) to typical Mexican breakfasts (chilaquiles, burritos, quesadillas) significantly improved (30%– 48% reduction) the postprandial glucose response in subjects with type 2 diabetes (68). Although the study was small (n < 12 per group) and not controlled for varying degrees of insulin resistance, overweight, or obesity, the results clearly support further study of a standardized extract to evaluate its potential clinical efficacy.

Mormordica charantia (Bitter Melon)

Mormordica charantia is reported to be the most popular plant used worldwide to treat diabetes (40, 41). It has many names depending on the geographic location of origin: in India, where it is widely used for diabetes (25), *M. charantia* is known as karela, bitter melon, and bitter gourd. In other parts of the world, it is also known as wild cucumber, ampalaya, and cundeamor (23). The glucose-lowering activity of *M. charantia* (administered as both fresh juice and unripe fruit) has been well documented in animal models of diabetes (25, 69, 70). Compounds possessing antidiabetic activity include charantin and vicine (30, 41, 71). In addition, other bioactive components of bitter melon extract appear to have structural similarities to animal insulin (e.g., polypeptide-p) (69, 71). Several modes of action have been proposed to account for the antidiabetic activity of *M. charantia*, including inhibition of glucose absorption in the gut, stimulation of insulin secretion, and stimulation of hepatic glycogen synthesis (23, 69). More recent work has identified additional potential modes of action including alteration of the expression of lipid enzymes (72, 73), increased insulin signaling (74), and activation of AMP-activated protein kinase (75).

Four clinical trials have reported bitter melon juice, fruit, and dried powder to have a moderate hypoglycemic effect (23, 30, 76). However, these studies were small, were not randomized or double-blind, and were of insufficient quality to recommend the use of *M. charantia* without careful monitoring. When used at typical doses, 300 to 600 mg of juice extract or 1 to 2 g of powdered leaf daily, *M. charantia* is generally well tolerated, although it should not be used by children or pregnant women (23, 71, 76).

Allium (*sativum* and *cepa*) (Garlic)

Allium sativum (garlic) had been used as a medicinal herb by the ancient Sumerians, Egyptians, Greeks, Chinese, Indians, and later the Italians and English (79). The leading Indian ancient medical text, *Charaka-Samhita*, recommended garlic for the treatment of heart disease and arthritis over many centuries (79). Compounds present in aqueous garlic extract or raw garlic homogenate thought to be the principal bioactive components include allicin (allyl 2-propenethiosulfonate or diallyl thiosulfonate), allyl methyl thiosulfonate, 1-propenyl allyl thiosulfonate, and γ-L-glutamyl-S-alkyl-L-cysteine.

In modern times, garlic preparations have been widely recognized as agents for prevention and treatment of cardiovascular and other metabolic diseases, atherosclerosis, hyperlipidemia, thrombosis, hypertension, and diabetes (80–83). Epidemiological evidence indicates an inverse correlation between garlic consumption and the reduced risk of the development of cardiovascular disease (84–86). The efficacy of garlic in cardiovascular diseases has been more evident in nonclinical models, thus prompting a variety of clinical trials (79). Many of these trials have reported beneficial effects of garlic on almost all cardiovascular conditions mentioned above (87); however, a number of studies have reported no beneficial effects, casting doubt on the reputed health benefits of garlic. These differences could have arisen as a result of methodological shortcomings, the use of different formulations or preparations of garlic, heterogeneity of patient populations, dietary inconsistencies, and different time scales of the studies. The glucose-lowering activity of garlic in humans with type 2 diabetes is not well studied. In the studies that have evaluated garlic, the data have been conflicting (30, 79, 88). Thus, the role of garlic in glucose control has yet to be established convincingly but is worthy of further study.

Gymnema sylvestre (Gurmar)

Gymnema sylvestre (also called gurmar), a woody plant that grows wild in India, has a long history of use in Ayurvedic medicine (25). The leaves of *G. sylvestre* contain glycosides and the peptide gurmarin (40, 41). Other plant constituents include resins, gymnemic acids, saponins, stigmasterol, quercitol, and several amino acid derivatives. A water-soluble acidic fraction called GS4 has been used in most clinical studies (see next paragraph). Several modes of action have been proposed to account for the antidiabetic activity of *G. sylvestre*, including increased glucose uptake and utilization, increased insulin secretion, and increased b-cell number (30, 77). The use of *G. sylvestre* for diabetes has been the subject of a recent review (78).

There have been several small clinical studies in individuals with type 1 and type 2 diabetes (reviewed in [23]). These studies have reported that *G. sylvestre* decreased fasting glucose and HbA$_{1c}$, lowered insulin requirements in individuals with type 1 diabetes, and lowered the dose of antihyperglycemic medications in individuals with type 2 diabetes. *G. sylvestre* also appears to facilitate endogenous insulin secretion, but it is not a substitute for insulin. There are no data from double-blind, placebo-controlled studies in humans that validate the efficacy of *G. sylvestre* in type 1 or type 2 diabetes. The extract (~400 mg daily) of *G. sylvestre* is well tolerated, and no significant side effects have been reported.

Panax (*ginseng, japonicus,* and *quinquefolius*) and *Eleutherococcus*

Ginseng, a member of the plant family *Aaraliaceae*, has been used in traditional Chinese medicine for thousands of years (33, 38, 89). The botanical name for Asian ginseng (Chinese or Korean) is *Panax ginseng*; Japanese ginseng is known as *Panax japonicus*; American ginseng is *Panax quinquefolius*. Siberian ginseng belongs to the genus *Eleutherococcus*. Many therapeutic claims have been ascribed to the use of ginseng root extract, including improved vitality and immune function along with beneficial effects on cancer, diabetes, cardiovascular disease, and sexual function (90). Bioactive compounds that have been identified in ginseng species include ginsenosides, polysaccharides, peptides, and fatty acids (40, 41). Most pharmacological actions are attributed to the ginsenosides, a family of steroids named saponins (40, 41). A comprehensive review of the randomized controlled trials (RCTs) evaluating ginseng extracts (mostly *Panax ginseng* and *Panax quinquefolius*) has been performed, and the authors concluded that there was insufficient evidence to support efficacy for any of the indications given above (90). However, in light of the extreme compositional variability of ginsenoside concentrations reported in a sampling of 32 studies, it is possible that the antihyperglycemic efficacy might be as variable as the ginsenoside content of the extract (91, 92). There are ample reports supporting the beneficial effects of various types of ginseng in rodent models of diabetes (93–95).

Two small clinical studies have evaluated the use of ginseng in diabetes. In a double-blind, placebo-controlled study, 36 patients with type 2 diabetes were treated for eight weeks with ginseng extract (species not specified) at 100 (n = 12) or 200 (n = 12) mg per day, or with a placebo (n = 12) (96). Ginseng (100 and 200 mg/day) but not placebo lowered fasting blood glucose by approximately 0.5–1 mmol/l ($P < 0.05$). Eight subjects who were given ginseng and two who were given placebo achieved normal fasting blood glucose. In response to an oral glucose challenge, the area under the two-hour blood glucose curve was reduced approximately 16% ($P < 0.001$) in the eight ginseng-treated patients who had normalized fasting blood glucose, without any concomitant change in immunoreactive insulin or C-peptide. The 200 mg dose improved HbA$_{1c}$ (~0.5% decrease; $P < 0.05$) and physical activity compared to placebo. Ginseng had no effect on plasma lipids.

More recently, the results of a double-blind, randomized, crossover-design clinical study evaluating a Korean red ginseng (*P. ginseng*) preparation was reported (97). Nineteen participants with well-controlled type 2 diabetes (sex: 11 M:8 F, age: 64±2 years, BMI: 28.9±1.4 kg/m^2, HbA$_{1c}$: 6.5%) received the selected Korean red ginseng preparation (rootlets) and placebo at the selected dose (2 g/meal = 6 g/day) for 12 weeks as an adjunct to their usual antidiabetic therapy (diet and/or medications). Although the participants remained well controlled (HbA1$_c$ = 6.5%) throughout the study, there was no significant change in the HbA$_{1c}$; however, an improvement in oral glucose tolerance and insulin sensitivity was reported.

Another small study reported the acute effects of *Panax quinquefolius* administration (single dose on four separate occasions; 3 g/treatment) or placebo on glucose tolerance in patients with type 2 diabetes (n = 9) and in nondiabetic subjects (n = 10) (98). In both groups, ginseng caused a significant reduction ($P < 0.05$) in the area under the blood glucose curve by approximately 20% compared to placebo. The potential clinical efficacy of ginseng extract is ambiguous but warrants further study using standardized extracts.

Aloe Vera

The dried sap of the aloe plant (aloes) is a traditional botanical remedy frequently used to treat dermatitis and burns and to enhance wound healing (99), and is one of a variety of plants used for diabetes in India (25) and the Arabian Peninsula (100). There is some evidence of efficacy of aloe extract in rodent models (101, 102).

The ability of aloe extract to lower the blood glucose was studied in five patients with type 2 diabetes (103). Following the ingestion of aloe (one-half a teaspoonful daily for 4 to 14 weeks), fasting serum glucose level decreased in every patient from a mean of 273 ± 25 (SE) to 151 ± 23 mg/dl ($P < 0.05$) with no change in body weight. This glucose-lowering activity has been confirmed in two other studies which reported that oral administration of the aloes juice (1 tablespoon twice daily) reduced fasting glucose and triglycerides in subjects with type 2 diabetes in both the absence and presence of concomitant sulfonylurea therapy (104, 105). No adverse effects were reported in these studies. Aloe gel also holds the potential for glucose-lowering activity, as it contains glucomannan, a water-soluble fiber that reportedly has glucose-lowering and insulin-sensitizing activities (106, 107). The potential clinical efficacy of this plant is unclear but warrants further study.

Cinnamomum cassia (Cinnamon)

Anderson and colleagues have previously reported that an ammonium hydroxide extract of cinnamon potentiated the effect of insulin on glucose oxidation in isolated rat adipocytes (108, 109). Close evaluation of these in vitro data reveals that the cinnamon extract actually possessed insulin mimetic activity, since the stimulatory effects were independent of insulin concentration and no added insulin was required to achieve maximal glucose oxidation (109). A water-soluble polyphenolic polymer from cinnamon has been isolated and shown to have insulin-like activity as well as antioxidant activity in vitro (110, 111). Additionally, enzyme inhibition studies have shown that the bioactive compound(s) isolated from cinnamon can stimulate autophosphorylation of a truncated form of the insulin receptor and can inhibit PTP-1, the rat homolog of the tyrosine phosphatase PTP-1B that inactivates the insulin receptor (110, 111).

Two small studies have reported beneficial effects of cinnamon extract on glucose tolerance in healthy, nondiabetic individuals. The intake of 6 g cinnamon with rice pudding was reported to reduce postprandial blood glucose and delay gastric emptying without affecting satiety (112). Cinnamon ingestion (5 g) reduced total plasma glucose responses in an oral glucose tolerance test (judged by the area under the curve) by 10% to 13%; $P < 0.05$, compared to placebo, as well as improving insulin sensitivity (113).

Five small studies (n < 50 subjects per group) yielded information on the use of cinnamon intervention in individuals with type 2 diabetes. Kahn et al. were the first to report a beneficial effect of cinnamon extract glycemic and lipid control (114). A total of 60 people with type 2 diabetes (30 men and 30 women aged 52.2 ± 6.32 years) were divided randomly into six groups. Groups 1, 2, and 3 consumed 1, 3, or 6 g of cinnamon daily, respectively, and groups 4, 5, and 6 were given placebo capsules corresponding to the number of capsules consumed for the three levels of cinnamon. The cinnamon was consumed for 40 days, followed by a 20-day washout period. After 40 days, all three doses of cinnamon significantly reduced the mean fasting serum glucose (18%–29%), triglyceride (23%–30%), LDL cholesterol (7%–27%), and total cholesterol (12%–26%) levels; no significant changes were noted in the placebo groups. Changes in HDL cholesterol were not significant, and no significant adverse events were reported. The results of this interesting study suggest that intake of 1, 3, or 6 g of cinnamon per day reduces serum glucose, triglyceride, LDL cholesterol, and total cholesterol.

A more recent trial examined an aqueous-purified cinnamon extract on long-term glycemic control and lipids in patients with type 2 diabetes with equivocal results (115). A total of 79 patients on insulin therapy but treated with oral antidiabetics or diet were randomly assigned to take either cinnamon extract or a placebo capsule three times a day for four months in a double-blind study. The amount of aqueous cinnamon extract corresponded to 3 g of cinnamon powder per day. The mean absolute and percentage differences between the pre- and postintervention fasting plasma glucose levels of the cinnamon and placebo groups were significantly different. There was a significantly higher reduction in the cinnamon group (10.3%) than in the placebo group (3.4%). No significant intragroup or intergroup differences were observed regarding HbA_{1c}, lipid profiles, or pre- and postintervention levels of these parameters. The decrease in plasma glucose correlated significantly with the baseline concentrations, indicating that subjects with a higher initial plasma glucose level exhibited a greater response from cinnamon intake. This observation is consistent with that observed for prescription oral antihyperglycemic agents (49). No adverse effects were observed.

In the third study, 25 postmenopausal patients with type 2 diabetes (aged 62.9 ± 1.5 y, BMI 30.4 ± 0.9 kg/m^2) participated in a six-week intervention, during which they were supplemented with either cinnamon (1.5 g/day) or a placebo (116). Before and after two and six weeks of supplementation, arterialized blood samples were obtained and oral glucose tolerance tests were performed. Blood lipid profiles and multiple indices of whole-body insulin sensitivity were determined. There were no Time × Treatment interactions for whole-body insulin sensitivity or oral glucose tolerance. The blood lipid profile of fasting subjects did not change after cinnamon supplementation. These results showed that cinnamon supplementation (1.5 g/day) did not improve whole-body insulin sensitivity or oral glucose tolerance and did not modulate blood lipid profile in postmenopausal patients with type 2 diabetes.

In the fourth study, 60 subjects with type 2 diabetes were randomized (single-blind) to either 1.5 g per day of cinnamon cassia powder or placebo, as add-on treatment in combination with their current therapy (metformin or sulfonylurea). The duration of treatment was 12 weeks. The primary end point was a reduction in HbA_{1c}. After a 12-week period, HbA_{1c} was decreased similarly in both groups, from 8.14% to 7.76% in the cinnamon group and from 8.06% to 7.87% in the placebo group. This change was not found to be statistically significantly different. No significant intergroup differences were observed in either fasting plasma glucose or lipid control. Thus, cinnamon cassia powder (1.5 g/day) was judged to be ineffective at improving either glycemic or lipid control in subjects with type 2 diabetes.

In the fifth study and the first to be conducted in the United States, it was reported that cinnamon taken at a dose of 1 g daily for three months produced no significant change in fasting glucose, HbA_{1c}, insulin, or lipid control (117). Recently, a meta-analysis of the randomized controlled trials evaluating cinnamon intervention has been published (118), and the conclusion of the authors was that cinnamon does not appear to improve HbA_{1c}, fasting glucose, or lipid parameters in patients with type 1 or type 2 diabetes. However, it is possible that differences between studies related to dose, type of cinnamon evaluated, method of extraction, and varying degrees of diabetes, overweight, obesity, insulin resistance, and concurrent medications could also contribute to the conflicting results (119). Thus, the ability of cinnamon to improve long-term glycemic or lipid control has yet to be confirmed, and its use for type 2 diabetes is not recommended.

Traditional Chinese Medicine

A discussion of botanical interventions for type 2 diabetes would not be complete without the thoughtful consideration of traditional Chinese medicine. Over the centuries, Chinese herbal "drugs" have served as a primary source for the prevention and treatment of many diseases, including diabetes. *Xiao-ke* is a term used to refer to wasting and thirsting syndrome (type 1 diabetes); the more modern term, *Tang-niao-bing*, means "sugar urine illness" (type 2 diabetes) (120). Unfortunately, a review of traditional Chinese medicine in the context of type 2 diabetes is beyond the scope of this chapter. However, several excellent reviews on this subject are available and will provide the reader with a more definitive evaluation of this subject than can be presented herein (121–127).

SUMMARY AND POSSIBILITIES FOR TREATMENT

Clearly, many natural products including botanicals and other nutraceuticals have hypoglycemic, antihyperglycemic, insulin-sensitizing, antihyperlipidemic, antihypertensive, and anti-inflammatory activities. There are published studies reporting the antidiabetic activity of well over a thousand different botanicals and nutraceuticals. The number of those treatments evaluated in clinical trials is approximately 100 (30). In the vast majority of these trials, the botanicals and nutraceuticals were evaluated as an adjunct to diet and prescription medications. Fifty-eight of the trials were controlled and conducted in individuals with diabetes or impaired glucose tolerance. Of these, statistically significant treatment effects were reported in 88% of trials (23 of 26) evaluating a single botanical and 67% of trials (18 of 27) evaluating individual vitamin or mineral supplements (reviewed in [30]). When reported, side effects were few and generally mild (gastrointestinal irritation and nausea).

However, many of the studies suffered from design flaws including small sample sizes (< 10 subjects), heterogeneity of subjects, and short duration of treatment. Furthermore, there is a lack of multiple studies for many of the individual supplements. Despite the apparent lack of side effects of these treatments, it would be prudent to be aware of the potential for dietary supplements, especially botanicals, to interact with a patient's prescription medication. One of the most important potential botanical-drug interactions is that of garlic, *Trigonella*, and *Ginkgo biloba* with nonsteroidal anti-inflammatory drugs (including aspirin) or warfarin, as these botanicals possess limited anticoagulant activity (53, 128). Another potential interaction of concern is one involving *G. biloba*, a botanical widely used for the treatment of memory and concentration problems, confusion, depression, anxiety, dizziness, tinnitus, and headache (129, 130). Ingestion of *G. biloba* extract by patients with type 2 diabetes may increase the hepatic metabolic clearance rate of not only insulin but also hypoglycemic medications, resulting in reduced insulin-mediated glucose metabolism and elevated blood glucose (131). Another issue to consider with botanicals is the potential for batch-to-batch variation caused by age of the plant, geographic source, time of harvest, and method of drying and preparation, all of which can dramatically impact the purity and potency of active ingredients. None of the agents discussed here are recommended for use in pregnant or lactating women or in children. Furthermore, patients should be advised on the proper use of any alternative treatment to avoid the risk of hypoglycemia.

That being stated, several botanical extracts merit consideration as complementary approaches for use in patients with type 2 diabetes. Botanical treatments with the strongest evidence of clinical safety and efficacy include *I. batas* (caiapo), *C. indica*, *T. foenum-graecum* (fenugreek), *M. charantia* (bitter melon), and *Opuntia* (prickly pear cactus; nopal).

REFERENCES

[1]Zimmet P, Alberti KG, Shaw J. Global and societal implications of the diabetes epidemic. *Nature.* 2001; 414:782–787.

[2]National Diabetes Information Clearinghouse. National Diabetes Statistics; http://diabetes.niddk.nih.gov/ dm/pubs/statistics/#1.

[3]International Diabetes Federation. Costs of Diabetes; www.eatlas.idf.org/Costs_of_diabetes/.

[4]Reaven GM. Insulin resistance and its consequences: type 2 diabetes mellitus and coronary heart disease. In: LeRoith D, Taylor SI, Olefsky JM, eds. *Diabetes Mellitus: A Fundamental and Clinical Text.* Philadelphia, PA: Lippincott Williams & Wilkins; 2000:604–615.

[5]Reaven GM. Role of insulin resistance in human disease. *Diabetes.* 1988;37:1595–1607.

[6]DeFronzo RA. Pathogenesis of type 2 diabetes: metabolic and molecular implications for identifying diabetes genes. *Diabetes Rev.* 1997;5:177–269.

[7]Hill JO, Wyatt HR, Reed GW, Peters JC. Obesity and the environment: where do we go from here? *Science.* 2003;299:853–855.

[8]Turner RC, Cull CA, Frighi V, Holman RR. Glycemic control with diet, sulfonylurea, metformin, or insulin in patients with type 2 diabetes mellitus: progressive requirement for multiple therapies (UKPDS 49). *JAMA.* 1999;281:2005–2012.

[9]DeFronzo RA. Pharmacologic therapy for type 2 diabetes mellitus. *Ann Intern Med.* 1999;131:281–303.

[10]Evans JL, Rushakoff RJ. Oral pharmacological agents for type 2 diabetes: sulfonylureas, meglitinides, metformin, thiazolidinediones, a-glucosidase inhibitors, and emerging approaches. In: Degroot L, Goldfine ID, Rushakoff RJ, eds. Endotext.com: Diabetes and Carbohydrate Metabolism. www.medtext.com: MDtext. com, 2007.

[11]Mizuno CS, Chittiboyina AG, Kurtz TW, Pershadsingh HA, Avery MA. Type 2 diabetes and oral antihyperglycemic drugs. *Curr Med Chem.* 2008;15:61–74.

[12]Bolen S, Feldman L, Vassy J, Wilson L, Yeh HC, Marinopoulos S, Wiley C, Selvin E, Wilson R, Bass EB, Brancati FL. Systematic review: comparative effectiveness and safety of oral medications for type 2 diabetes mellitus. *Ann Intern Med.* 2007;147:386–399.

[13]Evans JL. Antioxidants: do they have a role in the treatment of insulin resistance? *Indian J Med Res.* 2007;125:355–372.

[14]Krentz AJ, Bailey CJ. Oral antidiabetic agents: current role in type 2 diabetes mellitus. *Drugs.* 2005;65: 385–411.

[15]Fuhr JP, He H, Goldfarb N, Nash DB. Use of chromium picolinate and biotin in the management of type 2 diabetes: an economic analysis. *Dis Manag.* 2005;8:265–275.

[16]Altman SH, Parks-Thomas C. Controlling spending for prescription drugs. *N Engl J Med.* 2002;346:855–856.

[17]Dham S, Shah V, Hirsch S, Banerji MA. The role of complementary and alternative medicine in diabetes. *Curr Diab Rep.* 2006;6:251–258.

[18]Cicero AF, Derosa G, Gaddi A. What do herbalists suggest to diabetic patients in order to improve glycemic control? Evaluation of scientific evidence and potential risks. *Acta Diabetol.* 2004;41:91–98.

[19]Saxena A, Vikram NK. Role of selected Indian plants in management of type 2 diabetes: a review. *J Altern Complement Med.* 2004;10:369–378.

[20]Shekelle PG, Hardy M, Morton SC, Coulter I, Venuturupalli S, Favreau J, Hilton LK. Are Ayurvedic herbs for diabetes effective? *J Fam Pract.* 2005;54:876–886.

[21]Andrade-Cetto A, Heinrich M. Mexican plants with hypoglycemic effect used in the treatment of diabetes. *J Ethnopharmacol.* 2005;99:325–348.

[22]Johnson L, Strich H, Taylor A, Timmermann B, Malone D, Teufel-Shone N, Drummond R, Woosley R, Pereira E, Martinez A. Use of herbal remedies by diabetic Hispanic women in the southwestern United States. *Phytother Res.* 2006;20:250–255.

[23]Shapiro K, Gong WC. Natural products used for diabetes. *J Am Pharm Assoc (Wash).* 2002;42:217–226.

[24]Berman BM, Swyers JP, Kaczmarczyk J. Complementary and alternative medicine: herbal therapies for diabetes. *J Assoc Acad Minor Phys.* 1999;10:10–14.

[25]Grover JK, Yadav S, Vats V. Medicinal plants of India with anti-diabetic potential. *J Ethnopharmacol.* 2002;81:81–100.

[26]Murray MT, Pizzorno JE. Botanical medicine: a modern perspective. *Textbook of Natural Medicine.* Edinburgh: Churchill Livingstone; 1999.

[27]Modak M, Dixit P, Londhe J, Ghaskadbi S, Paul AD. Indian herbs and herbal drugs used for the treatment of diabetes. *J Clin Biochem Nutr.* 2007;40:163–173.

[28]Shane-McWhorter L. Botanical dietary supplements and the treatment of diabetes: what is the evidence? *Curr Diab Rep.* 2005;5:391–398.

[29]Evans JL. Non-pharmaceutical interventions for type 2 diabetes: nutrition, botanicals, antioxidants, minerals, and other dietary supplements. In: Degroot L, Goldfine ID, Rushakoff RJ, eds. Endotext.com: Diabetes and Carbohydrate Metabolism. www.medtext.com: MDtext.com, 2007.

[30]Yeh GY, Eisenberg DM, Kaptchuk TJ, Phillips RS. Systematic review of herbs and dietary supplements for glycemic control in diabetes. *Diabetes Care.* 2003;26:1277–1294.

[31]Dey L, Attele AS, Yuan CS. Alternative therapies for type 2 diabetes. *Altern Med Rev.* 2002;7:45–58.

[32]*Antioxidants in Diabetes Management.* 1st ed. New York, NY: Marcel Dekker; 2000.

[33]Griggs B. *Green Pharmacy: A History of Herbal Medicine.* 1st ed. London: Robert Hale; 1981.

[34]Bailey CJ, Turner RC. Metformin. *N Engl J Med.* 1996;334:574–579.

[35]Witters LA. The blooming of the French lilac. *J Clin Invest.* 2001;108:1105–1107.

[36]Cusi K, DeFronzo RA. Metformin: a review of its metabolic effects. *Diabetes Rev.* 1998;6:89–131.

[37]Oubre AY, Carlson TJ, King SR, Reaven GM. From plant to patient: an ethnomedical approach to the identification of new drugs for the treatment of NIDDM. *Diabetologia.* 1997;40:614–617.

[38]Ackerknecht EH. *A Short History of Medicine.* Rev. ed. Baltimore, MD: Johns Hopkins University Press; 1982.

[39]Bailey CJ, Day C. Traditional plant medicine as treatments for diabetes. *Diabetes Care.* 1989;12:553–564.

[40]Marles RJ, Farnsworth NR. Plants as sources of antidiabetic agents. *Economic and Medical Plant Research.* 1993;6:149–187.

[41]Marles RJ, Farnsworth NR. Antidiabetic plants and their active constituents. *Phytomed.* 1995;2:137–189.

[42]Haddad PS, Depot M, Settaf A, Cherrah Y. Use of antidiabetic plants in Morocco and Quebec. *Diabetes Care.* 2001;24:608–609.

[43]Jung M, Park M, Lee HC, Kang YH, Kang ES, Kim SK. Antidiabetic agents from medicinal plants. *Curr Med Chem.* 2006;13:1203–1218.

[44]Kusano S, Abe H. Antidiabetic activity of white skinned sweet potato (Ipomoea batatas L.) in obese Zucker fatty rats. *Biol Pharm Bull.* 2000;23:23–26.

[45]Kusano S, Abe H, Tamura H. Isolation of antidiabetic components from white-skinned sweet potato (Ipomoea batatas L.). *Biosci Biotechnol Biochem.* 2001;65:109–114.

[46]Ludvik BH, Mahdjoobian K, Waldhaeusl W, Hofer A, Prager R, Kautzky-Willer A, Pacini G. The effect of Ipomoea batatas (caiapo) on glucose metabolism and serum cholesterol in patients with type 2 diabetes: a randomized study. *Diabetes Care.* 2002;25:239–240.

[47]Ludvik B, Waldhausl W, Prager R, Kautzky-Willer A, Pacini G. Mode of action of ipomoea batatas (caiapo) in type 2 diabetic patients. *Metabolism.* 2003;52:875–880.

[48]Ludvik B, Neuffer B, Pacini G. Efficacy of Ipomoea batatas (caiapo) on diabetes control in type 2 diabetic subjects treated with diet. *Diabetes Care*. 2004;27:436–440.

[49]Bloomgarden ZT, Dodis R, Viscoli CM, Holmboe ES, Inzucchi SE. Lower baseline glycemia reduces apparent oral agent glucose-lowering efficacy: a meta-regression analysis. *Diabetes Care*. 2006;29:2137–2139.

[50]Ludvik B, Hanefeld M, Pacini G. Improved metabolic control by Ipomoea batatas (caiapo) is associated with increased adiponectin and decreased fibrinogen levels in type 2 diabetic subjects. *Diabetes Obes Metab*. 2007;Epub ahead of print.

[51]Azad Khan AK, Akhtar S, Mahtab H. Coccinia indica in the treatment of patients with diabetes mellitus. *Bangladesh Med Res Counc Bull*. 1979;5:60–66.

[52]Kuriyan R, Rajendran R, Bantwal G, Kurpad AV. Effect of supplementation of Coccinia cordifolia extract on newly detected diabetic patients. *Diabetes Care*. 2008;31:216–220.

[53]Anonymous. *PDR for Herbal Medicines*. 1st ed ed. Montvale, NJ: Medical Economics Co.; 1998.

[54]Brasch E, Ulbricht C, Kuo G, Szapary P, Smith M. Therapeutic applications of fenugreek. *Altern Med Rev*. 2003;8:20–27.

[55]Sauvaire Y, Petit P, Broca C, Manteghetti M, Baissac Y, Fernandez-Alvarez J, Gross R, Roye M, Leconte A, Gomis R, Ribes G. 4-Hydroxyisoleucine: a novel amino acid potentiator of insulin secretion. *Diabetes*. 1998;47:206–210.

[56]Broca C, Manteghetti M, Gross R, Baissac Y, Jacob M, Petit P, Sauvaire Y, Ribes G. 4-Hydroxyisoleucine: effects of synthetic and natural analogues on insulin secretion. *Eur J Pharmacol*. 2000;390:339–345.

[57]Broca C, Gross R, Petit P, Sauvaire Y, Manteghetti M, Tournier M, Masiello P, Gomis R, Ribes G. 4-Hydroxyisoleucine: experimental evidence of its insulinotropic and antidiabetic properties. *Am J Physiol*. 1999;277:E617–E623.

[58]Vijayakumar MV, Bhat MK. Hypoglycemic effect of a novel dialysed fenugreek seeds extract is sustainable and is mediated, in part, by the activation of hepatic enzymes. *Phytother Res*. 2008;22:500–505.

[59]Madar Z, Abel R, Samish S, Arad J. Glucose-lowering effect of fenugreek in non-insulin dependent diabetics. *Eur J Clin Nutr*. 1988;42:51–54.

[60]Sharma RD, Sarkar A, Hazra DK. Use of fenugreek seed powder in the management of non-insulin dependent diabetes mellitus. *Nutr Res*. 1996;16:1331–1339.

[61]Gupta A, Gupta R, Lal B. Effect of Trigonella foenum-graecum (fenugreek) seeds on glycaemic control and insulin resistance in type 2 diabetes mellitus: a double blind placebo controlled study. *J Assoc Physicians India*. 2001;49:1057–1061.

[62]Kochhar A, Nagi M. Effect of supplementation of traditional medicinal plants on blood glucose in non-insulin-dependent diabetics: a pilot study. *J Med Food*. 2005;8:545–549.

[63]Flammang AM, Cifone MA, Erexson GL, Stankowski LF, Jr. Genotoxicity testing of a fenugreek extract. *Food Chem Toxicol*. 2004;42:1769–1775.

[64]Roman-Ramos R, Flores-Saenz JL, Alarcon-Aguilar FJ. Anti-hyperglycemic effect of some edible plants. *J Ethnopharmacol*. 1995;48:25–32.

[65]El Kossori RL, Villaume C, El Boustani E, Sauvaire Y, Mejean L. Composition of pulp, skin and seeds of prickly pears fruit (Opuntia ficus indica sp.). *Plant Foods Hum Nutr*. 1998;52:263–270.

[66]Frati AC, Gordillo BE, Altamirano P, Ariza CR, Cortes-Franco R, Chavez-Negrete A. Acute hypoglycemic effect of Opuntia streptacantha Lemaire in NIDDM. *Diabetes Care*. 1990;13:455–456.

[67]Frati-Munari AC, Gordillo BE, Altamirano P, Ariza CR. Hypoglycemic effect of Opuntia streptacantha Lemaire in NIDDM. *Diabetes Care*. 1988;11:63–66.

[68]Bacardi-Gascon M, Duenas-Mena D, Jimenez-Cruz A. Lowering effect on postprandial glycemic response of nopales added to Mexican breakfasts. *Diabetes Care*. 2007;30:1264–1265.

[69]Nag B, Medicherla S, Sharma SD. Orally active fraction of momordica charantia, active peptides thereof, and their use in the treatment of diabetes. *US Patent*. 2002;6,391,854:1–14.

[70]Chen Q, Chan LL, Li ET. Bitter melon (Momordica charantia) reduces adiposity, lowers serum insulin and normalizes glucose tolerance in rats fed a high fat diet. *J Nutr*. 2003;133:1088–1093.

[71]Krawinkel MB, Keding GB. Bitter gourd (Momordica charantia): a dietary approach to hyperglycemia. *Nutr Rev*. 2006;64:331–337.

[72]Chan LL, Chen Q, Go AG, Lam EK, Li ET. Reduced adiposity in bitter melon (Momordica charantia)-fed rats is associated with increased lipid oxidative enzyme activities and uncoupling protein expression. *J Nutr*. 2005;135:2517–2523.

[73]Huang HL, Hong YW, Wong YH, Chen YN, Chyuan JH, Huang CJ, Chao PM. Bitter melon (Momordica charantia L.) inhibits adipocyte hypertrophy and down regulates lipogenic gene expression in adipose tissue of diet-induced obese rats. *Br J Nutr*. 2008;99:230–239.

[74]Sridhar MG, Vinayagamoorthi R, Arul S, V, Bobby Z, Selvaraj N. Bitter gourd (Momordica charantia) improves insulin sensitivity by increasing skeletal muscle insulin-stimulated IRS-1 tyrosine phosphorylation in high-fat-fed rats. *Br J Nutr*. 2008;99:806–812.

[75]Tan MJ, Ye JM, Turner N, Hohnen-Behrens C, Ke CQ, Tang CP, Chen T, Weiss HC, Gesing ER, Rowland A, James DE, Ye Y. Antidiabetic activities of triterpenoids isolated from bitter melon associated with activation of the AMPK pathway. *Chem Biol.* 2008;15:263–273.

[76]Basch E, Gabardi S, Ulbricht C. Bitter melon (Momordica charantia): a review of efficacy and safety. *Am J Health Syst Pharm.* 2003;60:356–359.

[77]Kanetkar P, Singhal R, Kamat M. Gymnema sylvestre: a memoir. *J Clin Biochem Nutr.* 2007;41:77–81.

[78]Leach MJ. Gymnema sylvestre for diabetes mellitus: a systematic review. *J Altern Complement Med.* 2007;13:977–983.

[79]Banerjee SK, Maulik SK. Effect of garlic on cardiovascular disorders: a review. *Nutr J.* 2002;1:4.

[80]Liu CT, Sheen LY, Lii CK. Does garlic have a role as an antidiabetic agent? *Mol Nutr Food Res.* 2007;51:1353–1364.

[81]Borek C. Garlic reduces dementia and heart-disease risk. *J Nutr.* 2006;136:810S–812S.

[82]Budoff M. Aged garlic extract retards progression of coronary artery calcification. *J Nutr.* 2006;136:741S–744S.

[83]Ahmad MS, Ahmed N. Antiglycation properties of aged garlic extract: possible role in prevention of diabetic complications. *J Nutr.* 2006;136:796S–799S.

[84]Kendler BS. Garlic (Allium sativum) and onion (Allium cepa): a review of their relationship to cardiovascular disease. *Prev Med.* 1987;16:670–685.

[85]Keys A. Wine, garlic, and CHD in seven countries. *Lancet.* 1980;1:145–146.

[86]Kris-Etherton PM, Etherton TD, Carlson J, Gardner C. Recent discoveries in inclusive food-based approaches and dietary patterns for reduction in risk for cardiovascular disease. *Curr Opin Lipidol.* 2002;13:397–407.

[87]Ashraf R, Aamir K, Shaikh AR, Ahmed T. Effects of garlic on dyslipidemia in patients with type 2 diabetes mellitus. *J Ayub Med Coll Abbottabad.* 2005;17:60–64.

[88]Sobenin IA, Nedosugova LV, Filatova LV, Balabolkin MI, Gorchakova TV, Orekhov AN. Metabolic effects of time-released garlic powder tablets in type 2 diabetes mellitus: the results of double-blinded placebo-controlled study. *Acta Diabetol.* 2008;45:1–6.

[89]Xie JT, Mchendale S, Yuan CS. Ginseng and diabetes. *Am J Chin Med.* 2005;33:397–404.

[90]Vogler BK, Pittler MH, Ernst E. The efficacy of ginseng: a systematic review of randomised clinical trials. *Eur J Clin Pharmacol.* 1999;55:567–575.

[91]Sievenpiper JL, Arnason JT, Vidgen E, Leiter LA, Vuksan V. A systematic quantitative analysis of the literature of the high variability in ginseng (Panax spp.): should ginseng be trusted in diabetes? *Diabetes Care.* 2004;27:839–840.

[92]Vuksan V, Sievenpiper JL. Herbal remedies in the management of diabetes: lessons learned from the study of ginseng. *Nutr Metab Cardiovasc Dis.* 2005;15:149–160.

[93]Xie JT, Wang CZ, Ni M, Wu JA, Mehendale SR, Aung HH, Foo A, Yuan CS. American ginseng berry juice intake reduces blood glucose and body weight in ob/ob mice. *J Food Sci.* 2007;72:S590–S594.

[94]Lee WK, Kao ST, Liu IM, Cheng JT. Ginsenoside Rh2 is one of the active principles of Panax ginseng root to improve insulin sensitivity in fructose-rich chow-fed rats. *Horm Metab Res.* 2007;39:347–354.

[95]Kim HY, Kang KS, Yamabe N, Nagai R, Yokozawa T. Protective effect of heat-processed American ginseng against diabetic renal damage in rats. *J Agric Food Chem.* 2007;55:8491–8497.

[96]Sotaniemi EA, Haapakoski E, Rautio A. Ginseng therapy in non-insulin-dependent diabetic patients. *Diabetes Care.* 1995;18:1373–1375.

[97]Vuksan V, Sung MK, Sievenpiper JL, Stavro PM, Jenkins AL, Di BM, Lee KS, Leiter LA, Nam KY, Arnason JT, Choi M, Naeem A. Korean red ginseng (Panax ginseng) improves glucose and insulin regulation in well-controlled, type 2 diabetes: results of a randomized, double-blind, placebo-controlled study of efficacy and safety. *Nutr Metab Cardiovasc Dis.* 2008;18:46–56.

[98]Vuksan V, Sievenpiper JL, Koo VY, Francis T, Beljan-Zdravkovic U, Xu Z, Vidgen E. American ginseng (Panax quinquefolius L) reduces postprandial glycemia in nondiabetic subjects and subjects with type 2 diabetes mellitus. *Arch Intern Med.* 2000;160:1009–1013.

[99]Vogler BK, Ernst E. Aloe vera: a systematic review of its clinical effectiveness. *Br J Gen Pract.* 1999;49:823–828.

[100]Al Rowais NA. Herbal medicine in the treatment of diabetes mellitus. *Saudi Med J.* 2002;23:1327–1331.

[101]Tanaka M, Misawa E, Ito Y, Habara N, Nomaguchi K, Yamada M, Toida T, Hayasawa H, Takase M, Inagaki M, Higuchi R. Identification of five phytosterols from Aloe vera gel as anti-diabetic compounds. *Biol Pharm Bull.* 2006;29:1418–1422.

[102]Beppu H, Shimpo K, Chihara T, Kaneko T, Tamai I, Yamaji S, Ozaki S, Kuzuya H, Sonoda S. Antidiabetic effects of dietary administration of Aloe arborescens Miller components on multiple low-dose streptozotocin-induced diabetes in mice: investigation on hypoglycemic action and systemic absorption dynamics of aloe components. *J Ethnopharmacol.* 2006;103:468–477.

[103]Ghannam N, Kingston M, Al Meshaal IA, Tariq M, Parman NS, Woodhouse N. The antidiabetic activity of aloes: preliminary clinical and experimental observations. *Horm Res.* 1986;24:288–294.

[104]Yongchaiyudha S, Rungpitarangsi V, Bunyapraphatsara N, Chokechaijaroenporn O. Antidiabetic activity of Aloe vera L. juice: I. clinical trial in new cases of diabetes mellitus. *Phytomed.* 1996;3:241–243.

[105]Bunyapraphatsara N, Yongchaiyudha S, Rungpitarangsi V, Chokechaijaroenporn O. Antidiabetic activity of Aloe vera L. juice: II. clinical trial in diabetes mellitus patients in combination with glibenclamide. *Phytomed.* 1996;3:245–248.

[106]Vuksan V, Jenkins DJA, Spadafora P, Sievenpiper JL, Owen R, Vidgen E, Brighenti F, Josse R, Leiter LA, Bruce-Thompson C. Konjac-Mannan Glucomannan improves glycemia and other associated risk factors for coronary heart disease in type 2 diabetes: a randomized controlled metabolic trial. *Diabetes Care.* 1999;22:913–919.

[107]Vuksan V, Sievenpiper JL, Owen R, Swilley JA, Spadafora P, Jenkins DJ, Vidgen E, Brighenti F, Josse RG, Leiter LA, Xu Z, Novokmet R. Beneficial effects of viscous dietary fiber from Konjac-mannan in subjects with the insulin resistance syndrome: results of a controlled metabolic trial. *Diabetes Care.* 2000;23:9–14.

[108]Khan A, Bryden NA, Polansky MM, Anderson RA. Insulin potentiating factor and chromium content of selected foods and spices. *Biol Trace Element Res.* 1990;24:183–188.

[109]Berrio LF, Polansky MM, Anderson RA. Insulin activity: stimulatory effects of cinnamon and brewer's yeast as influenced by albumin. *Horm Res.* 1992;37:225–229.

[110]Evans JL, Jallal B. Protein tyrosine phosphatases: their role in insulin action and potential as drug targets. *Exp Opin Invest Drugs.* 1999;8:139–160.

[111]Imparl-Radosevich J, Deas S, Polansky MM, Baedke DA, Ingebritsen TS, Anderson RA, Graves DJ. Regulation of PTP-1 and insulin receptor kinase by fractions from cinnamon: implications for cinnamon regulation of insulin signalling. *Horm Res.* 1998;50:177–182.

[112]Hlebowicz J, Darwiche G, Bjorgell O, Almer LO. Effect of cinnamon on postprandial blood glucose, gastric emptying, and satiety in healthy subjects. *Am J Clin Nutr.* 2007;85:1552–1556.

[113]Solomon TP, Blannin AK. Effects of short-term cinnamon ingestion on in vivo glucose tolerance. *Diabetes Obes Metab.* 2007;9:895–901.

[114]Khan A, Safdar M, li Khan MM, Khattak KN, Anderson RA. Cinnamon improves glucose and lipids of people with type 2 diabetes. *Diabetes Care.* 2003;26:3215–3218.

[115]Mang B, Wolters M, Schmitt B, Kelb K, Lichtinghagen R, Stichtenoth DO, Hahn A. Effects of a cinnamon extract on plasma glucose, HbA, and serum lipids in diabetes mellitus type 2. *Eur J Clin Invest.* 2006;36:340–344.

[116]Vanschoonbeek K, Thomassen BJ, Senden JM, Wodzig WK, van Loon LJ. Cinnamon supplementation does not improve glycemic control in postmenopausal type 2 diabetes patients. *J Nutr.* 2006;136:977–980.

[117]Blevins SM, Leyva MJ, Brown J, Wright J, Scofield RH, Aston CE. Effect of cinnamon on glucose and lipid levels in non insulin-dependent type 2 diabetes. *Diabetes Care.* 2007;30:2236–2237.

[118]Baker WL, Gutierrez-Williams G, White CM, Kluger J, Coleman CI. Effect of cinnamon on glucose control and lipid parameters. *Diabetes Care.* 2008;31:41–43.

[119]Anderson RA. Chromium and polyphenols from cinnamon improve insulin sensitivity. *Proc Nutr Soc.* 2008;67:48–53.

[120]Covington MB. Traditional Chinese medicine in the treatment of diabetes. *Diabetes Spectrum.* 2001;14:154–159.

[121]Zhao HL, Tong PC, Chan JC. Traditional Chinese medicine in the treatment of diabetes. *Nestle Nutr Workshop Ser Clin Perform Programme.* 2006;11:15–25.

[122]Li YJ, Xu HX. Research progress on anti-diabetic Chinese medicines. *Zhong Yao Cai.* 2006;29:621–624.

[123]Fan Z. A survey of treatment of diabetic complications with Chinese drugs. *J Tradit Chin Med.* 2005;25:153–159.

[124]Jia W, Gao W, Tang L. Antidiabetic herbal drugs officially approved in China. *Phytother Res.* 2003;17:1127–1134.

[125]Liu JP, Zhang M, Wang WY, Grimsgaard S. Chinese herbal medicines for type 2 diabetes mellitus. *Cochrane Database Syst Rev.* 2004;Issue 3:CD003642.

[126]Li WL, Zheng HC, Bukuru J, De KN. Natural medicines used in the traditional Chinese medical system for therapy of diabetes mellitus. *J Ethnopharmacol.* 2004;92:1–21.

[127]Jia W, Gao WY, Xiao PG. Antidiabetic drugs of plant origin used in China: compositions, pharmacology, and hypoglycemic mechanisms. *Zhongguo Zhong Yao Za Zhi.* 2003;28:108–113.

[128]Abebe W. Herbal medication: potential for adverse interactions with analgesic drugs. *J Clin Pharm Ther.* 2002;27:391–401.

[129]Canter PH, Ernst E. Ginkgo biloba: a smart drug? A systematic review of controlled trials of the cognitive effects of ginkgo biloba extracts in healthy people. *Psychopharmacol Bull.* 2002;36:108–123.

[130]Birks J, Grimley EV, Van Dongen M. Ginkgo biloba for cognitive impairment and dementia. *Cochrane Database Syst Rev.* 2002;CD003120.

[131]Kudolo GB. The effect of 3-month ingestion of Ginkgo biloba extract (EGb 761) on pancreatic beta-cell function in response to glucose loading in individuals with non-insulin-dependent diabetes mellitus. *J Clin Pharmacol.* 2001;41:600–611.

Botanical Medicine: From Bench to Bedside
Edited by R. Cooper and F. Kronenberg
© Mary Ann Liebert, Inc.

Chapter 3
Botanicals in Dermatology and Skin Health

Juliane Reuter,[1] *Irmgard Merfort,*[2] *Ute Wölfle,*[1] *Günter Seelinger,*[3] *and Christoph M. Schempp*[1,*]

Botanical extracts have been used for cosmetic and therapeutic purposes in the form of fresh plants or dried or extracted plant material since ancient times. These extracts are often registered as botanical medicine, also referred to as herbal medicine, phytotherapy, or phytomedicine (1). Today, increasing numbers of patients and consumers are asking for plant-based therapeutic preparations as a complementary dermatologic therapy. Botanical therapies are considered as therapeutic alternatives, as agents of safer choice in comparison to conventional therapy, or sometimes as the only effective therapeutic way remaining to treat a certain skin disease. The cosmetic industry is expanding the use of botanicals by introducing plant extracts, herbs, flowers, fruits, and seed oleates into their products, promising a gentler, more organic approach to beauty. Botanical-based cosmetics are well accepted by the consumers because they are said to possess the ability to detoxify, hydrate, strengthen, stimulate, relax, and balance the skin and hair. These products with active compounds are collectively referred to as "cosmeceuticals" (2)—a portmanteau of cosmetic and pharmaceutical.

Because the use of botanicals in dermatologic products is becoming increasingly popular, clinicians need to learn about their efficacy and possible side effects. The present chapter mainly focuses on botanicals that have been investigated in clinical trials. However, experimental research on botanicals was also considered to a limited extent when it seemed promising for product development in the near future.

The present chapter reviews the results of controlled clinical studies on botanicals used in dermatology. Plant-derived single compounds already established in dermatological therapy such as dithranol, salicylates, or podophyllotoxin are also discussed (Table 3.1). In the following sections, the botanicals are discussed under the dermatological indications where they have been studied or would be primarily indicated according to their mode of action (Table 3.2). Most of the studies on botanical extracts have been performed with

[1] Competence Center Skintegral, Department of Dermatology, University Medical Center Freiburg, Freiburg, Germany
[2] Institute of Pharmaceutical Sciences, University of Freiburg, Freiburg, Germany
[3] Medical and Pharmaceutical Services, Berlin, Germany
* Corresponding author: christoph.schempp@uniklinik-freiburg.de

Table 3.1. Plant-Derived Compounds Already Established in Dermatology

• Dithranol (Anthralin)	from *Andira arraroba*
• 8-Methoxypsoralen	from *Ammi majus*
• Podophyllin	from *Podophyllum peltatum*
• Salicylates	from *Salix alba*
• Tannins	from *Cortex quercus*

Table 3.2. Possible Claims and Targets for Botanicals in Dermatology According to Their Mode of Action (MOA)

MOA	
Cosmetological Claims/Targets	*Pharmacological Claims/Targets*
antimicrobial "impure skin,"	acne, infections
dandruff	seborrhoic eczema
anti-inflammatory "sensitive skin"	atopic dermatitis
antiproliferative dry, scaly skin	psoriasis
wound-healing "fragile skin" photoprotective	ulcers
anti-aging "mature skin"	solar keratoses, skin cancer

topical preparations. Where appropriate, studies with botanical food supplements are considered as well. Finally, the most important limitations for the use of botanicals in dermatology are outlined.

Literature references were obtained between December 2007 and June 2008 covering "botanicals," "phytomedicine," "phytotherapy," "herbal therapy," and "herbal medicine," combined with "dermatology" and "skin." This combination addresses specific skin disorders: "acne," "rosacea," "atopic dermatitis," "psoriasis," "chronic venous insufficiency," "skin infections," "alopecia," "vitiligo," "wounds," and "skin cancer," but also "UV-protection" and "sunscreen." To provide the reader with information on the quality of the studies, each study was classified according to the levels of evidence (LOE) A-D suggested by the U.K. National Health Service (3). In brief, LOE-A is assigned to consistent, randomized, controlled clinical trials and cohort studies; LOE-B is assigned to consistent retrospective cohorts, exploratory cohorts, outcome researches, case-control studies, or extrapolations from LOE-A studies; LOE-C is assigned to case-series studies or extrapolations from LOE-B studies; LOE-D is assigned to expert opinions without explicit critical appraisal or based on physiology, bench research, or first principles. Whenever possible, the level of evidence was indicated for each study in squared brackets, for example, as [LOE-A].

INFLAMMATORY SKIN DISEASES

Atopic Dermatitis

Atopic dermatitis (AD, atopic eczema, neurodermatitis) is a chronic inflammatory skin disease which is most abundant in children but may persist to adulthood or, more often, can be replaced by hay fever and asthma in later years ("atopic career"). It represents a hypersensitivity of the immune system with a strong hereditary component and increased responsiveness to environmental or food allergens or climate and to psychological factors like stress or fatigue. Prevalence of AD is increasing, with approximately 10% to 20% of children in industrial countries being affected and 1% to 3% of adults.

AD is characterized by red, itching skin with papulovesicles and oozing erosions in the acute stage and dry and scaly skin in chronic phases. Lesional skin is often subject to bacterial infections, especially with *Staphylococcus aureus*. Face, neck, bends of elbows, and hollows of the knees are primary sites, but any other skin areas may also be affected. There is no cure for AD, but relief from symptoms is possible and in children there is hope that it will vanish over the years. Prevention of atopic outbursts includes avoidance of food allergens or inhalative allergens but also optimized skin care, adequate clothing, and many other factors. Treatment includes stage-adequate skin care and anti-inflammatory, antipruritic, and antimicrobial treatment. The most important drugs are corticosteroids or calcineurin inhibitors that are usually applied topically but in severe cases also applied systemically.

Traditional herbal treatment of AD has to consider the actual stage of the disease. Acute, oozing eczema is covered (but not occluded) with cold wet packs made from oak bark (*Quercus spp.*), witch hazel (*Hamamelis virginiana*), black tea (*Camellia sinensis*), or chamomile (*Matricaria recutita*) decoctions. In subacute stages and intervals, ointments or creams with antiphlogistic and antipruritic drugs like balloon vine (*Cardiospermum halicacabum*), bittersweet (*Solanum dulcamara*), witch hazel, or oat straw are recommended. Oils from borage (*Borago officinalis*) or from evening primrose (*Oenothera biennis*) are rich in g-linoleic acid and used for systemic and topical application. Bacterial superinfections are treated topically with chamomile tea or oil from St. John's wort (*Hypericum perforatum*) (4, 5) [LOE-D].

Topical application: For most of these traditionally used herbal treatments, there is limited evidence from clinical studies (an overview of clinical studies in AD is given in Table 3.3). A partially double-blind, randomized study was carried out as a half-side comparison of a cream containing chamomile (*Matricaria recutita*) extract from the chemical race "Manzana" versus 0.5% hydrocortisone cream and the vehicle cream as placebo in 72 patients suffering from medium-degree AD. After two weeks of treatment, the chamomile cream displayed only a marginal superiority compared to 0.5% hydrocortisone and was not superior to placebo (6) [LOE-A].

Since bacterial colonization plays a role in the pathogenesis of AD, antimicrobial activity of a medical skin care product for AD would be beneficial. Recently, the antimicrobial property of a distillate of witch hazel (*Hamamelis virginiana*) and urea, formulated as a topical dermatological preparation that contains both active ingredients, has been investigated in vivo by using the simple occlusion test in 15 healthy volunteers.

The test revealed a significant antimicrobial activity of the product (7) [LOE-C]. Formulations containing *Hamamelis* distillate have mainly anti-inflammatory, hydrating, and

Table 3.3. Overview on Clinical Studies with Botanicals for Atopic Dermatitis

Botanicals	Patients (n)	Placebo Controlled	Study End Points	Route of Administration	Treatment Phase	Results	Ref. / LOE
Chamomile (*Matricaria recutita*)	72	+	itch, erythema, scaling	topical	2 weeks	mild superiority to placebo	6 / [LOE-A]
Witch hazel (*Hamamelis virginiana*)	72	+	itch, erythema, scaling	topical	2 weeks	not superior to placebo	8 / [LOE-A]
St. John's wort (*Hypericum perforatum*)	28	+	SCORAD	topical	4 weeks	AD improved	9 / [LOE-A]
Shiunko (Japanese Kampo medicine)	21	+	bacterial species	topical	3 weeks	bacterial isolates↓	12 / [LOE-B]
Oregon grape root	42 adults	–	EASI	topical	12 weeks	AD improved	15 / [LOE-B]
Oregon grape root (*Mahonia aquifolium*)	27 children	–	itch, erythema	topical	4 weeks	AD improved	16 / [LOE-B]
pansy (*Viola tricolor*), gotu kola (*Centella asiatica*)	88 adults	+	itch, erythema	topical	4 weeks	AD improved but not significantly	17 / [LOE-A]
Licorice (*Glycyrrhiza glabra*)	108	+	edema, itch, erythema	topical	2 weeks	AD improved	19 / [LOE-A]
Licorice (*Glycyrrhiza glabra*)	218	+	EASI, BSA, itch	topical	50 days	AD improved	21 / [LOE-A]
vine leaves (*Vitis vinifera*), allantoin and telmesteine	20	+	TEWL, itch, erythema	topical	72 hours	TEWL↓ erythema↓	22 / [LOE-B]
Oolong tea	30	+	EASI, itch	topical	5 weeks	AD improved	20 / [LOE-A]
Hochu-ekki-to (Japanese Kampo medicine)	121	–	itch, clinical signs	oral 3 × daily	6 months	AD improved	23 / [LOE-B]
	10	–	skin symptoms, eosinophils, IgE	oral 7.5g granules daily	3 months	AD improved, IgE↓, eosinophils↓	24 / [LOE-D]
Traditional Chinese herbal medicine (TCHM)	85 children	+	SCORAD, CDLQI	oral 3 capsules 2 × daily	12 weeks	Quality of life improved, AD not superior to placebo	26 / [LOE-A]
	40 adults	+	erythema, surface damage	oral decoction daily	5 months	AD improved	27 / [LOE-A]

LOE=level of evidence according to (3); SCORAD=scoring of atopic dermatitis score; EASI=Eczema Area and Severity Index; BSA=affected body surface area;
TEWL=trans-epidermal water loss; CDLQI=Children's Dermatology Life Quality Index

barrier-stabilizing effects that may be beneficial in AD maintenance therapy. However, *Hamamelis* is not efficient enough to treat severe AD, as shown in a double-blind, randomized paired trial in patients suffering from moderately severe AD. Seventy-two patients were treated with a *Hamamelis* distillate cream compared with the corresponding drug-free vehicle and 0.5% hydrocortisone cream over a period of 14 days. The *Hamamelis* preparation was not superior to the vehicle (8) [LOE-A].

In contrast, both antimicrobial activity and therapeutic efficacy have been demonstrated for St. John's wort (*Hypericum perforatum*) extract (9, 10). A medical skin care product in the form of a cream distributed in European countries was tested in a randomized, placebo-controlled, double-blind, half-side comparison study in 28 patients with AD. The efficacy of the *Hypericum* cream was significantly superior to its vehicle. The skin tolerance and cosmetic acceptability of the *Hypericum* cream was excellent (9) [LOE-A]. In addition to antimicrobial activity, one possible mode of action of St. John's wort and its major compound hyperforin might be the inhibition of the antigen-presenting capacity of epidermal Langerhans cells (11) [LOE-D].

Another placebo-controlled study with only seven AD patients was performed with Shiunko, a typical Japanese Kampo drug made from herbal extracts. The clinical effectiveness and the changes in bacterial species and cell numbers on the skin were evaluated. Bacterial counts were reduced with Shiunko in four of seven patients compared to one for placebo (12) [LOE-B].

No effect superior to placebo could be demonstrated in the following trials: a randomized, double-blind, placebo-controlled trial with 53 patients with mild to intermediate AD using 20% and 10% sea buckthorn (*Hippophae rhamnoides*) containing cream (13) [LOE-A]; a randomized, double-blind, placebo-controlled study with 20 AD patients using an ointment containing 15% black seed (*Nigella sativa L.*) oil (14) [LOE-A].

Oregon grape root: Besides displaying antimicrobial activity due to berberine and other constituents, Oregon grape root inhibits proinflammatory cytokines. A cream containing 10% *Mahonia* extract ("psorberine") has recently been evaluated in an open-label trial in 42 adult AD patients treated three times daily over a period of 12 weeks. There was a significant improvement of the Eczema Area and Severity Index (EASI) score (15) [LOE-B].

An open, noncontrolled study with 27 children suffering from AD was conducted with an over-the-counter herbal ointment containing 5% of homeopathic mother tinctures each of the botanicals Oregon grape root (*Mahonia aquifolium*), pansy (*Viola tricolor hortensis*), and gotu kola (*Centella asiatica*). Within the 2–4-week observation period, the symptoms resolved completely in 22% of the patients, an additional 60% reporting marked improvement (16) [LOE-B]. In a previously conducted, double-blind, clinically vehicle-controlled, randomized, half-side comparison with 88 adult patients suffering from mild to moderate AD, the same ointment was not superior to the vehicle after four weeks of treatment. However, a subanalysis indicated that the cream might be effective under conditions of cold and dry weather (17) [LOE-A].

Glycyrrhetinic acid as the most important compound from licorice has been shown to possess pronounced anti-inflammatory activity (18) [LOE-D]. A standardized extract of licorice (*Glycyrrhiza glabra*) in the form of a 1% and 2% gel has been investigated in the treatment of AD. In a double-blind, vehicle-controlled phase II trial, 2% licorice gel was more effective than 1% gel and the vehicle in reducing the scores for erythema, oedema, and itching after two weeks of treatment (30 patients in each group) (19) [LOE-A].

A new, pharmacy-sold, phytotherapeutic cream for the treatment of AD contains 2% glycyrrhetinic acid, an extract of the leaves of grape vine (*vitis vinifera*), allantoin, and telmesteine (3-ethylhydrogen-3,4-thiazolidine-dicarboxylate). The compound telmesteine and the *Vitis vinifera* extract display antiprotease activity that inhibits harmful enzymes produced by damaged skin (20) [LOE-D]. *Vitis vinifera* contains oligomeric proanthocyanidines, which are among the most potent antioxidants in nature. They scavenge and neutralize free radicals and prevent oxidative damage to vascular endothelium. In addition, proanthocyanidines form a barrier against enzymes involved in the destruction of elastin, collagen, and other substances that maintain skin integrity (21) [LOE-D]. Telmesteine has also been shown to possess free radical–scavenging activities. In a small, randomized, double-blind, vehicle-controlled trial with 20 subjects, this cream was superior to the vehicle in improving the sodium lauryl sulfate–induced irritant contact dermatitis as measured by parameters such as the transepidermal water loss (22) [LOE-B]. A European randomized, double-blind, vehicle-controlled study with 30 adult AD patients suffering from mild to moderate AD revealed that the above cream is safe and effective in the treatment of AD (20) [LOE-A]. This study was followed by a multicenter, randomized, vehicle-controlled clinical study over a period of five weeks with 218 AD patients in the United States, which confirmed the results of the pilot study, demonstrating highly significant superiority over placebo in all test parameters (21) [LOE-A].

Oral application: Oolong tea, a variety of black tea (*Camellia sinensis*), orally administered (1000 ml distributed to three serving sizes per day) seems to be effective in the treatment of recalcitrant AD. In an open study conducted over a period of six months with 121 patients, 63% of the subjects showed moderate to marked improvement of the skin after one month of treatment. Good treatment response was still observed in 54% of the patients after six months. The therapeutic efficacy of oolong tea in AD is attributed to the antiallergic properties of the oolong tea polyphenols (23) [LOE-B].

Japanese Kampo medicines have been investigated for efficacy and safety in 95 patients with recalcitrant AD (24) [LOE-C]. The most commonly used Kampo formula was Hochu-ekki-to containing astragalus root (*Astragalus membranaceus*), licorice (*Glycyrrhiza glabra*), jujube (*Ziziphus zizyphus*), ginseng (*Panax ginseng*), white *Atractylodes* rhizome (*Atractylodes macrocephalae*), fresh ginger (*Zingiber officinale*), and Chinese angelica root (*Angelica sinensis*). Since Kampo medicines are individually formulated for each patient, it was not possible to choose a defined Hochu-ekki-to formula as treatment for all types of AD in a randomized controlled study. The outcome of the study with 95 AD patients showed a slight (38%) to moderate (35%) or marked (20%) effect on the suppression of AD. The formula was ineffective in 4% of the patients (24) [LOE-C].

Japanese herbal medicine is thought to be useful as an alternative therapy of intractable AD in association with diet. It has been shown that increased blood eosinophil counts in patients with recalcitrant AD decreased significantly, and the serum-IgE levels also showed a tendency to decrease after administration of Hochu-ekki-to (25) [LOE-D].

Traditional Chinese herbal medicines (TCM) have been used to treat AD for many years, and their efficacy has attracted public attention. Several clinical trials have demonstrated the efficacy of TCM. Recently, a randomized, double-blind, placebo-controlled trial with 85 children suffering from AD has been conducted with twice daily dosing of three capsules of either TCM or placebo for 12 weeks. The daily dose corresponded to 9 g of an herbal formula consisting of *Lonicerae flos* (Jinyinhua) 2 g, *Menthae herba* (Bohe) 1 g, *Moutan cortex*

(Danpi) 2 g, *Atractylodis rhizoma* (Cangzhu) 2 g, and *Phellodendri cortex* (Huangbai) 2 g. The results of this study suggested that the TCM concoction is efficacious in improving quality of life and reducing topical corticosteroid use in children with moderate to severe AD. However, there was no significant difference in the improvement of symptoms as determined by SCORAD (Scoring of Atopic Dermatitis) (26) [LOE-A]. Another double-blind, placebo-controlled crossover trial investigated a formulation of ten orally administered Chinese medicinal plant extracts (*Clematis armandii, Dictamnus dasycarpus, Glycyrrhiza glabra, Ledebouriella saseloides, Lophatherum gracile, Rehmannia glutinosa, Paeonia lactiflora, Potentilla chinensis, Tribulus terrestris, and Schizonepeta tenuifolia*) in 40 adult patients. Patients had to drink 200 ml of freshly prepared decoction once a day, corresponding to 10 g of the above blend, or to a placebo blend of plants not estimated as helpful for AD. The extent and severity of erythema and surface damage were significantly reduced under verum compared to placebo. A subjective improvement of itching and sleep could be denoted during the treatment phase (27) [LOE-A]. Symptoms were significantly improved and stabilized during the one-year follow-up (28) [LOE-A].

A double-blind, placebo-controlled, randomized trial with 49 patients could not demonstrate that oral administration of a triherbal combination of Siberian ginseng (*Eleutherococcus senticosus*), yarrow (*Achillea millefolium*), and white deadnettle (*Lamium album*) in addition to topical treatments has an advantage over placebo in the treatment of AD (29) [LOE-A]. A randomized, double-blind, placebo-controlled, parallel group trial with 151 AD patients including children investigated the efficacy and tolerability of oral high-dosage treatment with borage oil, which contains a high concentration of g-linolenic acid (30) [LOE-A].

In summary, good scientific data are scarce for most traditionally used botanical treatments of AD, but their application seems justified on the basis of long-time clinical experience and theoretical considerations based on their active ingredients. However, their efficacy depends on good knowledge of drug quality, adequate preparation, and correct application. It is therefore desirable that more standardized preparations be developed and clinically proven. Of the plant species reported here, St. John's wort, Oregon grape root, licorice, and some traditional Chinese medicines are clearly on this path.

Psoriasis

Like AD, psoriasis represents an inflammatory erythematous and scaly skin disease but with a Th1 rather than Th2 cytokine pattern and an abnormal hyperproliferation of keratinocytes. Psoriasis also has a hereditary component, that is, when arthritis is present, and may be aggravated by lifestyle factors like alcohol and smoking. In severe stages, psoriasis may cover the whole body surface, and it can affect nails and joints. Mainly adult people are concerned, with a prevalence of about 2% to 3% in Western countries. Treatment strategies include topical application of anthralin, tar, and corticosteroids but also systemic immuno-modulatory and anti-inflammatory treatments with methotrexate, cyclosporine, or new biotechnological drugs like TNF or adhesion molecule antagonists. Phototherapy with ultraviolet B (UVB) or psoralen plus ultraviolet A (PUVA) is also effective.

Plant-derived standard therapies: The basic psoriasis therapy includes topical preparations containing salicylic acid (SA), originally derived from white willow bark (*Salix alba*). SA is ubiquitously found in plants, where it functions as a phenolic phytohormone.

SA-containing preparations have exfoliative effects on hyperkeratotic skin lesions and are therefore beneficial to "prepare" psoriatic skin for an anti-inflammatory treatment.

One of the most important topical psoriasis treatments is dithranol (in Germany, cignolin; in the United States, anthralin). Currently manufactured synthetically, dithranol was derived in former days from chrysarobin, a constituent of the bark of the araroba tree (*Andira araroba*) or goa tree found in the rain forests of the Amazon. Dithranol inhibits the release of proinflammatory cytokines and the growth of keratinocytes. Recently, a randomized, multicenter study with 106 patients revealed that topical dithranol, although difficult to use in an outpatient setting, is even superior to other established topical psoriasis drugs such as vitamin D3 analogues (31) [LOE-A].

The abnormal growth of keratinocytes is also inhibited by psoralens in combination with ultraviolet A irradiation (PUVA). The most potent psoralen is 8-methoxypsoralen (8-MOP, a furocoumarin from *Ammi majus*). Psoralens are photosensitizers that occur in different plant families such as Apiaceae, Rutaceae, and Moraceae (32) [LOE-D]. While PUVA was widely used as a systemic therapy in the United States and Europe, various studies have recently confirmed the antipsoriatic efficacy of 8-MOP as a bath additive or cream in combination with phototherapy for the topical treatment of psoriasis (33, 34) [LOE-A].

Traditional oral treatment of psoriasis with depurative teas has no scientific backup. The following antipsoriatic drugs are all applied topically. An overview of clinical studies on botanicals for psoriasis is given in Table 3.4. Oregon grape root (*Mahonia aquifolia* or *Berberis aquifolium*) is used not only for the treatment of acne but also for psoriasis. Recently, a report on three open clinical trials using *Mahonia aquifolium* cream and a review of earlier clinical data with *Mahonia aquifolium* for the treatment of plaque psoriasis has indicated that this botanical is a safe and possibly effective treatment for patients with mild to moderate psoriasis (35). A recent randomized, double-blind, placebo-controlled study in 200 patients yielded statistical proof of efficacy and safety of a 10% topical *Mahonia* cream standardized to 0.1% berberine in the treatment of psoriasis, with improvement in the Psoriasis Area Severity Index (PASI) as well as in the Quality of Life Index (36) [LOE-A].

Avocado oil combined with vitamin B12 in a cream has been shown in a randomized, prospective clinical trial to be equally beneficial as calcipotriol in the topical treatment of psoriasis without any adverse effects, especially with regard to long-term treatment (37) [LOE-A].

A double-blind, placebo-controlled clinical trial with 197 patients has shown that capsaicin (trans-8-methyl-N-vanillyl-6-nonenamide), the main ingredient in cayenne pepper (*Capsicum frutensis*), applied as an 0.025% cream four times daily for six weeks significantly decreases symptoms in psoriasis. The psoriasis severity score combined from scaling, thickness, erythema, and pruritus was different between both treatment groups from week 4 to week 6 (p=0.03) (38) [LOE-A]. These observations have already been established in former days in a double-blind, placebo-controlled study in 44 patients during a six-week treatment with topical capsaicin in moderate and severe psoriasis vulgaris; there was no difference in efficacy between 0.01% and 0.025% capsaicin cream but significant superiority of both to placebo (39) [LOE-A]. Transient burning at the site of application is the most frequent adverse effect reported in both trials. However, capsaicin is contraindicated on injured skin and should not be used on the face. Moreover, the time of application should be limited.

Table 3.4. Overview on Clinical Studies with Botanicals for Psoriasis

Botanicals	Patients (n)	Control	Study End Points	Route of Administration	Treatment Phase	Results	Ref. / [LOE]
Oregon grape root 10% (*Mahonia aquifolia*)	200	placebo	PASI, QLI	topical	12 weeks	superior to placebo	36 / [LOE-A]
Avocado (*Persea americana*) and vitamin B12	13	calcipotriol half-side	PASI, 20-MHz sonography	topical	12 weeks	slower, but finally equal efficacy of av.	37 / [LOE-B]
Capsaicin (from *Capsicum frutensis*)	197	placebo	combined psoriasis index	topical	6 weeks	superior to placebo (p = 0.03)	38 / [LOE-A]
	44	placebo, half-side	Scaling, erythema, overall improvement	topical	6 weeks	superior to placebo	39 / [LOE-A]
Aloe vera (*Aloe barbadensis* a. o. species)	60	placebo	PASI	topical	4 weeks	superior to placebo	41 / [LOE-A]
	41	placebo, half-side	score from erythema, infiltration, desquamation	topical	4 weeks	not superior to placebo	42 / [LOE-A]
Kukui nut oil (*Aleurites moluccana*)	30	mineral oil placebo	PASI, GSPS, plus develop. of one defined lesion	topical	12 weeks	not superior to placebo	43 / [LOE-A]

LOE=Level of evidence according to (3); PASI=Psoriasis Area Severity Index; QLI=Quality of Life Index; GSPS=Global Severity of Psoriasis Scale

The efficacy of bitter melon (*Momordica charantia*), another botanical that has been traditionally used for the treatment of psoriasis (40) [LOE-D], has not been proven yet in controlled clinical studies.

Aloe vera (*Aloe barbadensis*) is utilized as an ingredient in a myriad of health and cosmetic products, principally because of its valuable moisturizing emollient effects. Scientific literature yields conflicting reports on the efficacy of aloe vera in the treatment of psoriasis. A randomized, double-blind, placebo-controlled study with 60 patients treated with 0.5% aloe vera extract in a hydrophilic cream three times daily for up to four weeks showed the cream to be more effective than placebo without any side effects. Only 2 of 30 patients in the placebo group but 25 of 30 in the treatment group were rated as cured after four weeks, and the Psoriasis Area Severity Index (PASI) decreased from 8.9 to 8.2 in the placebo group and from 9.7 to 2.2 under verum treatment (41) [LOE-A]. In contrast, another double-blind, placebo-controlled study with 41 patients with slight to moderate psoriasis showed only a modest effect of a commercial, aloin-free aloe vera gel that was not superior to placebo. However, the high response rate of the placebo gel indicated a possible effect of the placebo in its own right, which could have made the aloe vera gel less effective (42) [LOE-A]. The difference may also be caused by the presence or absence of aloin, belonging to the anthranoids, which are known to have beneficial effects on psoriasis.

A double-blind, placebo-controlled pilot study with 30 patients was conducted to determine the effectiveness of the oil of the kukui nut tree (*Aleurites moluccana*) as a topical treatment for psoriasis. No significant beneficial effect of the oil could be demonstrated [LOE-A], although anecdotal reports existed from psoriasis patients visiting Hawaii who seemed to benefit from topical kukui nut oil (43).

In the treatment of psoriasis, traditional Chinese herbal medicines (TCM) are commonly used. Randomized, controlled clinical trials to assess the efficacy of Chinese herbs are difficult to undertake, because TCM, similar to Japanese Kampo medicines, consist of a mixture of herbs individually formulated for the patient. The specific combination utilized is often changed over time according to the clinical status of the patient. Therefore, scientific literature yields little with regard to controlled clinical trials to substantiate the effects of those herbal mixtures. However, a great number of uncontrolled studies have been performed with TCM in psoriasis. In these trials, a total of 174 Chinese herbs have been used. The ten most commonly used herbs are *Rhemannia glutinosa*, *Angelica sinensis*, *Salvia miltiorhiza*, *Dictamnus dasycarpus*, *Smilax glabra*, *Oldenlandia diffusa*, *Lithospermum erythrorhizon*, *Paeonia lactiflora*, *Carthamnus tinctorius*, and *Glycyrrhiza uralensis*. Most of the key actions of those botanicals, relevant to reduce psoriatic symptoms, reflect anti-inflammatory activities, modulation of cytokine production, or inhibition of angiogenesis (44) [LOE-D]. More experimental studies are needed to elucidate the exact mode of action of the specific herbs.

India madder root (*Rubia cordifolia*) is a Chinese herb with antiproliferative properties. There is evidence that induction of apoptosis of keratinocytes is the underlying mechanism for the observed antiproliferative action of Rubiae radix. Experimental results suggest that this drug is a promising source from which an herb-based topical agent could be developed for the treatment of psoriasis (45) [LOE-D].

In summary, there are some promising herbal treatments for psoriasis, which is a difficult-to-treat and chronic disease requiring a number of well-tolerated alternatives for individual therapy. In addition to the well-established plant-derived molecules, Oregon grape root and capsaicin are interesting candidates, and it is definitely reasonable to conduct more controlled clinical trials to substantiate positive effects of TCM in the treatment of psoriasis. However, psoriasis will require combination rather than monotherapy, and tolerability and cosmetic effects of botanical formulations are nearly as important as their therapeutic potency.

Acne

Acne is a common dermatological disease affecting about three of four juvenile people. It is characterized by numerous comedones which get inflamed at varying degrees, forming papules and pustules. Increase in androgenic steroids during puberty and a genetic disposition are the main causes, leading to overproduction of sebum and supranormal keratinization of hair follicles. Acne may be aggravated by external factors like smoking and use of inadequate cosmetics and especially by bacterial infection with *Propionibacterium acnes*. Severe acne ("acne conglobata") may cause serious social and psychological problems and leave scars in face and soul. Medical treatment aims at normalization of sebum production and keratinization and includes hygienic measures, peeling of hyperkeratinized skin, and anti-inflammatory and antibiotic drugs applied topically or systemically.

Traditional phytomedicines play an adjuvant role in acne therapy in Europe in addition to or in combination with intensive cosmetic care. A large number of herbs with anti-inflammatory, antihydrotic and/or antibacterial compounds are used for washings or steambaths. Examples are chamomile (*Matricaria recutita*), marigold (*Calendula officinalis*), and wheat bran (*Triticum aestivum*) (46). After cleaning, creams or aqueous decoctions with astringent compounds like tannins are applied topically. Witch hazel (*Hamamelis virginiana*) bark extract is most commonly used because it is considered to be very safe in topical administration. Other tannin-containing plants include white oak bark (*Quercus alba*), English walnut leaf (*Juglans regia*), agrimony (*Agrimonia eupatoria*), goldenrod (*Solidago virgaurea*), jambolan bark (*Syzygium cuminum cortex*), Labrador tea (*Ledum latifolium*), lady's mantle (*Alchemilla mollis*), lavender (*Lavandula angustifolia*), mullein (*Verbascum thapsus*), rhatany (*Krameria triandra*), Chinese rhubarb (*Rheum palmatum*), St. John's wort (*Hypericum perforatum*), and yellow dock (*Rumex crispus*) (47) [LOE-D]. Other herbs traditionally used topically or as depurative teas are daisy (*Bellis perennis*), pansy (*Viola tricolor*), quitch (*Elymus repens*), and dandelion (*Taraxacum officinale*) (46). Horsetail (*Equisetum spp.*) tea is recommended because of its high content of silicic acid, and topical application of yellow milk from fresh leaves of aloe (*Aloe ferox*) for its anthranoids [LOE-D].

Oral application: Vitex (*Vitex agnus-castus*) orally taken has been shown to be effective in the treatment of premenstrual acne (48) [LOE-D]. The whole-fruit extract increases progesterone levels and decreases estrogen levels by acting upon follicle-stimulating hormone and luteinizing hormone levels in the pituitary gland and decreases exceedingly high premenstrual prolactin levels via dopaminergic mechanisms (49). The German Commission E has recommended an intake of 40 mg per day. The agent should not be taken by pregnant or nursing women and adverse effects such as gastrointestinal tract upset and skin rashes are reported (49).

Topical effects: Besides the traditionally used antiacne botanicals, several herbs have been investigated for antimicrobial activities to evaluate their potential as herbal therapeutics for acne. *Propionibacterium acnes*, an anaerobic pathogen, plays an important role in the pathogenesis of acne and seems to initiate the inflammatory process by triggering the release of reactive oxygen species (ROS) and proinflammatory cytokines (50) [LOE-D]. Interestingly, the pronounced antibacterial effect of licorice (*Glycyrrhiza glabra*) against *Propionibacterium acnes* is not associated with the induction of resistance in the bacteria (51) [LOE-D]. A recent screening of plant extracts for antimicrobial activity against bacteria and yeasts with dermatological relevance revealed a strong inhibitory effect on *Propionibacterium acnes* of usnic acid, the major constituent of beard lichen (*Usnea barbata*). Bacterial growth was inhibited at concentrations from 1 μg/ml up. Moreover, *Usnea barbata* displays antioxidative and broad antimicrobial properties, making it a promising agent for the treatment of acne (52) [LOE-D]. A four-week open clinical trial compared essential oil from basil (*Ocimum gratissimum*) in four different concentrations (0.5% to 5%) and in four different bases to placebo and standard therapy (10% benzoyl peroxide). Two percent *Ocimum* essential oil in hydrophilic (alcohol or cetomacrogol) bases reduced lesions faster than standard and was well tolerated, while 5% was also highly effective but irritating. Although 126 students were included in the patient population, the number of treatment groups was too high for valid statistical proof of efficacy (53) [LOE-B]. Because of their antimicrobial effects, the German Commission E has also approved topically administered bittersweet nightshade (*Solanum dulcamara*) and systemically administered brewer's yeast (*Saccharomyces cerevisiae*) in the treatment of acne (48) [LOE-D]. Topical duckweed (*Lemna minor*) is used in China to treat acne (48) [LOE-D].

Oregon grape root (*Mahonia aquifolium* or *Berberis aquifolium*) is used for chronic skin eruptions or rashes associated with pustules in Western traditional medicine as well as in the Japanese Kampo medicines (Japanese traditional herbal medicines based on combinations of a number of individual medicinal plants). The main constituents of the crude mahonia extract are the two protoberberine alkaloids, berberine and jatrorrhizine, that display antimicrobial activity against various strains of coagulase negative staphylococci, *Propionibacterium acnes* and *Candida* species in vitro (54) [LOE-D]. It has been shown recently in an animal model that 100 μM berberine suppresses sebaceous gland lipogenesis by 63% (55) [LOE-D]. The alkaloid berberine is a bitter substance which displays antiadipogenic and anti-inflammatory effects on 3T3-L1 adipocytes in vitro, and the antiadipogenic effect seems to be caused by the down-regulation of adipogenic enzymes and transcription factors (56) [LOE-D]. However, the exact mode of action of berberine and berberine-rich botanicals in acne is still unknown.

The volatile oil of tea tree (*Melaleuca alternifolia*), a traditional herbal remedy of the Australian aborigines for bruises and skin infections, might also be beneficial in the treatment of acne. Besides its well-known antimicrobial properties, tea tree oil (TTO) displays anti-inflammatory activities by reducing histamine-induced inflammation of the skin (57) [LOE-D]. In a three-month, single-blind clinical trial with 124 patients, both 5% TTO and 5% benzoyl peroxide ameliorated acne, although the onset of action was slower for TTO; however, fewer patients in the TTO group complained of skin discomfort (58) [LOE-B]. While a placebo group was missing in this older report, recently, a 45-day, randomized, double-blind, placebo-controlled study with 60 patients has proven the efficacy of 5% topical TTO gel in mild to moderate acne vulgaris. TTO gel was 3.55 times more effective than placebo in terms of the total acne lesions counting test and 5.75 times more effective in the acne severity index (59) [LOE-A]. Although the study provided no evidence for differences in side effects and tolerability, the sensitizing potential of TTO and oxidized monoterpenes should be taken into account when using TTO for the treatment of acne (60) [LOE-C].

Gluconolactone is formed from a polyhydroxy acid synthesized by *Saccharomyces bulderi* (61) [LOE-D]. The results of a 150-patient, double-blind clinical study with topical application of 14% gluconolactone solution demonstrated a clearance of inflamed acne lesions that was significantly superior to placebo and comparable to 5% benzoyl peroxide but with fewer side effects (62) [LOE-A].

In summary, traditional herbal treatment in combination with cosmetic care is a well-established basis of acne therapy. Some botanicals, especially Oregon grape root, TTO, saccharomyces, and perhaps basil, may have the potential to replace chemical standard therapy in mild to moderate cases because of their efficacy and higher tolerability. Further valid controlled clinical studies that also consider optimization of pharmaceutical preparations are needed.

INFECTIOUS SKIN DISEASES

Bacteria, viruses, and fungi may not only cause primary infections of the skin like warts, herpes, folliculitis, onychomycosis, erysipelas, and many more but also complicate existing dermatological disorders like oozing eczema or intertrigo. Three factors suggest that infections of the skin will remain important in the future: increased mobility with dispersal of microorganisms across the world, susceptibility of the skin because of intensive hygiene, and development of resistant strains, for example, in *Staphylococcus aureus*. Plant extracts, juices, and decoctions have always been used to treat infections of the skin.

Bacterial infections: Numerous botanical compounds exhibit antimicrobial activities in vitro. Usually, antiseptic or antibiotic treatment is still the treatment of choice, and plant-derived antimicrobial therapeutics are rather used in an adjuvant manner or in mild cases of bacterial infections. For example, tea tree oil (*Melaleuca alternifolia*; TTO) not only is beneficial in the topical therapy of acne as mentioned before. It also functions as a topical antiseptic with an efficacy superior to that of phenol and displays broad-spectrum antimicrobial activity in vitro against gram-negative bacteria such as *Escherichia coli*, gram-positive bacteria such as *Staphylococcus aureus*, and the yeast *Candida albicans* (63) [LOE-D]. Disruption of plasma membrane barriers for ions and small molecules is discussed as a mode of action, monoterpenes being the active compounds.

Hyperforin, a major compound from St. John's wort (*Hypericum perforatum*), has been demonstrated to be highly effective against a panel of gram-positive bacteria, including multiresistant *Staphylococcus aureus* (10) [LOE-D].

Coriander oil (*Coriandrum sativum*) is another topical plant-derived agent with distinct antibacterial efficacy and good skin tolerance (32) [LOE-D]. It has been shown to be highly effective against *Escherichia coli* and other bacteria and fungi in vitro (64–68) [LOE-D]. Some isolated compounds (long-chain alcohols and aldehydes) may be very effective, but their combined effects in the crude oils are difficult to predict. Dodecenal from coriander had a minimum bactericidal concentration of 6.25 µg/ml against *Salmonella choleraesius* (68). Strength and spectrum of coriander oil fractions often exceeded those determined in the crude oil, but mixing of single fractions could result in additive, synergistic, or antagonistic effects. Recently, a topical lipolotio containing 1% v/v coriander oil has also been shown to inhibit UVB-induced erythema in humans to a significantly higher extent compared to placebo but less than 1% hydrocortisone (69) [LOE-A], making coriander oil an interesting treatment for inflammatory skin diseases with bacterial colonization.

Various plant extracts and isolated compounds have been screened for antimicrobial effects on bacteria and yeasts with dermatological relevance. Plant extracts from olibanum (*Boswellia serrata*), rosemary (*Rosmarinus officinalis*), sage (*Salvia officinalis*), and others have been shown to inhibit the growth of several gram-positive bacteria such as *Staphylococcus aureus* (including methicillin-resistant strains), *Propionibacterium acnes*, and *Corynebacterium* species (52) [LOE-D].

Japanese Kampo formulations have also been shown to possess antibacterial properties directed toward *Propionibacterium acnes*, *Staphylococcus epidermidis*, and *Staphylococcus aureus* (70) [LOE-D].

Fungal infections: Numerous botanicals, especially essential oils, exhibit antifungal activities in vitro. The essential oil of snow gum (*Eucalyptus pauciflora*) has been shown to possess strong antifungal properties against a broad spectrum of human pathogenic fungi, including *Epidermophyton*, *Microsporum*, and *Trichophyton* species. Within a non-vehicle-controlled clinical study, 1% essential oil formulated into an ointment was applied topically twice a day for three weeks to 50 patients suffering from tinea pedis, tinea corporis, or tinea cruris. After the second week of treatment, all patients were negative for fungal infection confirmed by microscopic evaluation of the scraping from the infected area after staining with 10% potassium hydroxide (KOH). After three weeks of treatment, 60% of the patients recovered completely as proven by microscopic evaluation and clinical signs such as erythema, scaling, itching, maceration, vesiculation, and pustulation, and 40% of the patients showed significant improvement of the clinical signs of tinea without any adverse effects. No KOH-negative cases relapsed at reexamination of the patients two months after the end of the treatment (71) [LOE-B].

Another antifungal plant is garlic (*Allium sativum*). Garlic contains the biologically active ingredient ajoene, a trisulphur compound that has been demonstrated to possess antifungal properties. In a clinical study with 34 patients suffering from tinea pedis, the use of an 0.4% ajoene cream resulted in complete clinical and mycological cure in 79% of the patients after seven days of treatment. The remaining 21% of patients achieved complete healing after seven additional days of treatment. All patients were evaluated for recurrence of mycotic infections 90 days after the end of treatment, yielding negative mycological cultures (72) [LOE-B].

Viral infections: Numerous botanicals exhibit antiviral properties in vitro. Only a few have been studied in vivo so far. Lemon balm (*Melissa officinalis*) formulated into a cream was investigated in a double-blind, placebo-controlled, randomized trial in 66 patients with recurrent *herpes simplex labialis*. The cream was used four times daily over a period of five days on the affected area. Lemon balm treatment resulted in significantly faster healing time and reduced spread of infection, blistering, and pain compared to placebo (73) [LOE-A].

A well-established dermatological therapy of *Condylomata acuminata*, which are caused by human papilloma viruses, is podophyllotoxin, extracted from the root of American mayapple (*Podophyllum peltatum*). Recently, in a randomized, double-blind study, 97 patients suffering from recurrent condylomata acuminata were treated with a podophyllotoxin solid lipid nanoparticles gel and a standard podophyllotoxin gel. The condyloma clearance rate in patients receiving podophyllotoxin solid lipid nanoparticle gel was 97.1%, close to that for patients treated with the routine preparation of 90.6%, but the nanoparticle preparation significantly reduced the recurrence rate and adverse side effects. It was concluded that podophyllotoxin delivered via solid lipid nanoparticle gel can effectively clear *Condylomata acuminata* and reduce the recurrence rate with only mild, tolerable side effects (74) [LOE-A].

An extract of arbor vitae (*Thuja occidentalis*) in the form of a tincture has traditionally been used as a topical treatment for common warts (*Verrucae vulgares*). Similarly, the application of fresh juice from greater celandine (*Chelidonium majus*) is said to be beneficial in the treatment of warts (52) [LOE-D]. Traditional systemic botanical treatment of warts includes immunostimulating plant extracts from purple coneflowers (*Echinacea purpurea*) or Siberian ginseng (*Eleutherococcus senticosus*) administered orally over a period of eight weeks (52) [LOE-D]. However, the efficacy of these traditional therapies has not been proven in controlled clinical trials so far.

In summary, there are effective botanicals for topical treatment of bacterial, fungal, and viral infections of the skin. They can be used adjuvant to other therapeutical measures or alone in mild to moderate cases. Especially when essential oils are used, possible contact sensitizations should be kept in mind. An important aspect is that garlic or aromatic herbs may be available when modern medicine is not, and this applies not only to the Third World but also to catastrophes in industrial nations, as we are experiencing them again and again. Some of these treatments are old house remedies that should not be forgotten.

CHRONIC VENOUS INSUFFICIENCY

Age, sedentary lifestyle, and obesity favor chronic venous insufficiency (CVI)—all factors with increasing importance in modern industrial societies. Primarily a vascular disease characterized by insufficient blood flow, edema, and heavy legs, CVI will cause itching, darkening, and hardening of lower leg skin and finally ulcera, thus entering the field of dermatology. Physical training is regarded as the best therapy, but many older patients are limited in this respect. Compression stockings and diuretics may give some relief, but their effect is only symptomatic. Topically applied creams and ointments have, apart from short-time relief from itching or inflammation, little effect beyond the physical massage process and often bear a risk of causing an allergic rush. There is, however, no convincing orally applied synthetic drug either.

Some botanicals reduce edema and inflammation, display antioxidative and proteolytic effects, and are able to seal the capillaries in CVI. Furthermore, they increase the venous tone and enhance the lymphatic flow. Orally administered botanicals for the venous system are especially used in the case of insufficiency, contraindication, or intolerance of compression therapy. Several botanicals are traditionally used to treat CVI and are first-line treatments for this indication today.

Extracts from the seeds of the horse chestnut (*Aesculus hippocastanum*) with the major constituent escin, a complex mixture of biologically active triterpenes, have traditionally been used to treat patients with CVI and to alleviate associated symptoms, including lower leg swelling. The efficacy of preparations containing horse chestnut seed extract is believed to be largely caused by an inhibitory effect on the catalytic breakdown of capillary wall proteoglycans (75) [LOE-D]. More than a dozen placebo- or reference-controlled clinical trials have shown that horse chestnut extract is superior to placebo and as effective as reference medications in improving objective symptoms of CVI like pain and leg volume (76) [LOE-A].

Flavonoid-containing drugs: Japanese pagoda tree (*Styphnolobium japonicum*) extract contains a high amount of the flavonoid rutin, which has pronounced antioxidative capacity

(77) [LOE-D]. The capacity of 1 to 2 g oxerutin (syn. 7-O-g-hydroxyethyl-rutosides) daily to improve symptoms of CVI stages I and II and to protect long-distance flyers from edema with ankle swelling and pain was reported in several controlled clinical trials, for example, (78–80) [LOE-A]. In a double-blind, randomized, placebo-controlled multicenter study, the efficacy of oxerutin has been evaluated in 120 female patients suffering from stage II CVI. The patients received 1 g oxerutin daily over a treatment period of 12 weeks with a follow-up period of 6 weeks. It turned out that the oxerutin treatment combined with compression therapy was significantly superior to compression therapy alone with regard to edema reduction. Moreover, the therapeutic effect of oxerutin was persistent even after cessation of the treatment (81) [LOE-A].

Rutin derivatives ("fagorutin") are also found in buckwheat (*Fagopyrum esculentum*); a randomized, double-blind, placebo-controlled clinical trial with 67 patients suffering from CVI found no change in leg edema during 12 weeks of treatment phase but a significant increase in the placebo group. Changes in other parameters were not significant (82) [LOE-A].

Red wine leaf (*Vitis viniferae folium*) extract is an herbal medicine containing various flavonoids, with quercetin-3-O-beta-glucuronide and isoquercitrin (quercetin-3-O-beta-glucoside) as the main components (83). Red wine leaf extract has been administered orally in once-daily doses of 360 mg and 720 mg in comparison to placebo in a 12-week, randomized, double-blind, placebo-controlled, parallel-group, multicenter study in patients with stage I and incipient stage II CVI. The extract was safe and effective in a dose-related manner in the treatment of mild CVI, significantly reducing edema and circumference of the lower leg and improving CVI-related symptoms to a clinically relevant extent. The edema reduction was at least equivalent to that reported for compression stockings and/or other edema-reducing agents (83) [LOE-A].

An extract from French maritime pine bark (*Pinus maritima*) (pycnogenol™) standardized for oligomeric proanthocyanidins has been shown to be beneficial at 150 mg daily in the treatment of CVI in a randomized, placebo-controlled, four-week trial with 39 patients; resting flux, rate of ankle swelling, edema, and a complex analogue scale for symptom rating all showed significant improvement versus start and versus placebo (84) [LOE-A]. In an open, controlled study with 40 patients comparing the efficacy of 360 mg pycnogenol daily to 600 mg horse chestnut seed extract over a period of four weeks, both medications were equally well tolerated, but French maritime pine bark extract was superior to the horse chestnut seed extract (85) [LOE-B]. Diosmin, a flavonoid glycoside found in citrus fruits, has also been shown in several randomized, controlled clinical studies to reduce edema and accelerate venous ulcer healing by anti-inflammatory action in patients suffering from CVI (86, 87) [LOE-A].

Butcher's broom (*Ruscus aculeatus*) is an orally used botanical medicine containing steroid saponines (ruscogenins) for the treatment of lower leg edema in patients with CVI. The efficacy and safety of a Ruscus extract has been confirmed in a multicenter, double-blind, randomized, placebo-controlled trial with 166 women suffering from CVI (88) [LOE-A].

Not directly aiming at CVI but nevertheless interesting, 400 mg daily of an extract of yellow sweet clover (*Melilotus officinalis*) containing 8 mg coumarin has been shown to be effective in reducing lymphedema of the upper arm caused by lymphadenectomy for breast cancer. A possible mode of action is the edema-preventing property of coumarines that results from the activation of macrophages and subsequent proteolysis in the tissue affected by chronic lymphedema (89) [LOE-C].

An uncontrolled clinical trial with a cream containing yellow sweet clover and Butcher's broom revealed improvement of edema, pain, heaviness, and itch of patients suffering from CVI. The cream was well tolerated (90) [LOE-C]. Another comparative controlled study suggests mild efficacy of the combination of a-tocopherol, rutin, *Melilotus officinalis*, and *Centella asiatica* administered orally in patients with CVI (91) [LOE-A].

In summary, there are some botanicals that are widely used and intensively investigated in CVI. Design and conductance of virtually all clinical trials have been criticized repeatedly, and clinical evidence for the use of oral botanicals in CVI was questioned (92). This, however, also applies to all other CVI therapies; high response to placebo may also be a reason why studies in venous insufficiency are difficult to perform (92). Nevertheless, the products are well accepted by the patients. Apart from minor or major shortcomings in individual studies, the broad data basis for chestnut and flavonoid drugs supports their usefulness as experienced by patients and therapists.

UV-INDUCED SKIN DAMAGE AND NONMELANOMA SKIN CANCER

Photoaging and the development of skin cancer are of increasing importance since changes in lifestyle have led to a significant increase of the individual cumulative ultraviolet (UV) doses. This trend is likely to continue. Therefore, the adverse effects of UV irradiation on the skin have become a major human health concern. New prevention strategies have to be developed to reduce UV exposure and delay photoaging processes aiming at reducing the incidence of skin cancer. Within this context, topically as well as orally administered botanicals are of interest. Basically all botanicals that have been shown to possess antioxidant properties can be considered beneficial in the prevention of photocarcinogenesis. It is suggested that routine consumption of those botanicals may provide protection against many harmful effects of UV irradiation. In combination with sunscreens or skin care lotions, they may provide an effective strategy for reducing UV-induced skin diseases (93).

UV-induced skin damage can be classified into three clinical stages. The acute stage of skin damage is sunburn, characterized by clinical signs of inflammation such as erythema, pain, and swelling and histologically by sunburn cells. In chronically UV-exposed skin, the elastic and collagenous fibers are rarefied and precancerous skin conditions such as actinic keratoses are present. Finally, in long-term UV-exposed skin, eventually nonmelanoma skin cancer such as squamous cell carcinoma and basal cell carcinoma may develop. The mechanisms, prevention, and therapy have been reviewed extensively by Yaar et al. (94). Various botanicals have been reported to prevent photocarcinogenesis by displaying anticarcinogenic and antimutagenic activities because of antioxidative and anti-inflammatory properties (95).

Protection from acute erythema: The extract of the tropical cabbage palm fern (CPF) (*Phlebodium aureum* or *Polypodium leucotomos*) is a plant-derived product that has been studied in vitro as well as in vivo. A clinical study with 21 healthy subjects exposed to UV irradiation before and after administration of CPF demonstrated that CPF, orally administered as well as topically used, displays significant photoprotective properties by preventing sunburn and psoralen-induced phototoxic reactions and immunohistochemically revealed photoprotection of epidermal Langerhans cells (96) [LOE-B]. In a recent small study with ten subjects, it was shown that CPF is an effective protector against PUVA-induced skin phototoxicity and protects the skin from damaging effects of PUVA as evidenced by histology (97) [LOE-C]. Another trial with nine volunteers assessed erythema reactions after UV irradiation without CPF and after oral administration of CPF. Clinical together with histological results revealed that oral CPF extract decreases UV-induced skin damage (98) [LOE-C]. One possible molecular mechanism for this protection seems to be the inhibition of UV-induced photoisomerization of trans-urocanic acid, a common photoreceptor located in the stratum corneum. The CPF extract also blocks its photodecomposition in the presence of oxidizing reagents such as H_2O_2 and titanium dioxide. Additionally, it was shown that CPF protects human fibroblasts from UV-induced death in vitro (99) [LOE-D].

Topical application of anti-inflammatory plant extracts immediately after irradiation can reduce symptoms of sunburn. In 40 human volunteers, an ointment containing 2% extract of sage (*Salvia officinalis*) rich in phenolic diterpenes inhibited UV-induced erythema in vivo to a similar extent as did 1% hydrocortisone (100) [LOE-A]. Anti-inflammatory efficacy in a UVB erythema test could also be demonstrated for a topical preparation containing 10% of a distillate from witch hazel (*Hamamelis virginiana*) (101) [LOE-A].

Dietary supplements that provide moderate protection against UV-induced erythema are carotenoids such as ß-carotene or lycopene. In a placebo-controlled, parallel group study design, 36 volunteers received ß-carotene, a carotenoid mix, or placebo for 12 weeks. Carotenoid levels in serum and skin of the palm and erythema intensity before and 24 hours after irradiation with a solar light simulator were measured at baseline and after 6 and 12 weeks of treatment. The results showed that long-term supplementation for 12 weeks with a carotenoid mix ameliorates UV-induced erythema in humans. The effect was comparable to a daily supplementation with 24 mg ß-carotene alone (102) [LOE-A]. Within a study of 36 healthy volunteers, the photoprotective effect of synthetic lycopene in comparison with a tomato extract and a drink containing the tomato extract in a solubilized form was evaluated. With these different carotenoid sources, the volunteers ingested similar amounts of lycopene (about 10 mg/day). After 12 weeks of supplementation, significant increases in lycopene serum levels and total skin carotenoids were observed in all groups. The induced erythema at week 0, week 4, and week 12 was most decreased at week 12, with a protective effect most pronounced in the group consuming the solubilized tomato extract (48% after 12 weeks) (103) [LOE-B].

EFFECTS OF LONG-TERM ORAL APPLICATION ON SKIN AGING AND CANCER PREVENTION

Green tea extract (manufactured from *Camellia sinensis*) with a high content of oligomeric proanthocyanidins is another UV damage–preventing agent. It mainly contains catechin and epicatechin derivatives with epigallocatechin gallate (EGCG) being the most important compound. It is able to scavenge free radicals and acts as a potent antioxidant. The anticarcinogenic properties of green tea have been thoroughly investigated in vitro as well as in vivo. Recently, a review of numerous studies with green tea has concluded that both oral and topical green tea consumption protects against inflammation and chemical and UV-induced carcinogenesis (104) [LOE-A]. Various cytokines involved in the inflammation process in the beginning of skin tumor development are inhibited by green tea extract. Moreover, biochemical markers of chemical carcinogenesis as well as UV-induced oxidative stress are counteracted by green tea extract. In addition, the UV-induced immunosuppression is prevented by green tea (104) [LOE-D]. Also, it has been shown that green tea protects against PUVA-induced photochemical damage to the skin (105) [LOE-D]. The in vitro photoprotective effects of tea polyphenols and caffeine as a component of tea have recently been evaluated within some reviews (106–108) [LOE-D]. However, tea polyphenols have yet to be evaluated in clinical intervention trials in humans.

Black tea (fermented *Camellia sinensis*) may also play a role in UV protection and chemoprevention due to theaflavins (109) [LOE-D]. It has been shown that theaflavins are as equally effective antioxidants as catechins in green tea (110) [LOE-D].

The extract of the fruits of the coffee plant (*Coffea arabica*) has been shown to exhibit antioxidant activity mediated by potent antioxidant polyphenols, especially chlorogenic acid, condensed proanthocyanidins, quinic acid, and ferulic acid (111) [LOE-D]. Because of these antioxidants, the extract might be valuable for photoprotection and chemoprevention. In a clinical study, 30 patients with actinic damage of the skin used a skin care system containing coffee extract. Twenty patients had full-face application of the test product, and ten patients had half-side application with the other side covered with a placebo cream. Compared to placebo, the test cream was significantly superior in improving fine lines, wrinkles, pigmentation, and overall appearance (112) [LOE-A]. In a double-blind, noncontrolled study, 24 women consumed either a high-flavonol or low-flavonol cocoa powder with epicatechin and catechin as major flavonol monomers dissolved in water for 12 weeks. UV-induced erythema was significantly decreased in the high-flavonol group by 15% and 25% after 6 and 12 weeks of treatment, respectively, whereas no changes occurred in the low-flavonol group. The ingestion of high-flavonol cocoa led to an increase in blood flow of cutaneous and subcutaneous tissues and to an increase in skin density and skin hydration (113) [LOE-B].

Silymarin, a flavonoid complex isolated from the seeds of milk thistle (*Silybum marianum*), has been demonstrated to possess anti-inflammatory, antioxidative, and anticarcinogenic properties in vivo in animal models. Experimental data suggest that silymarin may be a promising chemopreventive and pharmacologically safe agent that can be exploited or tested against skin cancer in humans. Moreover, silymarin may favorably supplement sunscreen protection and provide additional antiphotocarcinogenic protection (114) [LOE-D].

Some other interesting dietary botanicals mainly containing antioxidant polyphenols appear promising as UV-protection agents. Apigenin, a nontoxic botanical-derived flavonoid occurring in numerous herbs, fruits, and vegetables; curcumin obtained from the turmeric rhizome (*Curcuma longa*); proanthocyanidins from the seeds of grapes (*Vitis vinifera*); and resveratrol, a polyphenol found in numerous plant species including grapes, peanuts, fruits, red wine, and mulberries, have also been shown to possess the ability to protect the skin from harmful UV-induced effects by displaying antimutagenic, antioxidant, free radical–scavenging, anti-inflammatory, and anticarcinogenic properties (93). Other candidates are rosemary (*Rosmarinus officinalis*) extract (115); propolis (116), a resinous material produced by honeybees from the bud and bark of certain plants and trees; red ginseng (117); genistein, an isoflavone from soybeans (118); and pomegranate (*Punica granatum*) (119) [all LOE-D]. It has also been shown that the pomegranate extract protects human immortalized HaCaT keratinocytes against UVB-induced oxidative stress and markers of photoaging and might therefore be a useful supplement in skin care products (120) [LOE-D].

Therapeutic treatment of precancerous lesions: Recently, it has been shown in a nonrandomized comparison study that an ointment containing a highly purified triterpene extract from the outer bark of birch (*Betulae cortex*) might represent a new tool for the topical treatment of solar keratoses (121, 122) [LOE-B]. The high response rate of about 80% of the lesions was confirmed in a prospective randomized, placebo-controlled pilot study—partially with histological examination—but needs further substantiation on a larger scale (123) [LOE-A].

In summary, many botanicals containing antioxidant flavonoids or other polyphenols can contribute to skin protection from UV irradiation and prevent sunburn, nonmelanoma skin cancer, and early skin aging. Acute treatment before or after exposure to UV as well as long-time oral or topical applications seems appropriate depending on the specific drug used. Classical nutrients like green and black tea, fruits, and vegetables contain these antioxidants, which also have beneficial effects in other fields of health protection, but for effective UV protection higher amounts than taken with normal nutrition seem necessary. Botanicals may be used externally as cosmetics or part of sun protections or internally as food or food supplements. However, as shown above, the LOE from clinical trials is poor and many more large-scale studies are needed to rule out UV-protective effects for specific botanicals. Birch bark extract seems an interesting option for the treatment of in situ squamous cell carcinoma.

ALOPECIA

Diffuse thinning of scalp hair occurs when more than 100 hairs per day are regularly lost, which happens more often in women than in men; anamnestically, changes in hormonal state (e.g., after childbirth), metabolic disorders, or infectious diseases may be identified as causes, and no specific treatment is necessary when normal physiological conditions are reestablished. However, there may be other reasons, and hair loss cannot always be stopped. Two more specific types of hair loss are Alopecia androgenetica, male baldness, which is caused by high levels of dihydroxytestosterone and characterized by recession of the frontal hair line and/or a bald patch on the vertex; and Alopecia areata, an irregular pattern of one or several well-circumscribed hairless patches anywhere on the scalp, which is regarded as an inflammatory autoimmune deficiency and may occur in both sexes.

There is increasing interest of the cosmetic industry to develop products containing botanicals to treat or prevent hair loss and alopecia. Some botanical extracts are traditionally used to promote hair growth without scientific support, like birch sap in hair tonics. Garlic (*Allium sativum*) is used topically in India but associated with obvious olfactory side effects. A single-blinded clinical trial was designed to test the topical effectiveness of the juice of crude onion (*Allium cepa*), which has many sulphurous ingredients in common with garlic. Sixty-two male and female patients with patchy alopecia areata were treated with fresh onion juice in comparison with tap water, administered twice daily for two months. Only 23 patients in the active treatment group and 15 controls finished the study. However, the use of crude onion juice gave significantly higher results with regard to hair regrowth than did tap water (124) [LOE-B].

A standard medication for male androgenetic alopecia is finasteride, a potent inhibitor of 5-a-reductase (5AR), which converts testosterone to dihydrotestosterone. Finasteride was originally developed for treatment of benign prostatic hyperplasia (BPH). Plants containing phytosterols like b-sitosterol or phytosterol glycosides, like the palm tree saw palmetto (*Serenoa repens*), are traditionally used for BPH treatment, and the same mechanism is discussed as their mode of action. Therefore, it was intriguing to test botanical 5AR inhibitors in androgenetic alopecia. Recently, in a small, randomized, double-blind, placebo-controlled pilot study with 26 male subjects, the effectiveness of a combination of 50 mg b-sitosterol and 200 mg extract from the berries of saw palmetto twice daily was determined in the treatment of androgenetic alopecia. Ten patients were treated over five months with the active study formula. The blinded investigative staff assessment report showed that 60% of these study subjects were rated as improved at the final visit. In contrast, only 11% in the placebo group were rated as improved (125) [LOE-A]. Because of the small sample size, statistical significance was not the primary aim of the study. The formulation was well tolerated; one patient complained of loss of appetite possibly related to active treatment. In contrast to finasteride, the tested botanical 5AR inhibitors have no impact on prostate-specific antigen levels and do not interfere with cancer diagnostics (126). They are also widely used traditionally by women for a variety of indications without safety problems, so they may also be tested in androgenetic alopecia in women (127).

VITILIGO

Vitiligo, or leucodermia, describes a loss of skin pigmentation in sharply circumscribed, irregular patches. It occurs worldwide in about 1% to 2% of adult people, predominantly on face, neck, and outer sides of arms and legs. Melanin formation is disturbed in cells that contain unusually high concentrations of H_2O_2. Vitiligo is to some extent hereditary but also associated with hormonal and immune disorders. There is no convincing drug treatment. Phototherapy with narrow-band UVB and PUVA (psoralen plus UVA) are first-line treatments.

Treatment of vitiligo by UV exposure combined with oral or topical application of photosensitizing plant extracts goes back to the ancient times (1200 to 2000 B.C.), when *Ammi majus* was used in Egypt and *Psoralea corylifolia* in India for photochemotherapy (128). Modern oral 8-MOP PUVA of vitiligo therapy seems to be inferior to standard narrow-band UVB therapy (129), which nevertheless is not fully satisfactory. Combination of narrow-band UVB therapy with oral application of 250 mg cabbage palm fern (*Phlebodium aureum* or *Polypodium leucotomos*) extract, however, increased repigmentation on neck and hand areas significantly in comparison to placebo, as was recently shown in a double-blind, randomized trial with 50 patients treated twice weekly for 25 to 26 weeks. On trunk and extremites, the difference was less pronounced (130) [LOE-A].

Another clinical observation of 74 vitiligo patients investigated the therapeutic efficacy of Xiaobai mixture (XBM) in comparison to a control group treated with PUVA. The therapeutic effect of XBM was better than that of PUVA (131). Unfortunately, the ingredients of XBM are not clear because the reference of this study is only available in Chinese. A recent review of natural health product treatment for vitiligo criticizes the quality of studies performed with plant materials but acknowledges that l-phenylalanine in combination with phototherapy and oral application of Ginkgo are promising (132).

Recently, it has been shown in a double-blind, placebo-controlled trial with 52 patients suffering from vitiligo that the oral administration of an extract of 50 mg Gingko (*Gingko biloba* L.) three times daily over a six-month period is effective in treating limited, slowly spreading vitiligo (133) [LOE-A]. Ginkgo significantly induced cessation of active progression, and ten patients compared to only two in the placebo group showed marked to complete repigmentation. However, no information about a long-term follow-up was available.

Antioxidant and immunomodulatory properties of Ginkgo may be the underlying mechanisms. Since Ginkgo is one of the best-studied botanical medicines, this treatment appears to be safe.

WOUNDS, BURNS, AND INJURIES

With regard to herbal therapy, we should keep in mind that we talk about smaller and milder forms of wounds, burns, and injuries. All wound treatments must consider the many causes of wounds such as vascular diseases, diabetes, vasculitis, and others and should be stage adequate, with focus on cleaning, mechanical protection, and anti-infectious measures in fresh wounds, while in later stages stimulation of tissue growth without excessive keloid formation is required.

Widely used traditional European botanicals in wound care are chamomile (*Matricaria recutita*), marigold (*Calendula officinalis*), and arnica (*Arnica montana*). All are applied locally. Aqueous (teas, decoctions) extracts of chamomile or marigold are used as washings or wet packs for fresh wounds. Arnica should never be applied on open wounds and not as an undiluted tincture because of possible sensitization. However, arnica ointments are excellent on later stages of healing wounds, for contusions and bruises. Marigold is especially recommended for wounds with bacterial infections. Small, well-circumscribed lesions may be treated with oil of St. John's wort (*Hypericum perforatum*), which is also believed to reduce scars by inhibition of keloid formation. All of these drugs have anti-inflammatory and antimicrobial activities. Active compounds are diverse and complex within each plant. Chamomile contains essential oil with bisabolol and chamazulen as well as saponines and other ingredients; alcoholic extraction yields the most complete blend, which may be transferred to aqueous formulations or ointments (134) [LOE-D].

Marigold (*Calendula officinalis* L.) has been topically used for wound treatment since ancient times. It has been shown to display bactericide, antiseptic, and anti-inflammatory as well as free radical–scavenging properties (135) [LOE-D]. Marigold was approved by the former German Commission E as a wound-healing agent (136) [LOE-D]. A recent prospective randomized trial in 254 patients who underwent surgical treatment of breast cancer and received postsurgical radiation therapy compared the effectiveness of a 10% *Calendula* ointment versus the standard therapy trolamine in the prevention of radiodermatitis. Twice daily application of *Calendula* ointment over the whole period of radiotherapy was significantly superior to trolamine and highly effective in the prevention of acute radiodermatitis (137) [LOE-A].

Diluted alcoholic preparations from the flowers of arnica (*Arnica montana*) are applied externally for the treatment of bruises, sprains, inflammation caused by insect bites, gingivitis, and aphthous ulcers and for the symptomatic treatment of rheumatic complaints (138) [LOE-C]. The secondary metabolites mediating the anti-inflammatory effects are sesquiterpene lactones of the 10a-methylpseudoguaianolide type such as helenalin, 11a,13-dihydrohelenalin, and their ester derivatives (139) [LOE-D]. It was demonstrated that these compounds mainly exert their anti-inflammatory effect by inhibiting the transcription factor NF-κB (140, 141) [LOE-D].

Although arnica has a long history in folk medicine and is widely used among consumers, up to now only a few clinical studies with arnica preparations have been carried out. In the field of dermatology, the possible synergism of vein-typical hydrotherapy according to Kneipp and topical arnica treatment was investigated in a double-blind, randomized clinical trial with 100 patients suffering from CVI (142) [LOE-A]. Both hydrotherapy and combined therapy were found to be successful. However, the combined therapy showed a significantly better result than the monotherapy.

The gel of aloe vera (*Aloe barbadensis*) is said to be beneficial in the treatment of chronic wounds and thermal injury (143, 144) [LOE-D]. A recently conducted systematic review of scientific literature found four clinical trials with 371 patients (including two randomized controlled trials) that supported that aloe vera might be an effective agent used in wound healing of first- to second-degree burns (145) [LOE-A].

Wound-healing activity has been demonstrated in animal models for numerous botanical extracts—to name a few, teak (*Tectona grandis*) (146) [LOE-D], golden trumpet (*Allamanda cathartica*) (147) [LOE-D], vitex (*Vitex trifolia* and *Vitex altissima*) (148) [LOE-D], Madagascar periwinkle (*Catharanthus roseus*) (149) [LOE-D], gotu kola (*Centella asiatica*) (150) [LOE-D], and sacred basil (*Ocimum sanctum*) (151) [LOE-D]. Curcumin obtained from the turmeric rhizome (*Curcuma longa*) (152) [LOE-D] and pycnogenol™ from French maritime pine bark (*Pinus maritima*) (153) [LOE-D] seem to be promising agents in the treatment of wounds. However, the efficacy of these traditional therapies has not been proven in controlled clinical trials so far.

In summary, some classical wound-healing plants are still first-line treatments for trivial injuries. Marigold, arnica, and aloe have proven effective in recent controlled trials.

ADVERSE EFFECTS OF PLANT EXTRACTS ON THE SKIN

This section is not intended to address each commonly used botanical. It is intended to increase the awareness of clinicians for the eventuality of side effects and how they may present.

Virtually all herbal remedies may provoke allergic reactions, and several botanicals hold the risk of photosensitization. The prevalence of contact sensitization against some botanical compounds such as oxidization products of monoterpenes, terpinene, balsam of Peru, and compositae plants is quite high in Europe (154). Contact sensitization toward cosmetics containing plant extracts as a fragrance is increasingly reported. Such patients should avoid plant extracts in their personal care products (155). Therefore, clinicians should be informed not only on the beneficial effects of botanicals for dermatological disorders but also on specific side effects that the use of herbal remedies might cause.

Botanicals may cause phytodermatitis, which can be classified into nonimmunological such as toxic or phototoxic dermatitis and immunological phytodermatitis such as immediate-type hypersensitivity, allergic contact dermatitis, or photoallergic dermatitis (60) (Table 3.5). An example of toxic phytodermatitis is the irritant phorbol dermatitis caused by the sun spurge (*Euphorbia helioscopia* L.) (156). Furocoumarins represent the principal agents responsible for phototoxic phytodermatitis. They comprise psoralens such as 5-methoxypsoralen (5-MOP, bergapten) and 8-MOP (methoxalen, xanthotoxin), which possess distinct photosensitizing potential. Furocoumarins also occur in burning bush (*Dictamnus albus* L.) and garden rue (*Ruta graveolens* L.) belonging to the Rutaceae plant family (157, 158). Phototoxic skin reactions to psoralens include the Berlock-dermatitis caused by 5-MOP, contained in cosmetically used *Citrus bergamia* (bergamot oil). Dermatitis bullosa pratensis is frequently caused by 8-MOP that mainly occurs in the Apiaceae family (Umbelliferae), which

Table 3.5. The Various Forms of Phytodermatitis

Nonimmunological Phytodermatitis	
Irritant dermatitis	physical—mechanical (cactus spines)
	chemical—toxic (poison ivy, spurge)
Phototoxic dermatitis	psoralens (bullous-/ Berlock-dermatitis)
	furoquinolines (Rutaceae: rue, gas plant)
	naphtodianthrones (hypericin, fagopyrin)
Immunological Phytodermatitis	
Immediate-type allergy	contact urticaria, food allergy
Allergic contact eczema	dermatitis from compositae, monoterpenes
Photoallergic dermatitis	immediate or delayed type (rare)

includes plants such as the giant hogweed (*Heracleum mantegazzianum*) (159) and various vegetables or herbs such as celery, parsnip, and parsley (160).

Besides toxic and phototoxic phytodermatitis, some botanicals may cause allergic contact dermatitis sensitized to plants or plant products. The Asteraceae arnica (*Arnica montana*) has been classified as a strong allergen, according to sensitization studies with guinea pigs (161). Its sesquiterpene lactones (SLs), especially those with an a-methylene-g-lactone moiety, are the most important allergens responsible for inducing allergic contact dermatitis. In a recent clinical study, 443 patients were patch tested with Compositae mix, SL mix, arnica, marigold, and propolis. Other plant species from the Asteraceae family that also contain SLs, such as tansy (*Tanacetum vulgare*), feverfew (*Tanacetum parthenium*), yarrow (*Achillea millefolium*), and elecampane (*Inula helenium*), may also induce sensitization or elicitation of Compositae dermatitis. Chamomile (*Chamomilla recutita*) and marigold (*Calendula officinalis*) are different from the mentioned Asteraceae species (162). As extracts of these plants are frequently used in occupational and cosmetic products, patch testing with additional plant extracts or adjustment of the commercial Compositae mix to regional conditions has been recommended (163). However, the sensitizing potential of arnica may be overestimated. Recent studies have shown that arnica tinctures and SLs are only weak contact sensitizers. The potent anti-inflammatory effects of SLs are dominant and fail to overcome immune regulation, which prevents contact hypersensitivity (164).

In essential oils such as peel oil from citrus fruits or the tea tree oil from *Melaleuca alternifolia*, the allergens are oxidized degradation products of monoterpenes (165, 166). Tea tree oil has become one of the most common contact allergens. Moreover, tea tree oil and lavender oil have recently been reported to cause prepubertal gynecomastia (167). A recent review on the adverse effects of herbal drugs in dermatology summarizes the different sensitizing potential of herbal remedies such as aloe vera, chamomile, or curcumin and aromatherapy oils such as lavender or tea tree oil (168).

DISCUSSION

Botanicals applied to wounds and skin diseases are perhaps the oldest medicines of mankind, and they still have their place in modern medicine. Three mechanisms of botanical medicines are especially important in modern view: anti-inflammatory, antimicrobial, and antioxidant properties, which are often combined in a single plant extract and may be based on a number of ingredients rather than on single compounds. This combination is relevant for some actual trends in dermatology: the increasing number of inflammatory skin diseases in industrial nations, the emergence of microbial strains resistant to conventional antibiotics, and the increased challenge of skin by lifestyle and environmentally caused irradiation. Plants offer a huge range of substances and combinations that may be used for more and more specific and individual therapies. It is worthwhile to search for more valuable botanicals in folk medicines all over the world.

Botanicals are often used in trivial affections of the skin as home remedies or in skin care products before professional medical help is necessary. Although not all herbs used traditionally are clinically well documented in a modern sense, drugs like chamomile, marigold, arnica, and others seem well established empirically and supported by pharmacological understanding of their mechanisms of action. Dermatologists should not try to discredit this use but should know about indications, mode of application, and risks and limitations. In acute and serious cases, botanicals may often be not sufficient but still helpful as adjuvants. For example, astringent and wound-healing effects may complement measures to suppress acute inflammation, infection, or pain that require treatment with stronger remedies.

Scientific evidence for clinical efficacy of botanicals is often scarce. A number of controlled clinical trials have been conducted, for example, in atopic dermatitis, but only very few when a specific plant species is regarded, with limited numbers of patients, and not always with positive results. More investigations are necessary to confirm that *Mahonia*, *Glycyrrhiza*, and *Hypericum* are effective in atopic dermatitis, or *Mahonia* and capsaicin in psoriasis. Numerous trials have been conducted in chronic venous insufficiency with *Hippocastanum* and flavonoid drugs, but drug treatment of this disease is a matter of discussion in general. There is strong evidence for the use of botanicals in UV protection. This, however, is related only to a minor extent to medical treatment but rather to diet recommendations and cosmetic care. Nevertheless, plant-derived topical formulations can be used to treat sunburns, to ameliorate side effects in PUVA, or to enhance efficacy in UVB treatment. Birch extract even seems to be effective in therapy of precancerous skin deletions caused by long-time irradiation.

UV protection is also important for cosmetic purposes in antiaging treatment. Another field of cosmetic application is cellulite; many products are advertised as effective, but clinical evidence up to now supports only mild, short-time improvement (169, 170). Caffeine and other botanicals may be efficient, but delivery in special formulations seems necessary to reach the relevant tissues (171, 172). Redness of the face may also be a cosmetic problem but also associated with rosacea; there is first evidence that certain botanical treatment might help against rosacea, but more rigid application of diagnostic criteria is necessary in this field (173).

Efficacy of dermatological preparations with defined, single, active substances is modulated by choice of the base formulation; with botanicals, a further variable to be considered is the quality of the active substance itself, that is, the composition of the plant extract.

The quality of botanical extracts depends upon many factors such as extraction procedures, drug-to-extract relation, and the resulting concentration of active compounds but also upon plant growth conditions and the time of harvesting. It is also important to consider the plant subspecies and chemical races when selecting the appropriate plant material for a special skin condition (174). Botanical cosmeceuticals are largely unregulated and therefore often lack pharmaceutical quality and evidence of safety and efficacy. In the United States, botanical extracts are often distributed as dietary supplements without regulatory requirements for standardization, safety, and efficacy (175). In contrast, in Germany, a regulatory authority known as Commission E has conducted an extensive review of more than 300 botanicals with established traditional use (176). The level of scientific evidence, reporting of adverse events, and toxicological data were evaluated and resulted in positive or negative plant monographs. The Commission E monographs together with the European Scientific Cooperative on Phytotherapy (ESCOP) monographs and the monographs of the American Botanical Council (ABC) are often used as a basis for decision making by regulatory authorities in European countries and in the United States (176).

It is apparent from these considerations that clinical evidence of efficacy and safety can be attributed only to the specific formulation tested and not to the investigated plant species in general. Thus, future clinical studies should concentrate on well-defined, standardized extracts and adequate dermatological formulations thereof, which are clearly described in the publications. Otherwise, contradictory results can hardly be interpreted. Vice versa, negative results will not discredit a botanical medicine unless the quality of the investigated preparation is demonstrated.

CONCLUSIONS

Herbal remedies have been used for the treatment of skin diseases since ancient times. Some effects have been reported anecdotally; some have been confirmed in randomized, controlled clinical trials. Plant monographs such as the monographs of the former German Commission E or the ESCOP (European Scientific Cooperative on Phytotherapy) monographs provide specific recommendations for the use and efficacy of various botanicals for the therapy of specific diseases. Botanicals play an important role as home remedies or self-medication of trivial dermatological disorders, but extracts with anti-inflammatory, antimicrobial, and antioxidant capacities seem especially useful in diseases of high actual and increasing importance such as atopic dermatitis, psoriasis, and infections with resistant germs, for which some botanicals might become first-line treatments. Wounds, burns, and acne are examples of applications in which traditional use of botanicals is helpful, at least as adjuvant treatments. However, many more controlled clinical studies with well-defined botanical extracts and preparations are needed to figure out the efficacy and risks of popular plant-derived products in dermatology. Extensive use of botanicals in nutrition supplements and cosmetic care should also be accompanied by research, especially concerning long-time safety and tolerability.

REFERENCES

[1]Mantle D, Gok MA, Lennard TW. Adverse and beneficial effects of plant extracts on skin and skin disorders. *Adverse Drug React Toxicol Rev.* 2001 Jun;20(2):89–103.

No funding and no conflict of interest declared by the authors.

[2]Choi CM, Berson DS. Cosmeceuticals. *Semin Cutan Med Surg*. 2006 Sep;25(3):163–168.

[3]Medicine. OCfE-b. Oxford Centre for Evidence-based Medicine. Levels of Evidence and Grades of Recommendation. 2008 [cited; Available from: http://www.cebm.net/index.aspx?o=1025#levels.

[4]Kraft K. [Diseases of the skin (I). Psoriasis and atopic eczema.] *Z Phytotherapie*. 2007;28(2):76–78.

[5]Schilcher H, Kammerer S. [Phytotherapy manual]. Urban und Fischer, München und Jena; 2000.

[6]Patzelt-Wenczler R, Ponce-Poschl E. Proof of efficacy of Kamillosan(R) cream in atopic eczema. *Eur J Med Res*. 2000 Apr 19;5(4):171–175.

[7]Gloor M, Reichling J, Wasik B, Holzgang HE. Antiseptic effect of a topical dermatological formulation that contains Hamamelis distillate and urea. *Forsch Komplementarmed Klass Naturheilkd*. 2002 Jun;9(3):153–159.

[8]Korting HC, Schafer-Korting M, Klovekorn W, Klovekorn G, Martin C, Laux P. Comparative efficacy of hamamelis distillate and hydrocortisone cream in atopic eczema. *Eur J Clin Pharmacol*. 1995;48(6):461–465.

[9]Schempp CM, Hezel S, Simon JC. [Topical treatment of atopic dermatitis with Hypericum cream. A randomised, placebo-controlled, double-blind half-side comparison study]. *Hautarzt*. 2003 Mar;54(3):248–253.

[10]Schempp CM, Pelz K, Wittmer A, Schopf E, Simon JC. Antibacterial activity of hyperforin from St John's wort, against multiresistant Staphylococcus aureus and gram-positive bacteria. *Lancet*. 1999 Jun 19;353(9170):2129.

[11]Schempp CM, Winghofer B, Ludtke R, Simon-Haarhaus B, Schopf E, Simon JC. Topical application of St John's wort (Hypericum perforatum L.) and of its metabolite hyperforin inhibits the allostimulatory capacity of epidermal cells. *Br J Dermatol*. 2000 May;142(5):979–984.

[12]Higaki S, Kitagawa T, Morohashi M, Yamagishi T. Efficacy of Shiunko for the treatment of atopic dermatitis. *J Int Med Res*. 1999 May–Jun;27(3):143–147.

[13]Thumm EJ, Stoss M, Bayerl C. Randomized trial to study efficacy of a 20% and 10% Hippophaë rhamnoides containing cream used by patients with mild to intermediate atopic dermatitis. *Akt Dermatol*. 2000;26: 285–290.

[14]Stern T, Bayerl C. Black seed oil ointment: a new approach for the treatment of atopic dermatitis? *Akt Dermatol*. 2002;28:74–79.

[15]Donsky H, Clarke D. Relieva, a Mahonia aquifolium extract for the treatment of adult patients with atopic dermatitis. *Am J Ther*. 2007 Sep–Oct;14(5):442–446.

[16]Abeck D, Klövekorn W, Danesch U. Behandlung des atopischen Ekzems bei Kindern mit einer pflanzlichen Heilsalbe: Ergebnisse einer offenen Studie mit Ekzevowen® derma. *Akt Dermatol*. 2005;31:523–526.

[17]Klovekorn W, Tepe A, Danesch U. A randomized, double-blind, vehicle-controlled, half-side comparison with a herbal ointment containing Mahonia aquifolium, Viola tricolor and Centella asiatica for the treatment of mild-to-moderate atopic dermatitis. *Int J Clin Pharmacol Ther*. 2007 Nov;45(11):583–591.

[18]Inoue H, Mori T, Shibata S, Koshihara Y. Modulation by glycyrrhetinic acid derivatives of TPA-induced mouse ear oedema. *Br J Pharmacol*. 1989 Jan;96(1):204–210.

[19]Saeedi M, Morteza-Semnani K, Ghoreishi MR. The treatment of atopic dermatitis with licorice gel. *J Dermatolog Treat*. 2003 Sep;14(3):153–157.

[20]Belloni G, Pinelli S, Veraldi S. A randomised, double-blind, vehicle-controlled study to evaluate the efficacy and safety of MAS063D (Atopiclair) in the treatment of mild to moderate atopic dermatitis. *Eur J Dermatol*. 2005 Jan–Feb;15(1):31–36.

[21]Abramovits W, Boguniewicz M. A multicenter, randomized, vehicle-controlled clinical study to examine the efficacy and safety of MAS063DP (Atopiclair) in the management of mild to moderate atopic dermatitis in adults. *J Drugs Dermatol*. 2006 Mar;5(3):236–244.

[22]Abramovits W, Gover MD, Gupta AK. Atopiclair nonsteroidal cream. *Skinmed*. 2005 Nov–Dec;4(6):369.

[23]Uehara M, Sugiura H, Sakurai K. A trial of oolong tea in the management of recalcitrant atopic dermatitis. *Arch Dermatol*. 2001 Jan;137(1):42–43.

[24]Kobayashi H, Mizuno N, Teramae H, Kutsuna H, Ueoku S, Onoyama J, et al. Diet and Japanese herbal medicine for recalcitrant atopic dermatitis: efficacy and safety. *Drugs Exp Clin Res*. 2004;30(5–6):197–202.

[25]Kobayashi H, Mizuno N, Teramae H, Kutsuna H, Ueoku S, Onoyama J, et al. The effects of Hochuekki-to in patients with atopic dermatitis resistant to conventional treatment. *Int J Tissue React*. 2004;26 (3–4):113–117.

[26]Hon KL, Leung TF, Ng PC, Lam MC, Kam WY, Wong KY, et al. Efficacy and tolerability of a Chinese herbal medicine concoction for treatment of atopic dermatitis: a randomized, double-blind, placebo-controlled study. *Br J Dermatol*. 2007 Aug;157(2):357–363.

[27]Sheehan MP, Rustin MH, Atherton DJ, Buckley C, Harris DW, Brostoff J, et al. Efficacy of traditional Chinese herbal therapy in adult atopic dermatitis. *Lancet*. 1992 Jul 4;340(8810):13–17.

[28]Sheehan MP, Stevens H, Ostlere LS, Atherton DJ, Brostoff J, Rustin MH. Follow-up of adult patients with atopic eczema treated with Chinese herbal therapy for 1 year. *Clin Exp Dermatol*. 1995 Mar;20(2):136–140.

[29]Shapira MY, Raphaelovich Y, Gilad L, Or R, Dumb AJ, Ingber A. Treatment of atopic dermatitis with herbal combination of Eleutherococcus, Achillea millefolium, and Lamium album has no advantage over placebo: a double blind, placebo-controlled, randomized trial. *J Am Acad Dermatol*. 2005 Apr;52(4):691–693.

[30]Takwale A, Tan E, Agarwal S, Barclay G, Ahmed I, Hotchkiss K, et al. Efficacy and tolerability of borage oil in adults and children with atopic eczema: randomised, double blind, placebo controlled, parallel group trial. *BMJ.* 2003 Dec 13;327(7428):1385.

[31]van de Kerkhof PC, van der Valk PG, Swinkels OQ, Kucharekova M, de Rie MA, de Vries HJ, et al. A comparison of twice-daily calcipotriol ointment with once-daily short-contact dithranol cream therapy: a randomized controlled trial of supervised treatment of psoriasis vulgaris in a day-care setting. *Br J Dermatol.* 2006 Oct;155(4):800–807.

[32]Augustin M, Hoch Y. *Phytotherapie bei Hautkrankheiten. Grundlagen-Praxis-Studien.* Munich: Elsevier GmbH; 2004.

[33]Amornpinyokeit N, Asawanonda P. 8-Methoxypsoralen cream plus targeted narrowband ultraviolet B for psoriasis. *Photodermatol Photoimmunol Photomed.* 2006 Dec;22(6):285–289.

[34]Vongthongsri R, Konschitzky R, Seeber A, Treitl C, Honigsmann H, Tanew A. Randomized, double-blind comparison of 1 mg/L versus 5 mg/L methoxsalen bath-PUVA therapy for chronic plaque-type psoriasis. *J Am Acad Dermatol.* 2006 Oct;55(4):627–631.

[35]Gulliver WP, Donsky HJ. A report on three recent clinical trials using Mahonia aquifolium 10% topical cream and a review of the worldwide clinical experience with Mahonia aquifolium for the treatment of plaque psoriasis. *Am J Ther.* 2005 Sep–Oct;12(5):398–406.

[36]Bernstein S, Donsky H, Gulliver W, Hamilton D, Nobel S, Norman R. Treatment of mild to moderate psoriasis with Relieva, a Mahonia aquifolium extract: a double-blind, placebo-controlled study. *Am J Ther.* 2006 Mar–Apr;13(2):121–126.

[37]Stucker M, Memmel U, Hoffmann M, Hartung J, Altmeyer P. Vitamin B(12) cream containing avocado oil in the therapy of plaque psoriasis. *Dermatology.* 2001;203(2):141–147.

[38]Ellis CN, Berberian B, Sulica VI, Dodd WA, Jarratt MT, Katz HI, et al. A double-blind evaluation of topical capsaicin in pruritic psoriasis. *J Am Acad Dermatol.* 1993 Sep;29(3):438–442.

[39]Bernstein JE, Parish LC, Rapaport M, Rosenbaum MM, Roenigk HH, Jr. Effects of topically applied capsaicin on moderate and severe psoriasis vulgaris. *J Am Acad Dermatol.* 1986 Sep;15(3):504–507.

[40]Grover JK, Yadav SP. Pharmacological actions and potential uses of Momordica charantia: a review. *J Ethnopharmacol.* 2004 Jul;93(1):123–132.

[41]Syed TA, Ahmad SA, Holt AH, Ahmad SH, Afzal M. Management of psoriasis with aloe vera extract in a hydrophilic cream: a placebo-controlled, double-blind study. *Trop Med Int Health.* 1996 Aug;1(4): 505–509.

[42]Paulsen E, Korsholm L, Brandrup F. A double-blind, placebo-controlled study of a commercial aloe vera gel in the treatment of slight to moderate psoriasis vulgaris. *J Eur Acad Dermatol Venereol.* 2005 May;19(3): 326–331.

[43]Brown AC, Koett J, Johnson DW, Semaskvich NM, Holck P, Lally D, et al. Effectiveness of kukui nut oil as a topical treatment for psoriasis. *Int J Dermatol.* 2005 Aug;44(8):684–687.

[44]Tse TW. Use of common Chinese herbs in the treatment of psoriasis. *Clin Exp Dermatol.* 2003 Sep;28(5): 469–475.

[45]Tse WP, Cheng CH, Che CT, Zhao M, Lin ZX. Induction of apoptosis underlies the Radix Rubiae-mediated anti-proliferative action on human epidermal keratinocytes: implications for psoriasis treatment. *Int J Mol Med.* 2007 Nov;20(5):663–672.

[46]Kraft K. [Diseases of the skin (II). Other eczema types, acne and pruritus.] *Z Phytotherapie.* 2007;28(3): 129–133.

[47]Peirce A, Fargis P, Scordato E. *The American Pharmaceutical Association Practical Guide to Natural Medicines.* New York, NY: Stonesong Press; 1999.

[48]Bedi MK, Shenefelt PD. Herbal therapy in dermatology. *Arch Dermatol.* 2002 Feb;138(2):232–242.

[49]Wuttke W, Jarry H, Christoffel V, et al. Chaste tree (Vitex agnus-castus): pharmacology and clinical indications. *Phytomedicine.* 2003 May;10(4):348–357.

[50]Jain A, Basal E. Inhibition of Propionibacterium acnes-induced mediators of inflammation by Indian herbs. *Phytomedicine.* 2003 Jan;10(1):34–38.

[51]Nam C, Kim S, Sim Y, Chang I. Anti-acne effects of Oriental herb extracts: a novel screening method to select anti-acne agents. *Skin Pharmacol Appl Skin Physiol.* 2003 Mar–Apr;16(2):84–90.

[52]Weckesser S, Engel K, Simon-Haarhaus B, Wittmer A, Pelz K, Schempp CM. Screening of plant extracts for antimicrobial activity against bacteria and yeasts with dermatological relevance. *Phytomedicine.* 2007 Aug;14(7–8):508–516.

[53]Orafidiya LO, Agbanie EO, Oyedele AO, et al. Preliminary clinical tests on topical preparations of Ocimum gratissimum L. leaf essential oil for the treatment of acne vulgaris. *Clin Drug Investig.* 2002;22(5): 313–319.

[54]Slobodnikova L, Kost'alova D, Labudova D, Kotulova D, Kettmann V. Antimicrobial activity of Mahonia aquifolium crude extract and its major isolated alkaloids. *Phytother Res.* 2004 Aug;18(8):674–676.

[55]Seki T, Morohashi M. Effect of some alkaloids, flavonoids and triterpenoids, contents of Japanese-Chinese traditional herbal medicines, on the lipogenesis of sebaceous glands. *Skin Pharmacol*. 1993;6(1): 56–60.

[56]Choi BH, Ahn IS, Kim YH, Park JW, Lee SY, Hyun CK, et al. Berberine reduces the expression of adipogenic enzymes and inflammatory molecules of 3T3-L1 adipocyte. *Exp Mol Med*. 2006 Dec 31;38(6):599–605.

[57]Koh KJ, Pearce AL, Marshman G, Finlay-Jones JJ, Hart PH. Tea tree oil reduces histamine-induced skin inflammation. *Br J Dermatol*. 2002 Dec;147(6):1212–1217.

[58]Bassett IB, Pannowitz DL, Barnetson RS. A comparative study of tea-tree oil versus benzoylperoxide in the treatment of acne. *Med J Aust*. 1990 Oct;153(8):455–458.

[59]Enshaieh S, Jooya A, Siadat AH, Iraji F. The efficacy of 5% topical tea tree oil gel in mild to moderate acne vulgaris: a randomized, double-blind placebo-controlled study. *Indian J Dermatol Venereol Leprol*. 2007 Jan–Feb;73(1):22–25.

[60]Schempp CM, Schopf E, Simon JC. [Plant-induced toxic and allergic dermatitis (phytodermatitis)]. *Hautarzt*. 2002 Feb;53(2):93–97.

[61]van Dijken JP, van Tuijl A, Luttik MA, Middelhoven WJ, Pronk JT. Novel pathway for alcoholic fermentation of delta-gluconolactone in the yeast Saccharomyces bulderi. *J Bacteriol*. 2002 Feb;184(3):672–678.

[62]Hunt MJ, Barnetson RS. A comparative study of gluconolactone versus benzoyl peroxide in the treatment of acne. *Australas J Dermatol*. 1992;33(3):131–134.

[63]Cox SD, Mann CM, Markham JL, Bell HC, Gustafson JE, Warmington JR, et al. The mode of antimicrobial action of the essential oil of Melaleuca alternifolia (tea tree oil). *J Appl Microbiol*. 2000 Jan;88(1):170–175.

[64]Lo Cantore P, Iacobellis NS, De Marco A, Capasso F, Senatore F. Antibacterial activity of Coriandrum sativum L. and Foeniculum vulgare Miller Var. vulgare (Miller) essential oils. *J Agric Food Chem*. 2004 Dec 29;52(26):7862–7866.

[65]Elgayyar M, Draughon FA, Golden DA, Mount JR. Antimicrobial activity of essential oils from plants against selected pathogenic and saprophytic microorganisms. *J Food Prot*. 2001 Jul;64(7):1019–1024.

[66]Delaquis PJ, Stanich K, Girard B, Mazza G. Antimicrobial activity of individual and mixed fractions of dill, cilantro, coriander and eucalyptus essential oils. *Int J Food Microbiol*. 2002 Mar 25;74(1–2):101–109.

[67]Singh G, Kapoor IP, Pandey SK, Singh UK, Singh RK. Studies on essential oils: part 10; antibacterial activity of volatile oils of some spices. *Phytother Res*. 2002 Nov;16(7):680–682.

[68]Kubo I, Fujita K, Kubo A, Nihei K, Ogura T. Antibacterial activity of coriander volatile compounds against Salmonella choleraesuis. *J Agric Food Chem*. 2004 Jun 2;52(11):3329–3332.

[69]Reuter J, Huyke C, Casetti F, Theek C, Frank U, Augustin M, et al. Anti-inflammatory potential of a lipolotion containing coriander oil in the ultraviolet erythema test. *J Dtsch Dermatol Ges*. 2008 Mar 26.

[70]Higaki S, Morimatsu S, Morohashi M, Yamagishi T, Hasegawa Y. Susceptibility of Propionibacterium acnes, Staphylococcus aureus and Staphylococcus epidermidis to 10 Kampo formulations. *J Int Med Res*. 1997 Nov–Dec;25(6):318–324.

[71]Shahi SK, Shukla AC, Bajaj AK, Banerjee U, Rimek D, Midgely G, et al. Broad spectrum herbal therapy against superficial fungal infections. *Skin Pharmacol Appl Skin Physiol*. 2000 Jan–Feb;13(1):60–64.

[72]Ledezma E, DeSousa L, Jorquera A, Sanchez J, Lander A, Rodriguez E, et al. Efficacy of ajoene, an organosulphur derived from garlic, in the short-term therapy of tinea pedis. *Mycoses*. 1996 Sep–Oct;39(9–10):393–395.

[73]Koytchev R, Alken RG, Dundarov S. Balm mint extract (Lo-701) for topical treatment of recurring herpes labialis. *Phytomedicine*. 1999 Oct;6(4):225–230.

[74]Xie FM, Zeng K, Chen ZL, Li GF, Lin ZF, Zhu XL, et al. [Treatment of recurrent condyloma acuminatum with solid lipid nanoparticle gel containing podophyllotoxin: a randomized double-blinded, controlled clinical trial]. *Nan Fang Yi Ke Da Xue Xue Bao*. 2007 May;27(5):657–659.

[75]Suter A, Bommer S, Rechner J. Treatment of patients with venous insufficiency with fresh plant horse chestnut seed extract: a review of 5 clinical studies. *Adv Ther*. 2006 Jan–Feb;23(1):179–190.

[76]Pittler MH, Ernst E. Horse chestnut seed for chronic venous insufficiency. *Cochrane Database Syst Rev*. 2006 Jan; 25(1):CD003230.

[77]Ng TB, Liu F, Wang ZT. Antioxidative activity of natural products from plants. *Life Sci*. 2000 Jan 14;66(8):709–723.

[78]Cesarone MR, Belcaro G, Pellegrini L, Ledda A, Vinciguerra G, Ricci A, Di Renzo A, Ruffini I, Gizzi G, Ippolito E, Fano F, Dugall M, Acerbi G, Cornelli U, Hosoi M, Cacchio M. Venoruton vs Daflon: evaluation of effects on quality of life in chronic venous insufficiency. *Angiology*. 2006 Mar;57(2):131–138.

[79]Cesarone MR, Belcaro G, Pellegrini L, Ledda A, Vinciguerra G, Ricci A, Gizzi G, Ippolito E, Fano F, Dugall M, Acerbi G, Cornelli U, Cacchio M. HR, 0-(beta-hydroxyethyl)-rutosides, in comparison with diosmin+hesperidin in chronic venous insufficiency and venous microangiopathy: an independent, prospective, comparative registry study. *Angiology*. 2005 Jan;56(1):1–8.

[80]Belcaro G, Cesarone MR, Nicolaides AN, Geroulakos G, Acerbi G, Candiani C, Griffin M, Bavera P, Dugall M, Brandolini R, Di Renzo A, Ricci A, Ippolito E, Winford M, Golden G. The LONFLIT4-Venoruton

study: a randomized trial prophylaxis of flight-edema in normal subjects. *Clin Appl Thromb Hemost.* 2003 Jan;9(1):19–23.

[81]Großmann K. Vergleich der Wirksamkeit einer kombinierten Therapie mit Kompressionsstrümpfen und Oxerouton (Venorouton®) versus Kompressionsstrümpfen und Placebo bei Patienten mit CVI. *Phlebologie.* 1997;26:105–110.

[82]Ihme N, Kiesewetter H, Jung F, Hoffmann KH, Birk A, Muller A, et al. Leg oedema protection from a buckwheat herb tea in patients with chronic venous insufficiency: a single-centre, randomised, double-blind, placebo-controlled clinical trial. *Eur J Clin Pharmacol.* 1996;50(6):443–447.

[83]Kiesewetter H, Koscielny J, Kalus U, Vix JM, Peil H, Petrini O, et al. Efficacy of orally administered extract of red vine leaf AS 195 (folia vitis viniferae) in chronic venous insufficiency (stages I–II). A random-ized, double-blind, placebo-controlled trial. *Arzneimittelforschung.* 2000 Feb;50(2):109–117.

[84]Cesarone MR, Belcaro G, Rohdewald P, Pellegrini L, Ledda A, Vinciguerra G, et al. Rapid relief of signs/symptoms in chronic venous microangiopathy with pycnogenol: a prospective, controlled study. *Angiology.* 2006 Oct–Nov;57(5):569–576.

[85]Koch R. Comparative study of Venostasin and Pycnogenol in chronic venous insufficiency. *Phytother Res.* 2002 Mar;16 Suppl 1:S1–5.

[86]Bergan JJ. Chronic venous insufficiency and the therapeutic effects of Daflon 500 mg. *Angiology.* 2005 Sep–Oct;56(Suppl 1):S21–S24.

[87]Katsenis K. Micronized purified flavonoid fraction (MPFF): a review of its pharmacological effects, therapeutic efficacy and benefits in the management of chronic venous insufficiency. *Curr Vasc Pharmacol.* 2005 Jan;3(1):1–9.

[88]Vanscheidt W, Jost V, Wolna P, Lucker PW, Muller A, Theurer C, et al. Efficacy and safety of a Butcher's broom preparation (Ruscus aculeatus L. extract) compared to placebo in patients suffering from chronic ve-nous insufficiency. *Arzneimittelforschung.* 2002;52(4):243–250.

[89]Pastura G, Mesiti M, Saitta M, Romeo D, Settineri N, Maisano R, et al. [Lymphedema of the upper ex-tremity in patients operated for carcinoma of the breast: clinical experience with coumarinic extract from Melilotus officinalis]. *Clin Ter.* 1999 Nov–Dec;150(6):403–408.

[90]Consoli A. [Chronic venous insufficiency: an open trial of FLEBS Crema]. *Minerva Cardioangiol.* 2003 Aug;51(4):411–416.

[91]Cataldi A, Gasbarro V, Viaggi R, Soverini R, Gresta E, Mascoli F. [Effectiveness of the combination of alpha tocopherol, rutin, melilotus, and centella asiatica in the treatment of patients with chronic venous insuf-ficiency]. *Minerva Cardioangiol.* 2001 Apr;49(2):159–163.

[92]Ehrhardt M. *Qualitätssicherung in der hausärztlichen Behandlung der chronisch venösen Insuffizienz: Entwicklung einer evidenzbasierten Leitlinie.* Dissertation. University of Hamburg, 2004.

[93]Baliga MS, Katiyar SK. Chemoprevention of photocarcinogenesis by selected dietary botanicals. *Photo-chem Photobiol Sci.* 2006 Feb;5(2):243–253.

[94]Yaar M, Gilchrest BA. Photoageing: mechanism, prevention and therapy. *Br J Dermatol.* 2007 Nov;157(5): 874–887.

[95]Afaq F, Mukhtar H. Botanical antioxidants in the prevention of photocarcinogenesis and photoaging. *Exp Dermatol.* 2006 Sep;15(9):678–684.

[96]Gonzalez S, Pathak MA, Cuevas J, Villarrubia VG, Fitzpatrick TB. Topical or oral administration with an extract of Polypodium leucotomos prevents acute sunburn and psoralen-induced phototoxic reactions as well as depletion of Langerhans cells in human skin. *Photodermatol Photoimmunol Photomed.* 1997 Feb–Apr;13 (1–2):50–60.

[97]Middelkamp-Hup MA, Pathak MA, Parrado C, Garcia-Caballero T, Rius-Diaz F, Fitzpatrick TB, et al. Orally administered Polypodium leucotomos extract decreases psoralen-UVA-induced phototoxicity, pig-mentation, and damage of human skin. *J Am Acad Dermatol.* 2004 Jan;50(1):41–49.

[98]Middelkamp-Hup MA, Pathak MA, Parrado C, Goukassian D, Rius-Diaz F, Mihm MC, et al. Oral Poly-podium leucotomos extract decreases ultraviolet-induced damage of human skin. *J Am Acad Dermatol.* 2004 Dec;51(6):910–918.

[99]Capote R, Alonso-Lebrero JL, Garcia F, Brieva A, Pivel JP, Gonzalez S. Polypodium leucotomos extract inhibits trans-urocanic acid photoisomerization and photodecomposition. *J Photochem Photobiol B.* 2006 Mar 1;82(3):173–179.

[100]Reuter J, Jocher A, Hornstein S, Monting JS, Schempp CM. Sage extract rich in phenolic diterpenes in-hibits ultraviolet-induced erythema in vivo. *Planta Med.* 2007 Sep;73(11):1190–1191.

[101]Hughes-Formella BJ, Filbry A, Gassmueller J, Rippke F. Anti-inflammatory efficacy of topical prepara-tions with 10% hamamelis distillate in a UV erythema test. *Skin Pharmacol Appl Skin Physiol.* 2002 Mar–Apr;15(2):125–132.

[102]Heinrich U, Gartner C, Wiebusch M, Eichler O, Sies H, Tronnier H, et al. Supplementation with beta-carotene or a similar amount of mixed carotenoids protects humans from UV-induced erythema. *J Nutr.* 2003 Jan;133(1):98–101.

[103]Aust O, Stahl W, Sies H, Tronnier H, Heinrich U. Supplementation with tomato-based products increases lycopene, phytofluene, and phytoene levels in human serum and protects against UV-light-induced erythema. *Int J Vitam Nutr Res.* 2005 Jan;75(1):54–60.

[104]Katiyar SK, Ahmad N, Mukhtar H. Green tea and skin. *Arch Dermatol.* 2000 Aug;136(8):989–994.

[105]Zhao JF, Zhang YJ, Jin XH, Athar M, Santella RM, Bickers DR, et al. Green tea protects against psoralen plus ultraviolet A-induced photochemical damage to skin. *J Invest Dermatol.* 1999 Dec;113(6):1070–1075.

[106]Cooper R, Morre DJ, Morre DM. Medicinal benefits of green tea: part I. review of noncancer health benefits. *J Altern Complement Med.* 2005 Jun;11(3):521–528.

[107]Cooper R, Morre DJ, Morre DM. Medicinal benefits of green tea: part II. review of anticancer properties. *J Altern Complement Med.* 2005 Aug;11(4):639–652.

[108]Camouse MM, Hanneman KK, Conrad EP, Baron ED. Protective effects of tea polyphenols and caffeine. *Expert Rev Anticancer Ther.* 2005 Dec;5(6):1061–1068.

[109]Nomura M, Ma WY, Huang C, Yang CS, Bowden GT, Miyamoto K, et al. Inhibition of ultraviolet B-induced AP-1 activation by theaflavins from black tea. *Mol Carcinog.* 2000 Jul;28(3):148–155.

[110]Leung LK, Su Y, Chen R, Zhang Z, Huang Y, Chen ZY. Theaflavins in black tea and catechins in green tea are equally effective antioxidants. *J Nutr.* 2001 Sep;131(9):2248–2251.

[111]Baumann LS. Less-known botanical cosmeceuticals. *Dermatol Ther.* 2007 Sep–Oct;20(5):330–342.

[112]Farris P. Idebenone, green tea, and coffeeberry extract: new and innovative antioxidants. *Dermatol Ther.* 2007 Sep–Oct;20(5):322–329.

[113]Heinrich U, Neukam K, Tronnier H, Sies H, Stahl W. Long-term ingestion of high flavanol cocoa provides photoprotection against UV-induced erythema and improves skin condition in women. *J Nutr.* 2006 Jun;136(6):1565–1569.

[114]Katiyar SK. Silymarin and skin cancer prevention: anti-inflammatory, antioxidant and immunomodulatory effects (Review). *Int J Oncol.* 2005 Jan;26(1):169–176.

[115]Huang MT, Ho CT, Wang ZY, Ferraro T, Lou YR, Stauber K, et al. Inhibition of skin tumorigenesis by rosemary and its constituents carnosol and ursolic acid. *Cancer Res.* 1994 Feb 1;54(3):701–708.

[116]Mitamura T, Matsuno T, Sakamoto S, Maemura M, Kudo H, Suzuki S, et al. Effects of a new clerodane diterpenoid isolated from propolis on chemically induced skin tumors in mice. *Anticancer Res.* 1996 Sep–Oct; 16(5A):2669–2672.

[117]Xiaoguang C, Hongyan L, Xiaohong L, Zhaodi F, Yan L, Lihua T, et al. Cancer chemopreventive and therapeutic activities of red ginseng. *J Ethnopharmacol.* 1998 Feb;60(1):71–78.

[118]Wei H, Saladi R, Lu Y, Wang Y, Palep SR, Moore J, et al. Isoflavone genistein: photoprotection and clinical implications in dermatology. *J Nutr.* 2003 Nov;133(11 Suppl 1):3811S–3819S.

[119]Syed DN, Malik A, Hadi N, Sarfaraz S, Afaq F, Mukhtar H. Photochemopreventive effect of pomegranate fruit extract on UVA-mediated activation of cellular pathways in normal human epidermal keratinocytes. *Photochem Photobiol.* 2006 Mar–Apr;82(2):398–405.

[120]Zaid MA, Afaq F, Syed DN, Dreher M, Mukhtar H. Inhibition of UVB-mediated oxidative stress and markers of photoaging in immortalized HaCaT keratinocytes by pomegranate polyphenol extract POMx. *Photochem Photobiol.* 2007 Jul–Aug;83(4):882–888.

[121]Laszczyk M, Jager S, Simon-Haarhaus B, Scheffler A, Schempp CM. Physical, chemical and pharmacological characterization of a new oleogel-forming triterpene extract from the outer bark of birch (betulae cortex). *Planta Med.* 2006 Dec;72(15):1389–1395.

[122]Huyke C, Laszczyk M, Scheffler A, Ernst R, Schempp CM. [Treatment of actinic keratoses with birch bark extract: a pilot study]. *J Dtsch Dermatol Ges.* 2006 Feb;4(2):132–136.

[123]Huyke C, Reuter J, Rodig M, Kersten A, Laszczyk M, Scheffler A, Nashan D, Schempp CM. Treatment of actinic keratoses with a novel betulin-based oleogel. A prospective, randomized, comparative pilot study. *J Dtsch Dermatol Ges.* 2009; 7. DOI: 10.111/j.1610-0387.2008.06865.x.

[124]Sharquie KE, Al-Obaidi HK. Onion juice (Allium cepa L.), a new topical treatment for alopecia areata. *J Dermatol.* 2002 Jun;29(6):343–346.

[125]Prager N, Bickett K, French N, Marcovici G. A randomized, double-blind, placebo-controlled trial to determine the effectiveness of botanically derived inhibitors of 5-alpha-reductase in the treatment of androgenetic alopecia. *J Altern Complement Med.* 2002 Apr;8(2):143–152.

[126]Gerber GS, Zagaja GP, Bales GT, et al. Saw palmetto (Serenoa repens) in men with lower urinary tract symptoms. Effects on urodynamic parameters and voiding symptoms. *Urology.* 1998;51:1003–1007.

[127]Lee MM, Lin SS, Wrensch MR, et al. Alternative therapies used by women with breast cancer in four ethnic populations. *J Nat Cancer Inst.* 2000; 92:42–47.

[128]Parrish JA, Fitzpatrick, TB, Tanenbaum L, et al. Photochemotherapy of psoriasis with oral methoxsalen and longwave ultraviolet. *N Engl J Med.* 1974 Dec; 291(23):1207–1211.

[129]Yones SS, Palmer RA, Garibaldinos TM, Hawk JL. Randomized double-blind trial of treatment of vitiligo: efficacy of psoralen-UV-A therapy vs. narrowband-UV-B therapy. *Arch Dermatol.* 2007 May; 143(5): 578–584.

[130]Middelkamp-Hup MA, Bos JD, Rius-Diaz F, et al. Treatment of vitiligo vulgaris with narrow-band UVB and oral Polypodium leucotomos extract. a randomized double-blind placebo-controlled study. *J Eur Acad Dermatol Venereol*. 2007 Aug;21(7):942–950.

[131]Liu ZJ, Xiang YP. [Clinical observation on treatment of vitiligo with xiaobai mixture]. *Zhongguo Zhong Xi Yi Jie He Za Zhi*. 2003 Aug;23(8):596–598.

[132]Szczurko O, Boon HS. A systematic review of natural health product treatment for vitiligo. *BMC Dermatology* 2008; 8: 2. doi:10.1186/1471-5945-5945-8-2.

[133]Parsad D, Pandhi R, Juneja A. Effectiveness of oral Ginkgo biloba in treating limited, slowly spreading vitiligo. *Clin Exp Dermatol*. 2003 May;28(3):285–287.

[134]Kraft K. [Diseases of the skin. Wounds and blunt traumata]. *Z Phytotherapie*. 2007;28(4):178–180.

[135]Cordova CA, Siqueira IR, Netto CA, Yunes RA, Volpato AM, Cechinel Filho V, et al. Protective properties of butanolic extract of the Calendula officinalis L. (marigold) against lipid peroxidation of rat liver microsomes and action as free radical scavenger. *Redox Rep*. 2002;7(2):95–102.

[136]Bisset NG, Wichtl M. *Herbal Drugs and Phytopharmaceuticals*. 2nd ed. Boca Raton, FL: CRC Press; 2001.

[137]Pommier P, Gomez F, Sunyach MP, D'Hombres A, Carrie C, Montbarbon X. Phase III randomized trial of Calendula officinalis compared with trolamine for the prevention of acute dermatitis during irradiation for breast cancer. *J Clin Oncol*. 2004 Apr 15;22(8):1447–1453.

[138]ESCOP. *Monographs on the medicinal uses of plant drugs. Arnicae flos*. European Scientific Cooperative on Phytotherapy. Stuttgart: Georg Thieme Verlag; 1997.

[139]Willuhn G. Arnica flowers; pharmacology, toxicology and analysis of the sesquiterpene lactones: their main active substances. In: Lawson LD, Bauer R, eds. *Phytomedicines of Europe Chemistry and Biological Activity*. Washington, DC; 1998:118–132.

[140]Lyss G, Knorre A, Schmidt TJ, Pahl HL, Merfort I. The anti-inflammatory sesquiterpene lactone helenalin inhibits the transcription factor NF-kappaB by directly targeting p65. *J Biol Chem*. 1998 Dec 11;273(50): 33508–33516.

[141]Garcia-Pineres AJ, Castro V, Mora G, Schmidt TJ, Strunck E, Pahl HL, et al. Cysteine 38 in p65/NF-kappaB plays a crucial role in DNA binding inhibition by sesquiterpene lactones. *J Biol Chem*. 2001 Oct 26;276 (43):39713–39720.

[142]Brock FB. Additiver effekt venentypischer hydrotherapie nach kneipp und lokaler arnika-anwendung bei patienten mit chronisch-venöser insuffizienz: synergismus naturheilkundlicher therapien. *Erfahrungsheilkunde*. 2001:357–363.

[143]Avijgan M. Phytotherapy: an alternative treatment for non-healing ulcers. *J Wound Care*. 2004 Apr;13 (4):157–158.

[144]Somboonwong J, Thanamittramanee S, Jariyapongskul A, Patumraj S. Therapeutic effects of aloe vera on cutaneous microcirculation and wound healing in second degree burn model in rats. *J Med Assoc Thai*. 2000 Apr;83(4):417–425.

[145]Maenthaisong R, Chaiyakunapruk N, Niruntraporn S, Kongkaew C. The efficacy of aloe vera used for burn wound healing: a systematic review. *Burns*. 2007 Sep;33(6):713–718.

[146]Majumdar M, Nayeem N, Kamath JV, Asad M. Evaluation of Tectona grandis leaves for wound healing activity. *Pak J Pharm Sci*. 2007 Apr;20(2):120–124.

[147]Nayak S, Nalabothu P, Sandiford S, Bhogadi V, Adogwa A. Evaluation of wound healing activity of Allamanda cathartica. L. and Laurus nobilis. L. extracts on rats. *BMC Complement Altern Med*. 2006;6:12.

[148]Manjunatha BK, Vidya SM, Krishna V, Mankani KL, Singh SD, Manohara YN. Comparative evaluation of wound healing potency of Vitex trifolia L. and Vitex altissima L. *Phytother Res*. 2007 May;21(5): 457–461.

[149]Nayak BS, Pinto Pereira LM. Catharanthus roseus flower extract has wound-healing activity in Sprague Dawley rats. *BMC Complement Altern Med*. 2006;6:41.

[150]Shetty BS, Udupa SL, Udupa AL, Somayaji SN. Effect of Centella asiatica L (Umbelliferae) on normal and dexamethasone-suppressed wound healing in Wistar Albino rats. *Int J Low Extrem Wounds*. 2006 Sep;5(3): 137–143.

[151]Udupa SL, Shetty S, Udupa AL, Somayaji SN. Effect of Ocimum sanctum Linn. on normal and dexamethasone suppressed wound healing. *Indian J Exp Biol*. 2006 Jan;44(1):49–54.

[152]Panchatcharam M, Miriyala S, Gayathri VS, Suguna L. Curcumin improves wound healing by modulating collagen and decreasing reactive oxygen species. *Mol Cell Biochem*. 2006 Oct;290(1–2):87–96.

[153]Blazso G, Gabor M, Schonlau F, Rohdewald P. Pycnogenol accelerates wound healing and reduces scar formation. *Phytother Res*. 2004 Jul;18(7):579–581.

[154]Aberer W. Contact allergy and medicinal herbs. *J Dtsch Dermatol Ges*. 2008 Jan;6(1):15–24.

[155]Thomson KF, Wilkinson SM. Allergic contact dermatitis to plant extracts in patients with cosmetic dermatitis. *Br J Dermatol*. 2000;1:84–88.

[156]Wilken K, Schempp CM. [Toxic phytodermatitis caused by Euphorbia helioscopia L. (sun spurge)]. *Hautarzt.* 2005;10:955–957.

[157]Schempp CM, Sonntag M, Schopf E, Simon JC. [Dermatitis bullosa striata pratensis caused by Dictamnus albus L. (burning bush)]. *Hautarzt.* 1996; 9:708–710.

[158]Schempp CM, Schopf E, Simon JC. [Bullous phototoxic contact dermatitis caused by Ruta graveolens L. (garden rue), Rutaceae. Case report and review of literature]. *Hautarzt.* 1999;6:432–434.

[159]McGovern TW, Barkley TM. Botanical briefs: giant hogweed, Heracleum mantegazzianum. *Cutis.* 2000;65:71–72.

[160]Vale PT. Prevention of phytophotodermatitis from celery. *Contact Dermatitis.* 1993;29:108.

[161]Hausen BM. Identification of the allergens of Arnica montana L. *Contact Dermatitis.* 1978;5:308.

[162]Paulsen E. Contact sensitization from Compositae-containing herbal remedies and cosmetics. *Contact Dermatitis.* 2002;4:189–198.

[163]Reider N, Komericki P, Hausen BM, Fritsch P, Aberer W. The seamy side of natural medicines: contact sensitization to arnica (Arnica montana L.) and marigold (Calendula officinalis L.). *Contact Dermatitis.* 2001;5:269–272.

[164]Lass C, Vocanson M, Martin S, Wagner S, Schempp C, Merfort I. Anti-inflammatory and immune regulatory mechanisms prevent contact hypersensitivity to Arnica montana L. *Exp Dermatol.* 2008; (E-pub ahead of print, Mar 12, 2008).

[165]Matura M, Goossens A, Bordalo O, Garcia-Bravo B, Magnusson K, Wrangsjo K, Karlberg AT. Oxidized citrus oil (R-limonene): a frequent skin sensitizer in Europe. *J Am Acad Dermatol.* 2002;5:709–714.

[166]Hausen BM, Reichling J, Harkenthal M. Degradation products of monoterpenes are the sensitizing agents in tea tree oil. *Am J Contact Dermat.* 1999;2:68–77.

[167]Henley DV, Lipson N, Korach KS, Bloch CA. Prepubertal gynecomastia linked to lavender and tea tree oils. *N Engl J Med.* 2007;5:479–485.

[168]Ernst E. Adverse effects of herbal drugs in dermatology. *Br J Dermatol.* 2000;5:923–929.

[169]Wanner M, Avram M. An evidence-based assessment of treatments of cellulite. *J Drugs Dermatol.* 2008 Apr;7(4):341–345.

[170]Rawlings AV. Cellulite and ist treatment. *Int J Cosmet Sci.* 2006 Jun; 28(3):175–190.

[171]Bertin C, Zunino H, Pittet JC, et al. A double-blind evaluation of the activity of an anti-cellulite product containing retinol, caffeine, and ruscogenine by a combination of several non-invasive methods. *J Cosmet Sci.* 2001 Jul;52(4):199–210.

[172]Hexsel D, Orlandi C, Zechmeister do Prado D. Botanical extracts used in the treatment of cellulite. *Dermatol Surg.* 2005 Jul; 31(7):866–872.

[173]Wu J. Treatment of rosacea with herbal ingredients. *J Drugs Dermatol.* 2006 Jan;5(1):29–32.

[174]Dattner AM. From medical herbalism to phytotherapy in dermatology: back to the future. *Dermatol Ther.* 2003;16(2):106–113.

[175]Thornfeldt C. Cosmeceuticals containing herbs: fact, fiction, and future. *Dermatol Surg.* 2005 Jul;31(7 Pt 2):873–880; discussion 80.

[176]Blumenthal M, Gruenwald J, Hall T, Rister RS. *The Complete German Commission E Monographs: Therapeutic Guide to Herbal Medicine.* Boston, MA: Integrative Medicine Communications; 1998.

PART II

Botanical Preparations: Preclinical and Clinical Approaches

Botanical Medicine: From Bench to Bedside
Edited by R. Cooper and F. Kronenberg
© Mary Ann Liebert, Inc.

Chapter 4

St. John's Wort: Quality Issues and Active Compounds

Veronika Butterweck

St. John's wort (*Hypericum perforatum* L.) (SJW) contains numerous compounds with documented biological activity. Constituents that have stimulated the most interest include the naphthodianthrones, hypericin and pseudohypericin; a broad range of flavonoids, including rutin, quercetin, quercitrin, miquelianin, amentoflavone, and hyperoside; and the phloroglucinols hyperforin and adhyperforin. Although there are some contradictions, most data suggest that several groups of active compounds are responsible for the antidepressant efficacy of the plant extract. Thus, according to the current state of scientific knowledge, the total extract has to be considered as the active substance.

Data on efficacy and quality of SJW extracts have to be taken into consideration. Owing to the fast-growing SJW market in the United States, more and more SJW products (herb and extracts) are sold at varying levels of quality. Considerable differences exist in the composition of biologically active constituents among various commercially available preparations of SJW. Furthermore, the documented characterization of SJW preparations in published randomized controlled trials has been less than adequate. Future scientific and clinical publications about the efficacy of SJW would benefit from a full pharmaceutical and phytochemical description of the extract.

SJW is used for the treatment of mild to moderate depression. The antidepressant efficacy of SJW extracts has been confirmed in numerous clinical studies and was assessed in meta-analyses (1, 2). The pharmacological actions of SJW have likewise been extensively reviewed (3–6). Reports about the mechanism of antidepressant action of SJW extracts and their constituents both in vivo and in vitro have also been published. Antidepressant activity was reported for the phloroglucinol derivative hyperforin (for a review, see [7]), for the naphthodianthrones hypericin and pseudohypericin (8–10), and for several flavonoids (11–14). The role and the mechanisms of these different compounds are still a matter of debate. However, based on recent results, it appears that the prevailing simplistic view of one plant → one active compound → one mechanism of action is incorrect. It is more likely that the multiple bioactive compounds contribute to the antidepressant activity of the crude plant extract in a complex manner. This review focuses on the present knowledge about the active constituents of SJW and their contribution to antidepressant activity.

College of Pharmacy, Department of Pharmaceutics, University of Florida, Gainesville, Florida; butterwk@cop.udl.edu

SJW CONSTITUENTS IN PRECLINICAL STUDIES

Flavonoids and Biflavonoids

Flavonolglycosides based on the aglycone quercetin represent up to 4% of the extract and form the largest group of secondary metabolites in *H. perforatum*. The major components are the flavonolglycosides rutin, hyperoside, isoquercitrin, quercitrin, and miquelianin and in smaller amounts the aglycon quercetin (Figure 4.1). Other flavonoid aglycones such as dihydroquercetin, luteolin, kaempferol, and myricetin are reported in the literature (15), but clear-cut data about their characterization are missing or the compounds occur in the plant only in trace amounts. When compared to other active ingredients, the flavonol glycosides show release rates from the powdered drug material and extract between 70% and 100% (16).

MAO Inhibition of Flavonoids

Several early in vitro experiments with SJW focused on pathways that alter monoamine neurotransmission in the central nervous system. Initial reports suggested that inhibition of monoamine oxidase (MAO)—the enzyme that is responsible for the catabolism of biogenic amines—is the main mechanism of antidepressant action of SJW extract. Studies performed by Sparenberg et al. showed most activity for the flavonoid aglycones—quercetin, kaemperol, and luteolin—whereas the glycosides were less active (15). However, the concentration in *Hypericum* of these substances, especially that of the aglycones, is too low to be responsible for the therapeutic efficacy of SJW extract (16).

Together with the ubiquitously existing monomeric flavonoids, the biflavonoids such as I3,II8-biapigenin and amentoflavone have been detected and exclusively occur in the flowering part of SJW (17) (Figure 4.2).

Receptor Binding of the Flavonoids and Biflavonoids

Nielsen et al. and Baureithel et al. focused their investigations on the biflavone amentoflavone, which bound to the brain benzodiazepine receptors with an affinity comparable to diazepam (18, 19). However, the flavonoids rutin, hyperoside, and quercitrin did not inhibit benzodiazepine binding up to concentrations of $1\,\mu M$. This result was recently confirmed by Butterweck and colleagues (20). In the same study, amentoflavone had remarkable affinity for the d-opioid receptor subtype in the nanomolar range ($K_i = 36.5\,nM$) and significantly

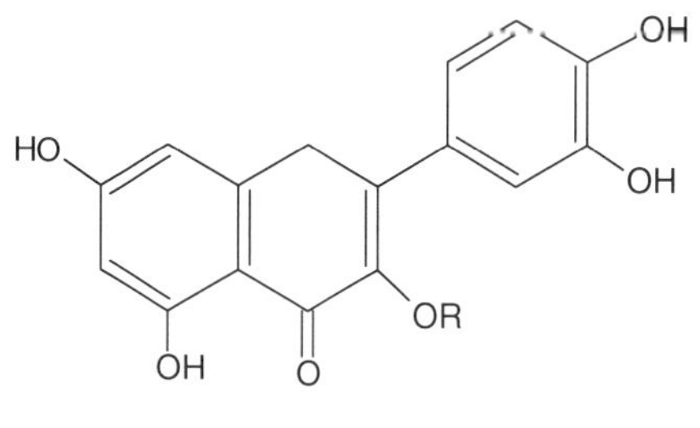

R = H	Quercetin
R = alpha-L-rhamnosyl	Quercitrin
R = beta-D-glycosyl	Isoquercitrin
R = beta-D-galactoside	Hyperoside
R = beta-D-rutinosyl	Rutin

Figure 4.1. Flavonoids from SJW

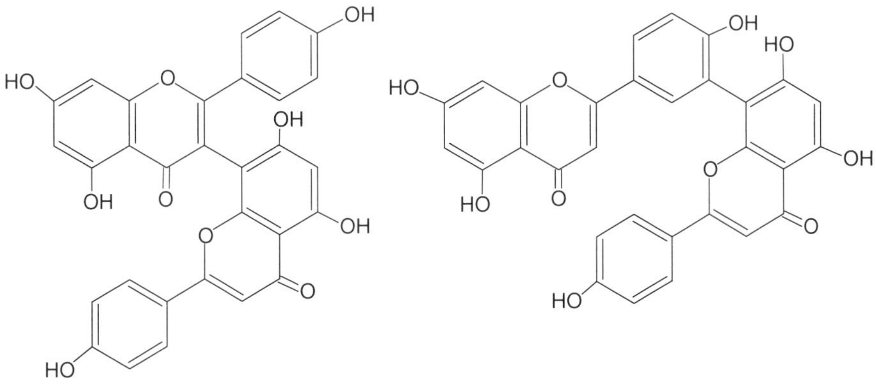

I3,II8-Biapigenin   Amentoflavone

Figure 4.2.   Biflavonoids from SJW

inhibited binding at 5-HT$_{1D}$, 5-HT$_{2C}$, and dopamine D$_3$ receptors. Further striking actions were observed for quercetin with an affinity to the D$_4$ receptor at Ki = 7.8 nM, miquelianin to the a$_{2C}$ receptor at 4 nM, and rutin to the a$_{2A}$ and a$_{2c}$ receptor at 9 nM (20).

In Vivo Tests on Flavonoids and Biflavonoids

Studies show that amentoflavone was able to pass the blood-brain barrier in vitro by passive diffusion (21). The potential antidepressant activity of some SJW flavonoids was confirmed in the forced swimming test, a well-established screening model for antidepressant activity (22). During bioassay-guided fractionation of SJW extract, a fraction was obtained that was mainly characterized by its high content of flavonoids. The fraction significantly reduced immobility time in the forced swimming test, and the effect was comparable to that of imipramine (12). The flavonoid fraction was further purified, and some flavonol glycosides such as hyperoside, quercitrin, isoquercitrin, and miquelianin, as well as the flavone glycoside astilbin, were isolated (16) and tested for activity in the forced swimming test at doses comparable to their amounts present in the crude drug material. Except for quercitrin and astilbin, all flavonoids (hyperoside, isoquercitrin, and miquelianin) were significantly active in the forced swimming test after acute, as well as after repeated, oral treatment.

The data obtained by Butterweck et al. (12) indicate certain flavonol-3-O-glycosides as active constituents of *Hypericum* extract. The activity seems to be bound to the sugar moiety of the aglycone quercetin, in that the glucoside, galactoside, and glucuronide forms are active compounds. It may be that these particular glycosides are absorbed from the intestine, whereas others are not.

Further evidence that flavonoids contribute to the antidepressant activity of SJW was recently provided by Butterweck et al. (11). The authors could show that hyperoside, isoquercitrin, and miquelianin significantly down-regulated plasma adrenocorticotropic hormone (ACTH) and corticosterone levels after two weeks of daily treatment. The effect was similar to the changes elicited by the prototypic synthetic antidepressant imipramine. Hypersecretion of ACTH and plasma cortisol have been reported in 40% to 50% of patients suffering from depression (23, 24). Normalization of the hyperactive hypothalamic-pituitary-adrenal (HPA) system occurs during successful antidepressant pharmacotherapy of depressive illness (25). These data clearly show that flavonoids represent a possible major active principle that may in turn contribute to the beneficial effect of SJW extract after oral dosing.

Potential Synergism of Flavonoids and Biflavonoids

It also could be shown that the flavonol-3-O-rutinoside rutin, which was inactive in the forced swimming test when administered orally as a pure compound, seems to play an important role in the SJW extract. Thus the addition of rutin to inactive extracts resulted in a strong pharmacological effect comparable to that of other extracts that contained a sufficient amount of rutin (14). Although the study provides sufficient quantitative data about the amount of flavonoids in the different SJW extracts, unfortunately no quantitative data are given for hypericin and hyperforin. Nevertheless, the experiments show that the pharmacological effects of an extract cannot directly be compared with the effects of single compounds. The authors suggest a modulation of phase I proteins for rutin, which would lead to an increased bioavailability of simultaneously administered active SJW compounds (14). However, this might also be achieved by an increased solubility of hypericin by rutin (see the following section on naphthodianthrones).

In a recent in vitro study, it could be demonstrated that miquelianin—besides crossing walls from the small intestine—was able to cross the blood-brain barrier, as well as the blood-cerebrospinal fluid barrier (26). This finding gives further evidence for the assumption that flavonoids are able to reach the central nervous system after oral administration. There might be synergistic or additive effects of single flavonoids, but this needs to be established in future investigations.

Naphthodianthrones

The naphthodianthrones hypericin and pseudohypericin occur in the flowers and leaves of the crude drug material in concentrations of 0.03% to 0.3%, depending on the developmental stage of the plant with significant variation (27) (Figure 4.3). The amount of pseudohypericin in SJW is approximately two to four times higher than that of hypericin (28). In some extracts this ratio may even be 10:1.

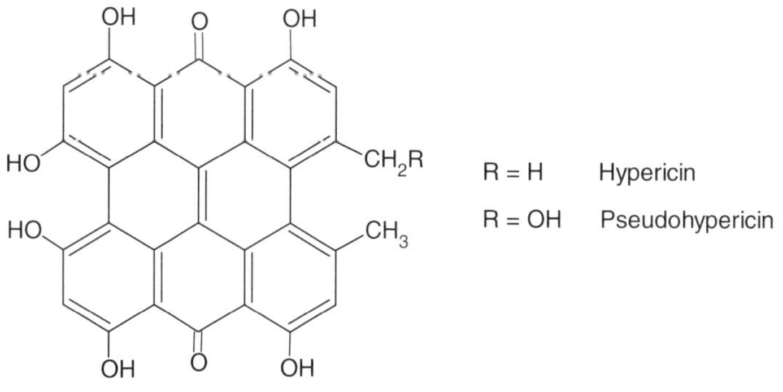

R = H   Hypericin

R = OH   Pseudohypericin

Figure 4.3. Naphthodianthrones from SJW

The naphthodianthrones show a restricted solubility in almost all solvents; the pure compounds, especially hypericin, are almost insoluble in water at ambient temperature. Nevertheless, more than 40% of the naphthodianthrone amount is extractable from the crude drug when preparing a tea with water at 60 to 80 °C (approx. 35% pseudohypericin and 6% hypericin) (29). The increase in solubility suggests the presence of coeffectors in the drug material that modify the solubility of the naphthodianthrones. The potassium salts of hypericin and pseudohypericin have been identified as "soluble" pigments of the *Hypericum* species (30).

Phototoxicity of the Naphthodianthrones

The naphthodianthrones attracted the attention of phytochemists early on because of their intense red color and their phototoxic properties (31, 32). Thus, toxicological concerns have centered on the potential photosensitizing effects of humans ingesting SJW extract, since this is a well-known toxic effect in animals consuming large amounts of the fresh plant material (1–4% of body weight). Calves receiving up to 3 g/kg of SJW herb have demonstrated no photosensitivity (33).

Bernd et al. (34) investigated the phototoxic activity of SJW extract (0.3% hypericin) using cultures of human keratinocytes. The authors cultivated human keratinocytes in the presence of different SJW extract concentrations and irradiated the cells with 150 mJ/cm2 UVB, 1 J/cm2 UVA, or 3 h with a white light of photon flux density 2.6 mmol m^{-2} s^{-1}. The determination of the bromodeoxyuridine incorporation rate showed a concentration- and light-dependent decrease in DNA synthesis with high hypericin concentrations ($\geq 50 \mu g/$ml) combined with UVA or visible light radiation. In the case of UVB irradiation, a clear phototoxic cell reaction was not detected. The researchers concluded that phototoxic reactions of the skin would not be expected from the amounts of SJW extract used in the treatment of depression because blood levels of hypericin would be below the phototoxic dose (34). Based on the hypericin content, others have estimated that the amount of a commercial extract of SJW required to increase the risk of phototoxicity is approximately 2 to 4g/d, or 5 to 10mg/d of hypericin (35, 36).

Receptor Interactions of the Naphthodianthrones

From a pharmacological standpoint, the hypericins are at present the most interesting compounds of SJW. Inhibition of monoamine oxidase (MAO) was considered as one of the key mechanisms used in conventional therapy for depression. Suzuki et al. (37) were the first to find that micromolar concentrations of hypericin could irreversibly inhibit MAO-A and MAO-B activity in vitro. However, the progress made in preparation and analytical techniques since 1984 has shown that the hypericin used in these experiments was impure and contained at least 20% of other constituents of the extracts—among these, the flavonoids are most noticeable. In fact, the MAO inhibitory effects of hypericin alone could not be confirmed in subsequent studies (38, 39).

The effects of hypericin in various receptor-screening models provide the most contradictory data: Raffa (40) found that hypericin had no affinity for traditional monoamine receptors or for adrenergic, gamma-aminobutyric acid (GABA), adenosine, or benzodiazepine receptors. The naphthodianthrone had modest affinity for muscarinic cholinergic receptors (subtype not measured) and similar affinity to σ receptors. Gobbi et al. (41) showed that hypericin inhibited ligand binding to NPY_1-, NPY_2-, and σ receptors. The authors found that these inhibitory effects were light dependent because they decreased or disappeared when binding assays were carried out in the dark.

Cott tested hypericin in a battery of 39 in vitro receptor assays, and hypericin showed affinity only for the N-methyl D-aspartate (NMDA) receptor (Ki ~ 1 μM) (39). These results could not be confirmed by Butterweck et al. (20). In Cott's study, hypericin showed high affinity for the D_3- dopamine receptor ($K_i = 34.5$ nM) and negligible affinities ($K_i > 1000$ nM) for nearly all other tested receptors and transporters. Interestingly, the affinity of hypericin for the D_3-receptor subtype was much higher than that of the atypical antipsychotic clozapine ($K_i = 372.3$ nM).

Simmen et al. showed that hypericin had the most potent binding inhibition of all tested constituents to human corticotropin-releasing factor 1 (CRF_1) receptor with an IC_{50} value of 300 nM (42). In a follow-up study, the same authors investigated the CRF-binding properties of both naphthodianthrones in greater detail by measuring their effect on CRF-stimulated cAMP formation in recombinant Chinese hamster ovary (CHO) cells (43). The authors found that only pseudohypericin selectively antagonized CRF (K(B) 0.76 μM).

In summary, the data from in vitro studies allocate interesting pharmacological properties to hypericin and similarly to the flavonoids. The therapeutic relevance of these findings needs verification by in vivo experiments. However, with regard to the contradictory effects of hypericin in various test models, it should be pointed out that the pharmacological evaluation of hypericin in most in vitro and in vivo studies is hampered by its poor solubility in aqueous solutions.

In Vivo Tests on the Naphthodianthrones

The in vivo effects of hypericin and pseudohypericin have been investigated by Butterweck et al. (10, 44, 45). During a bioassay-guided fractionation of a methanolic SJW extract, hypericin and pseudohypericin were detected as compounds that exerted antidepressant activity in the forced swimming test. Interestingly, pure hypericin and pseudohypericin did not reduce immobility time after acute pretreatment at doses comparable to the total extract, and only the exceptionally high dose of 0.23 mg/kg orally (p.o.) of hypericin was significantly active, whereas pseudohypericin indicated some nonsignificant activity at about 0.5 mg/kg (p.o.) (44).

A common biological alteration in patients with major depression is the activation of the HPA axis, manifested as hypersecretion of ACTH and cortisol. The hyperactivity of the HPA axis in depressed patients can be corrected during clinically effective therapy with standard antidepressant drugs such as imipramine, indicating that the HPA axis may be an important target for antidepressant action. Oral treatment of rats for two weeks with either SJW extract or hypericin significantly reduced plasma ACTH and corticosterone levels, suggesting a decrease in functional activity of the HPA axis (9).

In a more detailed study using in situ hybridization technique, it was shown that hypericin (0.2 mg/kg) given daily by gavage for eight weeks but not for two weeks significantly decreased levels of corticotropin-releasing hormone (CRH) mRNA by 16% to 22% in the hypothalamic paraventricular nucleus (PVN) and serotonin 5-HT$_{1A}$ receptor mRNA by 11% to 17% in the hippocampus (45). Thus, these results are of major interest because CRF_1 receptor antagonists as potential pharmacotherapies for depression and anxiety disorders are under current development (46).

Synergism Between Hypericins and Other Constituents

When a fraction of procyanidins, which was itself not active in the forced swimming test, was recombined with the naphthodianthrones, hypericin was significantly active at

0.028 mg/kg (p.o.), and pseudohypericin was active at 0.166 mg/kg (p.o.). The procyanidin fraction as well as the pure procyanidins B2 and C1 increased the water solubility of both hypericins, which may lead to a better bioavailability (10). When the octanol/water partition coefficient was being determined, it became obvious that the solubility of pure hypericin in water increased upon addition of some phenolic constituents typical for SJW extracts as well. Most effective in solubilizing hypericin was hyperoside (quercetin 3-O-beta-D-galactoside), which increased the concentration of hypericin in the water phase up to 400-fold in this model (26).

However, an improved solubility does not necessarily result in an improved bioavailability. In a pharmacokinetic study, Butterweck et al. investigated whether the improved water solubility in the presence or absence of procyanidin B2 or hyperoside is correlated to increased plasma levels of hypericin in rats, determined by reversed-phase high-performance liquid chromatography (HPLC) using fluorimetric detection (47). Both compounds increased the oral bioavailability of hypericin by ca. 58% (B2) and 34% (hyperoside). The authors concluded that a significant accumulation of hypericin in rat plasma in the presence of both polyphenols might be responsible for the observed increased in vivo activity. These interesting pharmacokinetic properties would also explain why hypericin was inactive or why conflicting data were obtained in most in vitro experiments. These results are also of general importance for the concept of phytotherapy because they qualitatively and quantitatively describe the superiority of herbal extracts over single active ingredients.

Phloroglucinols

The main representative of the phloroglucinol group of constituents is hyperforin. Together with adhyperforin, hyperforin occurs exclusively in the generative parts of the plant, especially in the unripe fruits (Figure 4.4). Consequently, plant material collected at the end of the flowering period, when fruits are developing, will contain more hyperforin than material collected during the flowering time (as requested by monographs) (48). Hyperforin occurs in amounts up to 2% to 5% in the crude drug material and can reach about 6% in some extracts.

Although this compound is quite unstable—especially in aqueous solutions and when exposed to light and heat—it is present in many commercial extracts but at highly varying concentrations of 0% to 6% (49). Products of degradation are 2-methyl-3-buten-2-ol and two oxidation products with an intact hyperforin carbon skeleton (50, 51).

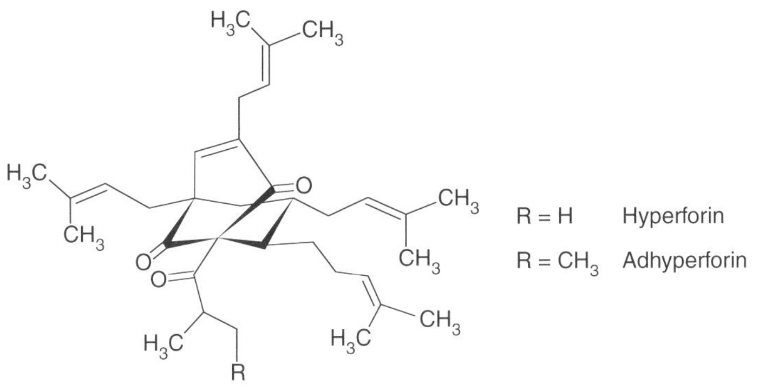

R = H   Hyperforin

R = CH₃   Adhyperforin

Figure 4.4. Phloroglucinols from SJW

Mechanisms of Action of Phloroglucinols Related to Neurotransmitters

Chatterjee and coworkers were the first who pointed to hyperforin as the major non-nitrogenous metabolite of SJW (52, 53). The authors have shown that a lipophilic CO_2-extract enriched in hyperforin as well as pure hyperforin in vitro inhibited serotonin-induced responses and uptake of neurotransmitters in peritoneal cells. The pharmacological work was continued by Müller et al., who detected that hyperforin was capable of inhibiting the reuptake of serotonin (5-HT), norepinephrine (NE), and dopamine (DA) at a potency comparable to that of conventional 5-HT and NE inhibitors (54). Moreover, the authors noted that the ability of hyperforin to inhibit the reuptake of 5-HT, NE, and DA at a nanomolar concentration sets it apart from any known synthetic antidepressant. Subsequent papers could confirm that hyperforin is a potent monoamine reuptake inhibitor, but all authors reported micromolar concentrations (55–57).

Buchholzer et al. first presented data on interactions of hyperforin with the cholinergic system (58). The authors found that hyperforin inhibited high-affinity choline uptake in rat synaptosomes. These results are of special interest and could form the basis for the use of hyperforin in cognitive disorders. To explain the mechanism of synaptosomal reuptake, several researchers focused therefore on the effects of SJW on monoamine transporters in intact neural cells. The neurotransmitter transporters have been proven to be important targets for drug discovery in the central nervous system, particularly for antidepressants (59). Gobbi et al. (55) reported that inhibition of 5-HT uptake by a methanolic hypericum extract and hyperforin is not due to a direct interaction with, and blockade of, the 5-HT transporters because both of them had no or only very slight inhibitory effect on [^{3}H]citalopram binding. The authors speculated that the inhibitory effects on synaptosomal 5-HT accumulation might be caused by a reserpine-like mechanism because similar results were obtained with Ro-04-1284, a reserpine-like compound, that also did not inhibit [^{3}H]citalopram binding. Their hypothesis was confirmed by the finding that SJW extract and hyperforin induced marked release from synaptosomes preloaded with [^{3}H]5-HT. The authors conclude that the apparent inhibition of uptake is an artifact from the interaction of the high concentration of the tested compounds with monoamine storage vesicles.

Jensen et al. found that the potency of hyperforin and adhyperforin on monoamine reuptake was comparable to that seen for imipramine, nomifensine, and fluoxetine (60). But contrary to the antidepressant drugs, the phloroglucinols potently inhibited all three transporter systems. Interestingly, the inhibition of DA-uptake by hyperforin and adhyperforin was not due to a direct interaction with the [^{3}H] WIN 35,428 (a cocaine analogue) binding site on the DA transporter as seen for imipramine, nomifensine, and fluoxetine. Therefore, the authors suggest a noncompetitive interaction of hyperforin and adhyperforin with the DA transporter.

Further Mechanistic Studies on Phloroglucinols

Another interesting hypothesis regarding the mechanism of synaptosomal reuptake is presented by Müller's group (57). The apparent inhibition of serotonin uptake observed with SJW extract and hyperforin in vitro might be caused by an increase in free intracellular sodium concentrations (57). Additional data suggested interactions of the compound with Na^+ channels or Na^+/H^+ exchangers (61). Such nonselective effects might explain why SJW extracts and hyperforin blocked the synaptosomal uptake of multiple neu-rotransmitters (52, 55, 57, 61).

Recent work indicated that hyperforin may also influence calmodulin-dependent mecha-nisms (62). Finally, hyperforin was reported to modulate several ionic conductances in cer-ebellar Purkinje cells including a P-type calcium channel that is known to be involved in neurotransmitter release (63). The authors also screened an ethanolic hypericum extract (hyperforin amount approx. 5%) on various voltage- and ligand-gated conductances (64). The plant extract inhibited almost all the ligand-gated ion channels; quercitrin was detected as a potent inhibitor of adenosine triphosphate (ATP)-induced conductance; biapigenin in-hibited both the acetylcholine- and ATP-induced conductance, whereas hyperoside blocked currents activated by ATP and alpha-amino-3-hydroxy-5-methyl-4-isoxazolepropionic acid (AMPA). The naphthodianthrone hypericin was inactive in all cases. The authors con-cluded that hyperforin is not the only active substance of SJW and that the extract contains several potentially neuroactive molecules, such as biapigenin, hyperoside, and quercitrin.

Relevance for the Situation In Vivo of Phloroglucinols

However, the concentration of hyperforin (micromolar range) used in these studies (64–66) was far higher than plasma concentrations reached in vivo. In human volunteers receiv-ing daily doses of 900 mg (3×300 mg) SJW extract, plasma steady-state concentrations of approximately 180 nM were measured (65). Reported IC_{50} values for hyperforin as an in-hibitor of synaptosomal uptake of serotonin have ranges from 120 nM to 3.300 nM. Accord-ing to the results of the studies mentioned above, the blood levels of hyperforin in human volunteers after a daily dose of 900 mg hypericum extract are within a concentration range needed to inhibit serotonin uptake in vitro, but the free drug concentration available for ac-tion at central ion channels in vivo is unclear.

In Vivo Tests on Phloroglucinols

The in vivo antidepressant effects of hyperforin, a hyperforin-enriched CO_2 extract, or more stable salts such as dicyclohexylammonium (DCHA), actetate, or sodium hyperforin were demonstrated in different animal models of depression. In the forced swimming test, triple administration of hyperforin acetate (5–20 mg/kg) significantly reduced the immo-bility time of rats, while in the learned helplessness test a daily treatment of 10 mg/kg for seven consecutive days was necessary to elicit an antidepressant effect (66). In the tail sus-pension test in mice, pure hyperforin significantly reduced immobility time in a dosage of 4 and 8 mg/kg, whereas it was inactive in dosages below or above that (67). In the same study, it was also shown that step-by-step removal of either hyperforin or hypericin did not result in a loss of pharmacological activity. The results clearly show that the crude SJW extracts contain several constituents with antidepressant activity.

In addition to the antidepressant effects, other behavioral effects of hyperforin have been described. Chatterjee and colleagues were the first to investigate two different SJW ex-tracts in the learned helplessness paradigm (52). According to this paradigm, the exposure to uncontrollable stress produces performance deficits in subsequent learning tasks, which can be reversed by subchronic treatment (4–7 days) with a variety of antidepressants in-cluding tricyclic antidepressants (TCAs), monoamine oxidase inhibitors (MAOIs), and atypical antidepressants, and in treatments related to electroconvulsive seizures (ECS) (68, 69). In the group treated with ethanolic extract (hyperforin amount 4.5%), escape deficits significantly and dose dependently decreased after 150 and 300 mg/kg/day (p.o.). Comparable effects were observed for the CO_2 extract (hyperforin amount 38.8%) in doses of 15 and 30 mg/kg/day (p.o.) (52).

A similar study was performed by Gambrana et al. (70), who used the escape deficit paradigm as a test model. When tested in the escape deficit paradigm, 25 mg, 50 mg, and 75 mg/kg (i.p.) of hyperforin significantly counteracted the effects of acute stress. Taken together, the results in the learned helplessness paradigm show that different SJW extracts (hydroalcoholic, CO_2) as well as hyperforin (pure or in salt form) could reduce behavioral deficits induced by uncontrollable shock. How far other constituents of SJW are active in this model needs to be further elucidated.

SJW CONSTITUENTS IN CLINICAL STUDIES

Most hypericum products were—and still are—standardized on the key compound hypericin. In most products, hypericin doses are applied in a range between 1 and 2 mg per day. A German study that analyzed 33 different SJW products showed that many extracts with a well-balanced ratio of the three main groups of components are standardized to an even higher upper limit of hypericin than that allowed by the proposed range of 0.1% to 0.3% (49). This upper limit can also not be derived from a photosensitizing potential associated to hypericin, as photosensitizing effects of SJW extracts are rare in clinical practice (35).

The flavonoids are mentioned as relevant for clinical efficacy in some clinical studies, but in most clinical studies, no information regarding the quantitative amount of this substance group in extracts of commercial preparations is found.

Several clinical studies with SJW extract were screened for information on the hyperforin content of the tested products. Unfortunately, information regarding the hyperforin content in all these publications is rare. Interestingly, in cases where data about the hyperforin content were provided, they were contradictory for the same extract in different studies. For example, Kalb et al. (71) indicate a hyperforin content of 1.5% for the extract with the brand name WS 5572 (Dr. Willmar Schwabe & Co. KG, Karlsruhe, Germany), whereas Laakmann et al. (72) declare a hyperforin content of 5% for the extract with the identical brand name, WS 5572. This is somewhat confusing, especially because the latter authors argue that hyperforin is important for the efficacy of SJW extract. For the extract WS 5570, Lecrubier et al. (73) report a hyperforin content of 3% to 6%. For another extract from the same manufacturer (WS 5573) that has been used as a reference extract by Laakmann et al. (72), a hyperforin content of 0.5% is stated in the publication. However, insufficient information is provided about the amount of other constituents (especially hypericin and flavonoids) in this specific extract. Thus, based on this study, no definite conclusion regarding the role of hyperforin for clinical efficacy can be drawn.

Further, in published studies using the product Neuroplant (Dr. Willmar Schwabe & Co. KG), neither the extract code name nor the hyperforin content is provided. In the case of older studies (74), it was still unclear which compound might play a role in clinical efficacy of SJW. Since then, many pharmacological studies have been performed, showing that hypericin, hyperforin, and flavonoids play a crucial role. Therefore, in ongoing current studies, it is imperative that the amount of those compounds be stated, in order to avoid contradictory and confusing results. In a recent study, Szegedi et al. (75) used the extract

WS 5570, but unfortunately, information regarding the hyperforin content is missing. Interestingly, heterogeneities regarding Neuroplant can be found in the phytochemical literature. While Melzer et al. (49) stated a hyperforin content of 5.0%, in a later publication (describing the extract as having a stabilized hyperforin content), only 4.1% hyperforin was found (76).

The largest number of clinical studies exists for the extract LI 160 (Lichtwer GmbH & Co. KG). However, even though some of these studies have been published up to four times, none of these publications contain any information about the hyperforin content of the extract.

In summary, the information provided about these extracts does not allow any conclusion about the relevance of the hyperforin content for clinical efficacy.

Data from Phytochemical Studies

Interestingly, whereas most clinical studies do not provide data about the hyperforin content, this information can be accessed from several phytochemical screening studies. A German study including 33 different commercial SJW products showed that their hyperforin contents varied between < 0.02% and 5.85% of extract (49); several products are within the range of 1.5% and 2.5%, which would be within the limit of 2% proposed in the draft monograph:

BardoH: 1.5%
Helarium: 2.5%
Hypericum Stada: 1.9%
Johanniskraut-Dragees SN: 2.3%
Neurovegetalin 425: 2.5%
Texx 300: 2.5% (span according to Wurglics et al.: 1.7% to 3.2%)
Tonizin forte: 1.7%

Another screening of different batches of several products was published by Wurglics et al. (76, 77). The measurements in some cases confirm the data of Melzer et al. (49); in other cases, the authors find different values. This difference is most obvious in the case of the extract LI 160, for which Melzer et al. state a hyperforin content of 4.3%, while Wurglics et al. found only 2.2% to 3.1%. A similar tendency is found in the product Felis, where Melzer et al. (49) found 4.9% hyperforin, while Wurglics et al. found only 1.9% to 3.5%. The reason for this discrepancy remains unclear.

For the extract STW3-VI, for which clinical data have been published (78), a hyperforin amount of 1.8% is stated, which is well within the range of 1.5% to 2.4% found by Wurglics et al. (76, 77). However, these values are also not compatible with the classes of hyperforin content proposed by the draft monograph.

Hyperforin Levels for Clinical Efficacy

Based on the present data, the question arises, is hyperforin necessary for the antidepressant activity of SJW? Data from in vitro or animal studies are either pro or contra hyperforin and do not help answer the question appropriately. Interestingly, a recent study showed that step-by-step elimination of hyperforin and hypericin from a hydroalcoholic SJW extract did not result in any loss of pharmacological activity (67). An extract free of hyperforin and hypericin but enriched in flavonoids (~12%) showed antidepressant activity in valid animal models. The results indicate that flavonoids are also involved in the therapeutic efficacy of SJW.

This question can be answered only by clinical studies. As mentioned above, a study approach to compare extracts directly with different hyperforin contents was conducted by Laakmann et al. (72). On the one hand, a statistically significant superiority between an extract with 5% hyperforin (WS 5572) in reducing the Hamilton depression score and placebo was demonstrated; on the other hand, no statistical differences were found between an extract with 0.5% hyperforin (WS 5573) and placebo and between the two extracts WS 5572 and WS 5573. Because of this result, it has been suggested that hyperforin may be relevant for the clinical efficacy of the extract, but this is not convincing because of (a) the lack of statistical power and (b) the lack of quantitative data for additional constituents (such as flavonoids and biflavones). Thus, it cannot be excluded that constituents other than hyperforin may have caused the small differences in efficacy of both extracts. Therefore, the outcome does not give convincing proof for the activity of hyperforin but indicates that there are extracts that show clinical efficacy and others that are inactive.

However, three clinical trials performed using an SJW extract with a low hyperforin amount (<0.2%) showed that the efficacy of this SJW extract was superior to placebo and as effective as imipramine and fluoxetine (79–81), thus showing that hyperforin is not necessarily needed for the antidepressive efficacy of SJW.

Taken together, the collected data from the clinical studies with SJW extracts allow only the conclusion that hyperforin is no convincing parameter for a prediction of the clinical efficacy.

The available analytical data show a large range of different hyperforin content for different extracts with clinically proven efficacy. Even for the same extract, the hyperforin content can differ considerably, as exemplified by the extract WS 5572, for which in different publications values of 5% (72) and 1.5% (71) are given, as already mentioned.

SJW SAFETY ISSUES

SJW and Drug Interactions

Besides the data on clinical efficacy, data on clinical safety of SJW extracts have to be considered. Recently, interactions of herbal medicines with synthetic drugs have come into focus. In the past three years, more than 50 papers were published regarding interactions between SJW and prescription drugs. Comedication with SJW resulted in decreased plasma concentrations of a number of drugs including amitriptyline, cyclosporine, digoxin, indinavir, irinotecan, warfarin, phenprocoumon, alprazolam, dextromethorphan, simvastatin, and oral contraceptives. Sufficient evidence from interaction studies and case reports indicate that SJW is a potent inducer of cytochrome P450 enzymes (particularly CYP3A4) and/or P-glycoprotein. Recent studies could show that the degree of enzyme induction by SJW correlates strongly with the amount of hyperforin found in the product. Products that do not contain substantial amounts of hyperforin (<1%) have not been shown to produce clinically relevant enzyme induction. As mentioned above, a German study that analyzed 33 different SJW products showed that the hyperforin content varied from < 0.5 mg per unit (< 0.02% of extract) to 24.87 mg per unit (5.85% of extract) (49). Data for the extract ZE 117, marketed as Remotive, indicate hypericin in an amount of 0.2% and negligible amounts of hyperforin (0.2%) (82). In the past, this also was most likely the case for extract LI 160, marketed as Jarsin or a similar extract, marketed as Neuroplant, before the extraction process was modified (83, 84). With the modified method, a hyperforin content of 4% to 5% has been reported for products containing LI 160 (49). This is equivalent to a daily dose of approximately 50 mg of hyperforin, based on a 300 mg extract administered three times daily. The widely differing amounts of hyperforin in SJW preparations should be taken into account when drug interactions with SJW are discussed. Most of the current cases that report a specific product involved SJW products that are rich in hyperforin (up to 5%). No drug interaction has been reported with products that have low contents of hyperforin (82, 85, 86). Furthermore, it is interesting to note that reports of drug interactions with SJW have not been reported before 1998, when a modified extraction method was introduced that led to products with a higher content of hyperforin (83, 84).

The most frequently documented drug interactions of SJW extract, which have been extensively reviewed in recently published articles (87, 88), are initially discussed in brief before dealing in detail with the role of hyperforin in these interactions.

Influence of SJW on P-glycoprotein and Several Cytochrome P-450 Enzyme Activities in Humans

CYP3A4, the most abundant cytochrome P-450 (CYP450) isoenzyme, is responsible for the metabolism of more than 73 medications and numerous endogenous compounds (89–91). Substrates for this isoenzyme include protease inhibitors, nonsedating antihistamines, calcium channel blockers, 3-hydroxy-3-methylglutaryl coenzyme A reductase inhibitors, benzodiazepines, estrogens, macrolide antibiotics, cyclosporine, carbamazepine, ketoconazole, and corticosterone (89–91). One method to determine the in vivo effect of medications on CYP3A4 activity is through the evaluation of the urinary 6-ß-hydroxycortisol/cortisol ratio. 6-ß-hydroxycortisol has been shown to be a nonspecific marker of CYP3A4 activity (92–94). Roby et al. (95) could show that reagent-grade SJW taken for 14 days (Hypericum Byers Club, Lot 180632, 0.3% hypericin, 3×300 mg/d, hyperforin amount not provided) at the dose recommended for the treatment of mild to moderate depression was associated with a significant increase in the mean urinary 6-ß-hydroxycortisol/cortisol ratio. The ratio increased from 7.1 to 13.0, suggesting a CYP3A4 induction after intake of SJW at the recommended dosage.

Besides an induction of CYP3A4 enzyme activities in the liver and small intestine, the involvement of the P-glycoprotein/MDR1 system in the intestine was also discussed. P-glycoprotein (P-gp), an ATP-dependent primary active transporter belonging to the ABC transporter superfamily, occurs in plasma membranes of many tissues, where it serves as an efflux transporter of xenobiotics (96). In the intestine, P-gp is located at the apical surface of epithelial cells and interferes with drug absorption by pumping out a variety of orally administered drugs, such as cyclosporine, into the intestinal lumen (97). After uptake by the enterocyte, many lipophilic drugs are either metabolized by CYP3A4 or pumped back into

Table 4.1. Reported Drug Interactions with St. John's Wort Preparations

Reported Pharmacokinetic Interactions

Drug Category	Drug(s)	Possible Mechanism of Interaction
Cystostatic drugs	Imatinib, Irinotecan	CYP3A4 induction
HIV drugs	Indinavir, Nevirapine	CYP3A4 and MDR1 induction
Immunosuppressants	Cyclosporine, Tacrolimus	CYP3A4 and MDR1 induction
Anticoagulants	Warfarin, Phenprocoumon	CYP2C9 induction
Cardiovascular drugs	Digoxin	MDR1 efflux activity induced
Opiates	Methadone	CYP3A4 induction
Oral contraceptives	Ethinylestradiol (EE) / Desogestrel, EE/Norethisterone, Levonorgestrel, Norethisterone*	CYP3A4 induction
Antiepileptic drugs	Carbamazepine*	CYP3A4 induction
Anti-asthma drugs	Theophylline *	CYP1A2 induction
HMG-CoA reductase inhibitors	Simvastatin, Atorvastatin*	Intestinal CYP3A4 induction

the lumen by the P-gp transporter. Therefore, CYP3A4 and P-gp may act in tandem as a barrier to oral delivery of many drugs.

This hypothesis could be confirmed in animal experiments as well as in clinical studies (98). The administration of SJW extract to rats during 14 days resulted in a 3.8-fold increase of intestinal P-glycoprotein/MdR1 expression and in a 2.5-fold increase in hepatic CYP3A4 expression (98). In a clinical study, the administration of SJW extract resulted in 1.4- and 1.5-fold increased expressions of duodenal P-glycoprotein/MDR and CYP3A4, respectively (98). These results indicate direct inducing effects of SJW on intestinal P-glycoprotein/MDR1 and intestinal and hepatic CYP3A4. In both studies, the extract LI 160 (80% methanol v/v, 0.3% hypericin, batch 99100400, 3×300 mg/d, unknown amount of hyperforin) was used.

In contrast to short-term administration (1×900 mg SJW in 24h), long-term SJW administration (3×300 mg/d for 14 days) resulted in a significant and selective induction of CYP3A4 (midazolam) activity in the intestinal wall (99). There was no change in CYP2C9 (tolbutamide), CYP1A2 (caffeine), or CYP2D6 (dextromethorphan) activities as a result of SJW administration. In contrast to the >50% decrease in the area under the plasma-concentration time curve (AUC) when midazolam was administered orally, long-term SJW administration caused a 20% decrease in AUC when midazolam was given intravenously. This result confirms the involvement of intestinal as well as hepatic CYP3A4. In this study, an SJW extract from Rexall Sundown Pharmaceuticals was used (0.3% hypericin, unknown hyperforin content, 3×300 mg) (99). The authors concluded that the reduced therapeutic efficacy of drugs metabolized by CYP3A4 should be anticipated during long-term administration of SJW.

Several reports have documented clinically relevant drug interactions between SJW and coadministered drugs such as indinavir, cyclosporine, and digoxin (100–102), attributing induction of hepatic CYP3A4 as the likely mechanism (95, 103). However, interactions with digoxin and indinavir are unlikely to be fully explained by this mechanism, as they are not only a CYP3A4 substrate but also a substrate for P-gp. Hennessy and coworkers (104) could show that SJW increased expression and enhanced the drug efflux function of P-gp in peripheral blood lymphocytes of healthy volunteers. P-gp expression increased 4.2-fold from baseline in subjects treated with SJW (Good n' Natural, 0.15% hypericin, 600 mg extract 3×daily) over a period of 16 days; there was no effect observed in patients receiving placebo.

In another pharmacokinetic study in healthy volunteers, changes in plasma pharmacokinetics of alprazolam as a probe for CYP3A4 activity and the ratio of dextromethorphan to its metabolite dextrorphan were measured after 14 days of comedication with SJW extract (LI 160, 2×300 mg/d; each tablet contained 1398 µg hyperforin, 151 µg hypericin, and 279 µg pseudohypericin) (105). A twofold decrease in the area under the curve for alprazolam plasma concentration versus time and a twofold increase in alprazolam clearance were observed following SJW administration. Alprazolam elimination half-life was shortened from a mean (SD) of 12.4 (3.9) hours to 6.0 (2.4) hours. The mean (SD) urinary ratio of dextromethorphan to its metabolite was 0.006 at baseline and 0.014 after SJW administration (105). These findings indicate that long-term administration of SJW may result in diminished clinical efficacy or increased dosage requirements for CYP3A4 substrates.

Recently, the authors Rengelshausen et al. (106) investigated the short-term and long-term effects of SJW on the pharmacokinetics of voriconazole. The metabolism of this new antifungal triazole is mediated by CYP2C19 and CYP3A4, as well as by CYP2C9 to a lesser extent. The authors could show that coadministration of the hyperforin-rich methanolic extract LI 160 with voriconazole increased the plasma AUC of the antifungal drug (by 22%) during the first ten hours of the first day of SJW administration when compared to the control. After 15 days of SJW intake, the AUC from hour 0 to infinity was reduced by 59% compared with control with a corresponding increase in oral voriconazole clearance. Thus, it is reasonable that SJW might induce the metabolism of voriconazole, depending on both CYP3A4 and CYP2C19.

Based on the studies listed above, it can be concluded that SJW induces hepatic and intestinal CYP3A4 and intestinal P-gp. Thus, it is likely that SJW will interact with drugs that are metabolized via CYP3A4 or P-gp. Interactions (until 2004) of SJW and synthetic drugs have been systematically reviewed (87, 88, 107, 108). These reviews clearly show that interactions between xenobiotics and the plant extract particularly occur with drugs that are metabolized and eliminated by both CYP3A4 and P-gp. It also becomes evident that not all drugs have the potential to interact with SJW. Table 4.1 gives an overview about drugs with which an interaction with SJW is likely to occur.

Pharmacological Evaluation of Interactions with Hyperforin

The mechanism for the apparent increase in drug metabolism by SJW extracts was examined by Moore et al. (109). They showed that hyperforin, a constituent of SJW, is a potent ligand ($K_{(i)} = 27$ nM) for the pregnane X receptor, an orphan nuclear receptor that regulates expression of the cytochrome P450 (CYP) 3A4 monooxygenase. Treatment of primary human hepatocytes with hypericum extracts or hyperforin resulted in a marked induction of CYP3A4 expression. The authors cautioned that because CYP3A4 is involved in the oxidative metabolism of > 50% of all drugs, their findings provide a molecular mechanism for the interaction of SJW with drugs and suggest that hypericum extracts would be likely to interact with numerous drugs (109). Interestingly, a study using alcoholic extracts of SJW prepared with methods that did not stabilize hyperforin reported CYP3A4 inhibition (103).

A study in mice investigated the role of components of hypericum extracts on CYP3A induction (110). This study explored whether hyperforin accounts for the inductive effects on CYP3A enzymes of SJW extracts. A hydroalcoholic extract containing 4.5% hyperforin was given at a dose of 300 mg/kg twice daily for 4 and 12 days. Hyperforin was given as dicyclohexylammonium (DCHA) salt (18.1 mg/kg) on the basis of its content in the extract, to ensure comparable exposure to hyperforin. The extract increased hepatic erythromycin-N-demethylase (ERND) activity, which is cytochrome P450 enzyme (CYP) 3A-dependent, about 2.2-fold after 4 days of dosing, with only slightly greater effect after 12 days (2.8 times controls). Hyperforin similarly increased ERND activity within 4 days, to 1.8 times the activity of controls, suggesting that hyperforin behaves qualitatively and quantitatively like the extract as regards induction of CYP3A activity. This effect was confirmed by Western blot analysis of hepatic CYP3A expression. Exposure to hyperforin at the end of the 4-day treatment was still similar to that with SJW extract, although it was variable and lower than after the first dose in both cases, further suggesting that hyperforin plays a key role in CYP3A induction by the SJW extract in the mouse. The authors proposed standardizing the extracts based on the hyperforin content in addition to hypericin content.

Clinical Evaluation of Interactions with Hyperforin

A recently completed four-period study in ten stable kidney transplant patients examined the influence of two SJW preparations with different hyperforin content on cyclosporine pharmacokinetic parameters (86). Test periods included baseline with cyclosporine alone, 14 days of treatment with low-hyperforin SJW comedication (< 1 mg hyperforin/day), a 4-week washout with cyclosporine doses alone, and 14 days of treatment with high-hyperforin SJW comedication (> 40 mg hyperforin/day). Cyclosporine kinetic parameters (AUC, C_{max}, and t_{max}) were determined at the end of each period.

Pharmacokinetic parameters were adjusted for cyclosporine dose, and plasma creatinine was monitored for safety. As shown in Table 4.2, there was no significant effect of low hyperforin on cyclosporine. However, high-hyperforin SJW decreased dose-adjusted exposure to cyclosporine, and increased doses of the immunosuppressant were required to maintain plasma creatinine. Serum creatinine was not different among treatment periods.

The results are consistent with a role for hyperforin in decreasing cyclosporine exposure. Induction of the intestinal drug transporter, P-glycoprotein, as well as induction of CYP3A4 could explain decreased bioavailability of cyclosporine in the presence of hyperforin-rich SJW preparations. The increased mean cyclosporine daily dose from 225 to 362 mg when patients were comedicated with the high-hyperforin preparation indicates that the change in cyclosporine levels was considered clinically significant by the medical investigator and required a dose increase. Thus, the dose-adjusted decrease in cyclosporine exposure of

Table 4.2. Influence of Different Preparations of St. John's Wort on Cyclosporine Dose–Corrected Pharmacokinetic Parameters in Ten Renal Transplant Patients (86)

Parameter	Baseline	Low:Hyperforin	Washout	High:Hyperforin
Dose (mg/day)	216±58	223±54	225±54*	362±63**
AUC (ng*h/mL)	3663±678	3109±527	3442±741	1671±313**
Cmax (ng/mL)	995±284	894±187	986±201	532±117**

p<0.05 vs. baseline; **p<0.01 vs. baseline

approximately 50% that is reflected by AUC and C_{max} values should be considered clinically significant.

Another study (111) compared effects of different SJW preparations containing different amounts of hyperforin on CYP3A4 activity using a midazolam probe (Study No. 786, Pilotstudie1: Midazolam-Interaktion) (Table 4.3). The approach provides a means to evaluate whether drugs affect CYP3A enzymes and thus would be likely to alter the clearance of other substances metabolized by this important isoenzyme. Hydroxylation of the benzodiazepine, midazolam, to 1-OH-midazolam is mediated almost exclusively by CYP3A isoenzymes. Midazolam plasma clearance that is reflected from plasma profiles of the benzodiazepine can be used as a marker for CYP3A activity. Drugs that are substrates, inducers, or inhibitors of CYP3A enzymes would be expected to alter the plasma profiles of midazolam.

The study included 42 healthy subjects randomized to six groups of seven subjects each (111). Midazolam plasma profiles were characterized following a 7.5 mg oral dose on day 1 prior to SJW exposure and 14 days later after repeated daily dosing with one of six SJW preparations. The test groups included the following different SJW preparations: Extract LI160 (drug-extract ratio 4–7:1; hyperforin content 4.6%, Lichtwer Berlin, Germany); hypericum herb powder A, which was used to explore dose-response relationship with hyperforin (hyperforin content 0.4%, Kneipp-Werke, Wuerzburg, Germany); and hypericum herb powder B with a very low hyperforin content (<0.1%, Kneipp-Werke, Wuerzburg, Germany). The decrease in midazolam AUC was highest in the LI160-treated group exposed to the highest hyperforin concentrations with a mean decrease of 79%, indicating induction of CYP3A enzymes. Using the herb powder A, the highest concentration (2700 mg/d,

Table 4.3. Effect of 14 Days of Different St. John's Wort Preparations on Percent Change in Midazolam AUC_{0-12h} Compared to Baseline (111)

SJW Preparation	Extract Dose (mg/d)	Hyperforin Dose (mg/d)	Mean % Change	95%-CI
LI 160 extract	900	41.25	−79.4	−88.6; −70.1
Hypericum powder A	2700	12.06	−47.9	−59.7; −36.2
Hypericum powder A	1800	8.04	−37.0	−58.2; −15.8
Hypericum powder A	1200	5.36	−31.3	−45.3; −17.3
Hypericum powder A	600	2.68	−20.4	−40.0; −0.8
Hypericum powder B	2700	0.13	−21.1	−33.9; −8.3

hyperforin amount 12.1 mg/d) showed the strongest decrease on midazolam AUC (-47.9%), when compared to the further dilutions of the powdered herb. A limited effect was noted after 14 days of dosing with the SJW herb powder B with a mean decrease in midazolam AUC values of 20.4% compared to baseline. Interestingly, the upper limit of the calculated 95% confidence intervals approached 0 for the two lowest hyperforin preparations, indicating little clinical significance. The results indicate induction of CYP3A4 varies between SJW products. SJW products with low hyperforin content induce CYP3A4 significantly less than those preparations with a high hyperforin amount. The degree of induction depends on the hyperforin dose.

CONCLUSIONS

Considerable differences exist in the composition of biologically active constituents among various commercially available preparations of SJW. Although several reports fail to rigorously define the specific herbal product used in clinical studies, investigators are increasingly aware that significant differences in outcome are likely to be product specific. However, a major change was made since 1998, when the quite unstable component of SJW, hyperforin, became stabilized in many products, leading to a 10- to 20-fold amount of hyperforin in the product. Moreover, the first reports of clinically significant drug interactions of SJW coincided with availability of hyperforin-enriched products. Further laboratory investigations demonstrated that CYP3A4 induction with SJW preparations was associated with hyperforin content, suggesting that this component plays a major role in clinically significant drug interactions. Clinical studies with traditional SJW extracts and products with low hyperforin content found low enzyme induction using midazolam probes that consistently had AUC decreases that were less than 50% compared to baseline. Since "hyperforin-free" extracts have been proven to be effective in clinical therapy, it is recommended to set an upper limit (1%) for the amount of hyperforin in SJW extracts in order to prevent clinically significant interactions with other comedicated drugs. It is further suggested that products used for clinical studies should be characterized by the extraction solvent, the drug-extract ratio, and the amount of hyperforin, hypericin, and total flavonoids. This information should allow a more substantial discussion of the data and would help to better explain discrepancies between studies.

REFERENCES

[1]Clement K, Covertson CR, Johnson MJ, Dearing K. St. John's wort and the treatment of mild to moderate depression: a systematic review. *Holist Nurs Pract.* 2006;20:197–203.

[2]Linde K, Mulrow CD, Egger M. St. John's wort for depression. In: *Cochrane Database Syst Rev.* 2005; CD000448.

[3]Butterweck V. Mechanism of action of St. John's wort in depression: what is known? *CNS Drugs.* 2003; 17(8):539–562.

[4]Greeson JM, Sanford B, Monti DA. St. John's wort (*Hypericum perforatum*): a review of the current pharmacological, toxicological, and clinical literature. *Psychopharmacology (Berl).* 2001;153(4):402–414.

[5]Mennini T, Gobbi M. The antidepressant mechanism of *Hypericum perforatum. Life Sci.* 2004;75(9): 1021–1027.

[6]Nathan PJ. *Hypericum perforatum* (St. John's Wort): a non selective reuptake inhibitor? A review of the recent advances in its pharmacology. *J Psychopharmacol.* 2001;15(1):47–54.

[7]Zanoli P. Role of hyperforin in the pharmacological activities of St. John's Wort. *CNS Drug Rev.* 2004;10(3):203–218.

[8]Butterweck V, Bockers T, Korte, B, Wittkowski W, Winterhoff H. Long-term effects of St. John's wort and hypericin on monoamine levels in rat hypothalamus and hippocampus. *Brain Res.* 2002;930(1–2): 21–29.

[9]Butterweck V, Korte B, Winterhoff H. Pharmacological and endocrine effects of *Hypericum perforatum* and hypericin after repeated treatment. *Pharmacopsychiatry.* 2001;34(Suppl 1):S2-S7.

[10]Butterweck V, Petereit F, Winterhoff H, Nahrstedt A. Solubilized hypericin and pseudohypericin from *Hypericum perforatum* exert antidepressant activity in the forced swimming test. *Planta Med.* 1998;64(4): 291–294.

[11]Butterweck V, Hegger M, Winterhoff H. Flavonoids of St. John's Wort reduce HPA axis function in the rat. *Planta Med.* 2004;70(10):1008–1011.

[12]Butterweck V, Jürgenliemk G, Nahrstedt A, Winterhoff H. Flavonoids from *Hypericum perforatum* show antidepressant activity in the forced swimming test. *Planta Med.* 2000;66:3–6.

[13]Calapai G, Crupi A, Firenzuoli F, Costantino G, Inferrera G, Campo G, Caputi A. Effects of *Hypericum perforatum* on levels of 5-hydroxytryptamine, noradrenaline and dopamine in the cortex, diencephalon and brainstem of the rat. *J Pharm Pharmacol.* 1999;51:723–728.

[14]Nöldner M, Schotz K. Rutin is essential for the antidepressant activity of *Hypericum perforatum* extracts in the forced swimming test. *Planta Med.* 2002;68(7):577–580.

[15]Sparenberg BL, Demisch J, Hölzl J. Untersuchungen über die antidepressiven Wirkstoffe von Johanniskraut. *Pharm Ztg Wiss.* 1993;138:239–254.

[16]Jurgenliemk G, Nahrstedt A. Phenolic compounds from *Hypericum perforatum. Planta Med.* 2002;68(1): 88–91.

[17]Berghöfer R Hölzl J. Johanniskraut (*Hypericum perforatum* L.): Prüfung auf Verfälschung. *Deutsche Apotheker Zeitung.* 1986;47(126):2569–2573.

[18]Baureithel KH, Buter KB, Engesser A, Burkard W, Schaffner W. Inhibition of benzodiazepine binding in vitro by amentoflavone, a constituent of various species of Hypericum. *Pharm Acta Helv.* 1997;72(3): 153–157.

[19]Nielsen M, Frokjaer S, Braestrup C. High affinity of the naturally-occurring biflavonoid, amentoflavon, to brain benzodiazepine receptors in vitro. *Biochem Pharmacol.* 1988;37(17):3285–3287.

[20]Butterweck V, Nahrstedt A, Evans J, Rauser L, Savage J, Popadak B, Ernsberger P, Roth BL. In vitro receptor screening of pure constituents of St. John's wort reveals novel interaction with a number of GPCR's. *Psychopharmacology.* 2002;162:193–202.

[21]Gutmann H, Brugisser R, Schaffner W, Bogman K, Botomino A, Drewe J. Transport of amentoflavone across the blood-brain barrier in vitro. *Planta Med.* 2002;68(9):804–807.

[22]Porsolt R, Le Pichon M, Jalfre M. Depression: A new animal model sensitive to antidepressant treatments. *Nature.* 1977;266:730–732.

[23]Gold PW, Licinio J, Wong ML, Chrousos GP. Corticotropin releasing hormone in the pathophysiology of melancholic and atypical depression and in the mechanism of action of antidepressant drugs. *Ann N Y Acad Sci.* 1995;771:716–729.

[24]Holsboer F, Barden N. Antidepressants and hypothalamic-pituitary-adrenocortical regulation. *Endocr Rev.* 1996;17:187–205.

[25]Barden N, Reul JM, Holsboer F. Do antidepressants stabilize mood through actions on the hypothalamic-pituitary-adrenocortical system? *Trends Neurosci.* 1995;18(1):6–11.

[26]Jurgenliemk G, Nahrstedt A. Dissolution, solubility and cooperativity of phenolic compounds from *Hypericum perforatum* L. in aqueous systems. *Pharmazie.* 2003;58(3):200–203.

[27]Cellarova E, Daxnerova Z, Kimakova K, Haluskova J. The variability of the hypericin content in the regenerants of *Hypericum perforatum. Act Biotechnol.* 1994;14:267–274.

[28]Brantner A, Kartnig TH, Quehenberger F. Vergleichende phytochemische Untersuchungen an *Hypericum perforatum* L. und *Hypericum maculatum* Crantz. *Scient Pharm.* 1994;62:261–276.

[29]Niesel S, Schilcher H. Vergleich der Freisetzung von Hypericin und Pseudohypericin in Abhängigkeit verschiedener Extraktionsbedingungen. *Arch Pharm.* 1990;323:755.

[30]Falk H, Schmitzberger W. On the nature of "soluble" hypericin in *Hypericum* species. *Monatshefte Chem.* 1992;123:731–739.

[31]Brockmann H. Phyotodynamisch wirksame Pflanzenfarbstoffe. In: Fortschr. Chem. Org. Naturst., Zechmeister, L., ed. Vienna: Springer, 1957, Vol. XIV:141–185.

[32]Lavie G, Mazur Y, Lavie D, Meruelo D. The chemical and biological properties of hypericin: a compound with a broad spectrum of biological activities. *Med Res Rev.* 1995;15(2):111–119.

[33]Southwell IA, Campbell MH. Hypericin content variation in *Hypericum perforatum* in Australia. *Phytochemistry.* 1991;30:475–478.

[34]Bernd A, Simon S, Ramirez Bosca A, Kippenberger S, Diaz Alperi J, Miquel J, Villalba Garcia JF, Pamies Mira D, Kaufmann R. Phototoxic effects of Hypericum extract in cultures of human keratinocytes compared with those of psoralen. *Photochem Photobiol*. 1999;69(2):218–221.

[35]Schulz V. Incidence and clinical relevance of the interactions and side effects of Hypericum preparations. *Phytomedicine*. 2001;8(2):152–160.

[36]Siegers CP, Biel S, Wilhelm KP. Zur Frage der Phototoxizität von *Hypericum. Nervenheilkunde*. 1993; 12:320–322.

[37]Suzuki O, Katsumata Y, Oya M. Inhibition of monoamine oxidase by hypericin. *Planta Med*. 1984;50: 272–274.

[38]Bladt S, Wagner H. Inhibition of MAO by fractions and constituents of hypericum extract. *J Geriatr Psychiatry Neurol*. 1994;7(Suppl 1):S57-S59.

[39]Cott JM. In vitro receptor binding and enzyme inhibition by *Hypericum perforatum* extract. *Pharmacopsychiatry*. 1997;30(Suppl 2):108–112.

[40]Raffa RB. Screen of receptor and uptake-site activity of hypericin component of St. John's wort reveals sigma receptor binding. *Life Sci*. 1998;62(16):L265–L270.

[41]Gobbi M, Moia M, Pirona L, Morazzoni P, Mennini T. In vitro binding studies with two *Hypericum perforatum* extracts—hyperforin, hypericin and biapigenin—on 5-HT_6, 5-HT_7, GABA_A/benzodiazepine, Sigma, NPY-Y1/Y2 Receptors and dopamine transporters. *Pharmacopsychiatry*. 2001;34(Suppl 1): S45–S48.

[42]Simmen U, Burkard W, Berger K, Schaffner W, Lundstrom K. Extracts and constituents of *Hypericum perforatum* inhibit the binding of various ligands to recombinant receptors expressed with the Semliki Forest virus system. *J Recept Signal Transduct Res*. 1999;19(1–4):59–74.

[43]Simmen U, Higelin J, Berger-Büter K, Schaffner W, Lundstrom K. Neurochemical studies with St. John's wort in vitro. *Pharmacopsychiatry*. 2001;34(Suppl 1):S137-S142.

[44]Butterweck V, Wall A, Lieflaender-Wulf U, Winterhoff H, Nahrstedt A. Effects of the total extract and fractions of *Hypericum perforatum* in animal assays for antidepressant activity. *Pharmacopsychiatry*. 1997; 30(Suppl):117–124.

[45]Butterweck V, Winterhoff H, Herkenham M. St. John's wort, hypericin, and imipramine: a comparative analysis of mRNA levels in brain areas involved in HPA axis control following short-term and long-term administration in normal and stressed rats. *Mol Psychiatry*. 2001;6(5):547–564.

[46]Vandenbogaerde A, Zanoli P, Puia G, Truzzi C, Kamuhabwa A, De Witte P, Merlevede W, Baraldi M. Evidence that total extract of *Hypericum perforatum* affects exploratory behavior and exerts anxiolytic effects in rats. *Pharmacol Biochem Behav*. 2000;65(4):627–633.

[47]Butterweck V, Lieflander-Wulf U, Winterhoff H, Nahrstedt A. Plasma levels of hypericin in presence of procyanidin B2 and hyperoside: a pharmacokinetic study in rats. *Planta Med*. 2003;69(3):189–192.

[48]Beerhues L. Hyperforin. *Phytochemistry*. 2006;67:2201–2207.

[49]Melzer M, Fuhrken D, Kolkmann R. Hyperforin im Johanniskraut. *Dt Apoth Ztg*. 1998;138(49):56–62.

[50]Orth HC, Rentel C, Schmidt PC. Isolation, purity analysis and stability of hyperforin as a standard material from *Hypericum perforatum* L. *J Pharm Pharmacol*. 1999;51(2):193–200.

[51]Trifunovic S, Vajs V, Macura S, Juranic N, Djarmati Z, Jankov R, Milosavljevic S. Oxidation products of hyperforin from *Hypericum perforatum. Phytochemistry*. 1998;49(5):1305–1310.

[52]Chatterjee S, Bhattacharya S, Wonnemann M, Singer A, Muller W. Hyperforin as a possible antidepressant component of hypericum extracts. *Life Sci*. 1998;63:499–510.

[53]Chatterjee SS, Noldner M, Koch E, Erdelmeier C. Antidepressant activity of *hypericum perforatum* and hyperforin: the neglected possibility. *Pharmacopsychiatry*. 1998;31(Suppl 1):7–15.

[54]Müller WE, Singer A, Wonnemann M, Hafner U, Rolli M, Schaefer C. Hyperforin represents the neurotransmitter reuptake inhibiting constituent of Hypericum extract. *Pharmacopsychiatry*. 1998;31(Suppl): 16–21.

[55]Gobbi M, Dalla Valle F, Ciapparelli C, Diomede L, Morazzoni L. *Hypericum perforatum* L. extract does not inhibit 5-HT transporter in rat brain cortex. *Naunyn-Schmiedeberg's Arch Pharmacol*. 1999;360: 262–269.

[56]Neary JT, Whittemore SR, Bu Y, Mehta H, Shi YF. Biochemical mechanisms of action of Hypericum LI 160 in glial and neuronal cells: inhibition of neurotransmitter uptake and stimulation of extracellular signal regulated protein kinase. *Pharmacopsychiatry*. 2001;34(Suppl 1):S103–S107.

[57]Singer A, Wonnemann M, Müller W. Hyperforin, a major antidepressant constituent of St. John's Wort, inhibits serotonin uptake by elevating free intracellular Na^+. *J Pharmacol Exp Ther*. 1999;290: 1363–1368.

[58]Buchholzer ML, Dvorak C, Chatterjee SS, Klein J. Dual modulation of striatal acetylcholine release by hyperforin, a constituent of St. John's wort. *J Pharmacol Exp Ther*. 2002;301(2):714–719.

[59]Amara SG, Kuhar MJ. Neurotransmitter transporters: recent progress. *Annu Rev Neurosci*. 1993;16:73–93.

[60]Jensen AG, Hansen SH, Nielsen EO. Adhyperforin as a contributor to the effect of *Hypericum perforatum* L. in biochemical models of antidepressant activity. *Life Sci.* 2001;14:1593–1605.

[61]Wonnemann M, Singer A, Müller WE. Inhibition of synaptosomal uptake of ^{3}H-L-glutamate and ^{3}H-GABA by hyperforin, a major constituent of St. John's wort: the role of amiloride sensitive sodium conductive pathways. *Neuropsychopharmacology.* 2000;23(2):188–197.

[62]Fisunov A, Lozovaya N, Tsintsadze T, Chatterjee S, Nöldner M, Krishtal O. Hyperforin modulates gating of P-type Ca^{2+} current in cerebellar Purkinje neurons. *Eur J Physiol.* 2000;440:427–434.

[63]Chatterjee S, Filippov V, Lishko P, Maximyuk O, Nöldner M, Krishtal O. Hyperforin attenuates various ionic conductance mechanisms in the isolated hippocampal neurons of the rat. *Life Sci.* 1999;65(22):2395–2405.

[64]Krishtal O, Lozovaya N, Fisunov A, Tsintsadze T, Pankratov Y, Kopanitsa M, Chatterjee SS. Modulation of ion channels in rat neurons by the constituents of *Hypericum perforatum. Pharmacopsychiatry.* 2001;34(Suppl 1):S74–S82.

[65]Biber A, Fischer H, Römer A, Chatterjee SS. Oral bioavailability of hyperforin from hypericum extracts in rats and human volunteers. *Pharmacopsychiatry.* 1998;31(Suppl 1):36–43.

[66]Zanoli P, Rivasi M, Baraldi C, Baraldi M. Pharmacological activity of hyperforin acetate in rats. *Behav Pharmacol.* 2002;13(8):645–651.

[67]Butterweck V, Christoffel V, Nahrstedt A, Petereit F, Spengler B, Winterhoff H. Step by step removal of hyperforin and hypericin: activity profile of different Hypericum preparations in behavioral models. *Life Sci.* 2003;73(5):627–639.

[68]Martin P, Soubrie P, Puech AJ. Reversal of helpless behaviour by serotonin uptake blockers in rats. *Psychopharmacology.* 1990;101:403–407.

[69]Martin P, Soubrie P, Simon P. The effect of monoamine oxidase inhibitors compared with classical tricyclic antidepressants on learned helplessness paradigm. *Progress in Neuropsychopharmacology and Biological Psychiatry.* 1987;11:1–7.

[70]Gambrana C, Ghiglieri O, Tolu P, De Montis G, Giachetti D, Bombardelli E, Tagliamonte A. Efficacy of an *Hypericum perforatum* (St. John's wort) extract in preventing and reverting a condition of escape deficit in rats. *Neuropsychopharmacology.* 1999;21(2):247–254.

[71]Kalb R, Trautmann-Sponsel RD, Kieser M. Efficacy and tolerability of Hypericum extract WS 5572 versus placebo in mildly to moderately depressed patients. *Pharmacopsychiatry.* 2001;34:96–103.

[72]Laakmann G, Schule C, Baghai T, Kieser M. St. John's wort in mild to moderate depression: the relevance of hyperforin for the clinical efficacy. *Pharmacopsychiatry.* 1998;31(Suppl 1):54–59.

[73]Lecrubier Y, Clerc C, Didi R, Kieser M. Efficacy of St. John's wort extract WS 5570 in major depression: A double-blind, placebo-controlled trial. *Am J Psychiatry.* 2002;159:1361–1366.

[74]Reh C, Laux P, Schenk N. Hypericum-Extrakt bei Depressionen: eine wirksame Alternative. *Therapiewoche.* 1992;42:1576–1581.

[75]Szegedi A, Kohnen R, Dienel A, Kieser M. Acute treatment of moderate to severe depression with hypericum extract WS 5570 (St. John's wort): randomised controlled double blind non-inferiority trial versus paroxetine. *BMJ.* 2005;330:503.

[76]Wurglics M, Westerhoff K, Kaunzinger A, Wilke A, Baumeister A, Dressman J, Schubert-Zsilovecz M. Batch-to-batch reproducibility of St. John's wort preparations. *Pharmacopsychiatry.* 2001;34(Suppl 1):S152–S156.

[77]Wurglics M, Westerhoff K, Kaunzinger A, Wilke A, Baumeister A, Dressman J, Schubert-Zsilavecz M. Comparison of German St. John's wort products according to hyperforin and total hypericin content. *J Am Pharm Assoc (Wash).* 2001;41(4):560–566.

[78]Gastpar M, Singer A, Zeller K. Comparative efficacy and safety of a once-daily dosage of hypericum extract STW3-VI and citalopram in patients with moderate depression: a double-blind, randomised, multicentre, placebo-controlled study. *Pharmacopsychiatry.* 39;2006:66–75.

[79]Schrader E. Equivalence of St. John's wort extract (Ze 117) and fluoxetine: a randomized, controlled study in mild-moderate depression. *Int Clin Psychopharmacol.* 2000;15(2):61–68.

[80]Schrader E, Meier B, Brattstrom A. Hypericum treatment of mild-moderate depression in a placebo-controlled study: a prospective, double-blind, randomized, placebo-controlled, multicentre study. *Human Psychopharmacology.* 1998;13:163–169.

[81]Woelk H. Comparison of St. John's wort and imipramine for treating depression: randomised controlled trial. *BMJ.* 2000;321(7260):536–539.

[82]Brattstroem A. Der Johanniskrautextrakt ZE 117: Wirksamkeit und Sicherheit. *DAZ.* 2002;30:97–99.

[83]Willmar Schwabe GC. Stable extract of *Hypericum perforatum* L., process for preparing the same and pharmaceutical composition. *International Patent.* 1997;WO 97/13489.

[84]Willmar Schwabe GC. Stable extract of *Hypericum perforatum* L., a method for producing the same, and corresponding pharmaceutical preparations. *International Patent.* 1998;WO 98/44936.

[85]Arold G, Donath F, Maurer A, Diefenbach K, Bauer S, Henneicke-von Zepelin HH, Friede M, Roots I. No relevant interaction with alprazolam, caffeine, tolbutamide, and digoxin by treatment with a low-hyperforin St. John's wort extract. *Planta Med.* 2005;71(4):331–337.

[86]Mai I, Bauer S, Perloff E, Johne A, Uehleke B, Frank B, Budde K, Roots I. Hyperforin content determines the magnitude of the St. John's wort-cyclosporine drug interaction. *Clin Pharmacol Ther.* 2004; in press.

[87]Mannel M. Drug interactions with St. John's wort: mechanisms and clinical implications. *Drug Saf.* 2004;27(11):773–797.

[88]Zhou S, Chan E, Pan SQ, Huang M, Lee EJ. Pharmacokinetic interactions of drugs with St. John's wort. *J Psychopharmacol.* 2004;18(2):262–276.

[89]Landrum-Michalets E. Update: clinically significant cytochrome P450 drug interactions. *Pharmacotherapy.* 1998;18:84–112.

[90]Smith DA, Abel SM, Hyland R, Jones BC. Human cytochrome P450's: selectivity and measurment in vivo. *Xenobiotica.* 1998;28:1095–1128.

[91]Smith S, Stubbins MJ, Harries LW, Wolf CR. Molecular genetics of human cytochrome P450 monooxygenase superfamily. *Xenobiotica.* 1998;28:1129–1165.

[92]Bienvenu T, Rey E, Pons G, d'Athis P, Olive G. A simple non-invasive procedure for the investigation of cytochrome P-450 IIIA dependent enzymes in humans. *Int J Clin Pharmacol Ther Toxicol.* 1991;29(11): 441–445.

[93]Dolara P, Lodovici M, Salvadori M, Zaccara G, Muscas GC. Urinary 6-beta-OH-cortisol and paracetamol metabolites as a probe for assessing oxidation and conjugation of chemicals in humans. *Pharmacol Res Commun.* 1987;19(4):261–273.

[94]Ged C, Rouillon JM, Pichard L, Combalbert J, Bressot N, Bories P, Michel H, Beaune P, Maurel P. The increase in urinary excretion of 6 beta-hydroxycortisol as a marker of human hepatic cytochrome P450IIIA induction. *Br J Clin Pharmacol.* 1989;28(4):373–387.

[95]Roby CA, Anderson GD, Kantor E, Dryer DA, Burstein AH. St. John's Wort: effect on CYP3A4 activity. *Clin Pharmacol Ther.* 2000;67(5):451–457.

[96]Gatmaitan ZC, Arias IM. Structure and function of P-glycoprotein in normal liver and small intestine. *Adv Pharmacol.* 1993;24:77–97.

[97]Lown KS, Mayo RR, Leichtman AB, Hsiao HL, Turgeon DK, Schmiedlin-Ren P, Brown MB, Guo W, Rossi SJ, Benet LZ, Watkins PB. Role of intestinal P-glycoprotein(*mdr1*) in interpatient variation in the oral bioavailability of cyclosporine. *Clin Pharmacol Ther.* 1997;62:248–260.

[98]Durr D, Stieger B, Kullak-Ublick GA, Rentsch KM, Steinert HC, Meier PJ, Fattinger K. St. John's Wort induces intestinal P-glycoprotein/MDR1 and intestinal and hepatic CYP3A4. *Clin Pharmacol Ther.* 2000; 68(6):598–604.

[99]Wang Z, Gorski JC, Hamman MA, Huang SM, Lesko LJ, Hall SD. The effects of St. John's wort (*Hypericum perforatum*) on human cytochrome P450 activity. *Clin Pharmacol Ther.* 2001;70(4):317–326.

[100]Johne A, Brockmoller J, Bauer S, Maurer A, Langheinrich M, Roots I. Pharmacokinetic interaction of digoxin with an herbal extract from St. John's wort (*Hypericum perforatum*). *Clin Pharmacol Ther.* 1999;66(4): 338–345.

[101]Piscitelli SC, Burstein AH, Chaitt D, Alfaro RM, Falloon J. Indinavir concentrations and St. John's wort. *Lancet.* 2000;355(9203):547–548.

[102]Ruschitzka F, Meier PJ, Turina M, Luscher TF, Noll G. Acute heart transplant rejection due to Saint John's wort [letter] [see comments]. *Lancet.* 2000;355(9203):548–549.

[103]Obach RS. Inhibition of human cytochrome P450 enzymes by constituents of St. John's Wort, an herbal preparation used in the treatment of depression. *J Pharmacol Exp Ther.* 2000;294(1):88–95.

[104]Hennessy M, Kelleher D, Spiers JP, Barry M, Kavanagh P, Back D, Mulcahy F, Feely J. St. John's Wort increases expression of P-glycoprotein: implications for drug interactions. *Br J Clin Pharmacol.* 2002; 53:75–82.

[105]Markowitz JS, DeVane CL, Boulton DW, Carson SW, Nahas Z, Risch SC. Effect of St. John's wort (*Hypericum perforatum*) on cytochrome P-450 2D6 and 3A4 activity in healthy volunteers. *Life Sci.* 2000;66(9): L133–L139.

[106]Rengelshausen J, Banfield M, Riedel KD, Burhenne J, Weiss J Thomsen T, Walter-Sack I, Haefeli WE, Mikus G. Opposite effects of short-term and long-term St. John's wort intake on voriconazole pharmacokinetics. *Clin Pharmacol Ther.* 2005;78(1):25–33.

[107]Izzo AA, Ernst E. Interactions between herbal medicines and prescribed drugs: a systematic review. *Drugs.* 2001;61(15):2163–2175.

[108]Mills E, Montori VM, Wu P, Gallicano K, Clarke M, Guyatt G. Interaction of St. John's wort with conventional drugs: systematic review of clinical trials. *BMJ.* 2004;329(7456):27–30.

[109]Moore LB, Goodwin B, Jones SA, Wisely GB, Serabjit-Singh CJ, Willson TM, Collins JL, Kliewer SA. St. John's wort induces hepatic drug metabolism through activation of the pregnane X receptor. *Proc Natl Acad Sci USA.* 2000;97(13):7500–7502.

[110]Cantoni L, Rozio M, Mangolini A, Hauri L, Caccia S. Hyperforin contributes to the hepatic CYP3A-inducing effect of *Hypericum perforatum* extract in the mouse. *Toxicol Sci.* 2003;75(1):25–30.

[111]Mueller SC, Majcher-Peszynska J, Klammt S, Uehleke B, Miekisch B, Kundt G, Drewelow B. Induction of CYP3A by St. Johns Wort (SJW) depends on hyperforin (HYF) dose. ABSTRACT. *Clinical Pharmacology & Therapeutics.* 2005;77(2):P36.

Botanical Medicine: From Bench to Bedside
Edited by R. Cooper and F. Kronenberg
© Mary Ann Liebert, Inc.

Chapter 5

Preclinical and Clinical Development of the Green Tea Catechin, Epigallocatechin Gallate, in Treating HIV-1 Infection

Christina L. Nance and William T. Shearer*

Since the first report of the acquired immunodeficiency syndrome (AIDS) caused by the human immunodeficiency virus (HIV) infection over two decades ago, more than 60 million people worldwide have been infected by HIV and more than one-third have died of AIDS (1). A reduction in deaths due to AIDS has also occurred globally over the past several years coincident with broader access to antiretroviral (ARV) therapy (2). Because a safe and effective vaccine treatment is still far away, in the near term, the continual development of effective, safe, and affordable anti-HIV drugs is critical to save the lives of people who have been and will be infected by HIV. Next to malaria, AIDS is the leading infectious cause of death in the world. Untreated disease caused by HIV has a case fatality rate that approaches 100%.

A new infection occurs somewhere in the world approximately every six seconds, resulting in 6,500 new infections daily (3). Heterosexual transmission of HIV-1 continues to be the predominant mode of the pandemic spread of HIV or AIDS. Worldwide, more than 90 percent of all adolescent and adult HIV infections have resulted from heterosexual intercourse (4).

With more than 95% of new infections occurring in developing countries where limited resources and cultural factors make containment of the epidemic difficult, the impact of the current level of HIV seroprevalence is enormous in terms of mortality, resource depletion, and human suffering (5). There is clearly an unmet need for treatment of individuals already infected. However, there is also a desperate need to prevent further infection.

HIV-1 infection ultimately results in impaired specific immune function by virtue of the initial binding of the HIV-1 virion envelope glycoprotein 120 (gp120) to the CD4 receptor in complex with a chemokine receptor on the T-cell surface (6). HIV-1 isolates

Department of Pediatrics, Baylor College of Medicine, Houston, Texas
*Corresponding author: clnance@texaschildrenshospital.org

are distinguishable by the main coreceptor used for cell entry, chemokine receptors CXCR4 or CCR5 (6). Virions utilizing CCR5 as a coreceptor (R5 viruses) are macrophage-tropic (M-tropic) (7, 8). Those using CXCR4 (X4 viruses) are T-cell-tropic (T-tropic) and perhaps more cytopathic. Most of the viruses observed soon after transmission (97%) utilize CCR5 coreceptors (7). Thus, the corresponding phenotypes of the viruses are X4, R5, or R5X4 if they use CXCR4, CCR5, or both coreceptors, respectively (9). Even though gp120 elicits virus-neutralizing antibodies, HIV-1 eludes the immune system and leads to the onset of AIDS. Ever since the discovery of the virus as the causative agent, there has been an intense effort to develop therapeutic methods to inhibit or prevent infection (10–12). Among the immune-based strategies designed to prevent the fateful initial binding event between the HIV-1 virion and target cell are chemokine analogs, chemokine receptor inhibitors, anti-HIV-1 monoclonal antibodies, fusion proteins, and vaccines (13).

Several natural products, such as ribosome inactivating proteins, alkaloids, flavonoids, and lignans, have been found to inhibit unique enzymes and proteins crucial to the life cycle of HIV, including the reverse transcription (RT) process, virus entry, and integrase or protease (14–17).

At present, because of the continuous emergence of drug resistance and side effects of currently available drugs, significant efforts have been spent on searching for more effective anti-HIV drugs (18). Medicinal plants are chemically complex and diverse. They produce botanical compounds that provide a wide spectrum of biological and pharmacological properties (18, 19). Therefore, screening anti-HIV agents from natural products may be a more effective approach for drug discovery.

Although many natural products have been reported to exhibit anti-HIV activities, to date, none of these compounds are found in the list of conventional ARV drugs. Many natural products have not been further investigated for their actual usefulness in combating the epidemic (20). Nevertheless, it should be stressed that a number of natural products mainly derived from plants have proven effective in suppressing HIV replication and progress. For example, calanolide derivatives, pokeweed antiviral proteins, and sulphated polysaccharides are some of the compounds with excellent and promising antiviral activities (17, 20). It is very much anticipated that anti-HIV cures and prophylactic preparations containing these natural products would soon be available.

Specifically, (+)-calanolide A and related coumarins isolated from various *Calophyllum* spp. represent a novel and distinct subgroup of nonnucleoside reverse transcriptase inhibitors (NNRTI). (+)-Calanolide A has already been the subject of a phase II clinical study in healthy, HIV-negative individuals. Studies have demonstrated that (+)-calanolide A has a favorable safety profile in both animal and human subjects (20).

In this chapter, we wish to review the evidence for another promising natural product from green tea, namely, epigallocatechin gallate (EGCG), and related polyphenols.

GREEN TEA CATECHIN, EPIGALLOCATECHIN GALLATE (EGCG)

There has been recently a significant research emphasis on identifying nutrients or food factors from natural sources for the prevention or treatment of diseases. In particular, there has been a long history of tea consumption in the world, and much attention has been placed on the medicinal benefits of green tea. Epidemiological studies suggest that the consumption of tea may reduce cancer and cardiovascular disease risk, resulting from its polyphenol components (21–27).

Flavonoids and related polyphenols possess promising anti-HIV activity. Several of these compounds inhibit RT, induce interferons which inactivate viral protease (28), and down-regulate the expression of HIV coreceptors such as CCR2b, CCR3, and CCR5 (29). However, the molecular mechanisms underlying the anti-HIV effects of flavonoids and polyphenolic compounds still need to be clearly elucidated (29).

Catechins and theaflavins are two groups of natural polyphenols found in green tea and black tea, respectively (30). Catechins account for 6% to 16% of the dry green tea leaves and contain four main catechin derivatives, including (–)-epicatechin (EC), (–)-epicatechin gallate (ECG), (–)-epigallocatechin (EGC), and (–)-epigallocatechin gallate (EGCG) (31) (Figure 5.1).

These tea polyphenols have recently received much attention, as they possess a broad spectrum of biological functions such as antioxidative, antibacterial, antitumor, antiviral, anti-inflammatory, and cardiovascular protection activities (21, 27, 42–47). EGCG is found to be the most prevalent and active catechin of green tea with respect to anticancer activity when tested in animals carrying several human cancer types, such as breast (32, 33), bladder (34), prostate (35), lung (36, 37), skin (38), and liver (39–41).

Cytotoxicity by these tea polyphenols was shown to be low on MRC-5, MT-2, and CEM cells. The safety of these catechin and theaflavin derivatives is attested to by a long history of tea consumption by people all over the world (31).

EGCG accounts for approximately 50% of the total amount of catechins in green tea (46). EGCG binds strongly to many biological molecules and affects a variety of enzyme activities and signal transduction pathways at micromolar or nanomolar levels attributable to

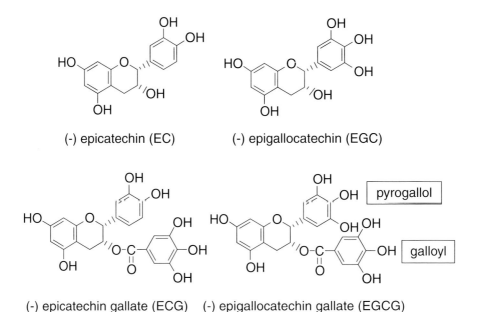

Figure 5.1. Structure of the Polyphenolic Catechins Found in Green Tea

its pyrogallol and galloyl moieties (48, 49). This specific component of green tea is thought to be responsible for the vast array of presumed health benefits. Among the properties ascribed to EGCG are antitumorigenic, anti-inflammatory, antioxidative, antiproliferative, antibacterial, and antiviral effects (33, 46, 48, 50, 51).

There have been no reports of clinical toxicity when green tea is consumed as a beverage throughout the day. Consumption of up to 20 cups of green tea per day is not uncommon in certain populations (52). A crucial aspect of translating the observed effects of EGCG to clinically relevant strategies is the necessity of achieving physiologically relevant concentrations. As tea catechins have poor bioavailability, most of the ingested EGCG does not reach the blood as a significant fraction and is eliminated presystemically (53). Phase I clinical trials involving pharmacokinetic studies of EGCG have shown that only a small percentage of the orally administered catechin appeared in the blood. Drinking the equivalent of two cups of green tea resulted in a mean peak plasma EGCG level of 170 nM after 1.5 hours (20, 49, 54). Thus, EGCG represents a potential low-cost inhibitor of HIV infection that could be associated with current anti-HIV therapy.

EGCG IN HIV-1 INFECTION

In HIV-1 infection, EGCG is responsible for the reported antiviral effects of green tea (31, 45, 46, 55–57). EGCG inhibits HIV-1 replication in human peripheral blood mononuclear cells (PBMCs) in vitro with a resultant decrease in HIV-1 p24 antigen concentration and reverse transcriptase (31, 45, 57).

At high concentrations (i.e., nonphysiologic; 50–200 μmol/L), EGCG has been shown to prevent the attachment of HIV-1–gp120 to CD4 molecules on T-cells (57). Also, recently it has been discovered that EGCG, at the nonphysiologic concentration of 200 μmol/L, blocked formation of the HIV-1 fusion-active core conformation, gp41 6-helix bundle (31).

Thus, the elucidation of the mechanism of action of the natural anti-HIV product, EGCG, on HIV-1 inhibition specifically at physiologically attainable concentrations appeared to be the missing link to a translational product in the fight against AIDS.

TRANSLATIONAL MEDICINE: EGCG AND THEORETICAL MODELING OF EGCG-CD4 BINDING CAPABILITIES

HIV-1 entry depends on the sequential interaction of the gp120 exterior envelope glycoprotein with the receptors on the cell, CD4, and members of the chemokine receptor family. Initial binding of the HIV-1 virions to cells involves the interaction of the viral envelope protein gp120 with CD4 (Figure 5.2) (6). Recombinant soluble CD4 proteins bind to the HIV-1 envelope glycoprotein gp120 and inhibit viral infection (58). High-affinity binding to gp120 occurs at the D1 domain of CD4 (58). The primary sites for HIV-1 interactions are on loops that protrude from the variable-like D1 domain in analogy with immunoglobulin complementarity-determining regions. The D2 domain is intimately associated with D1 but is variable-like (58). Therefore, there has been interest in finding molecules that block the binding of gp120 to CD4 (entry inhibitors) as a way of reducing HIV-1 infectivity.

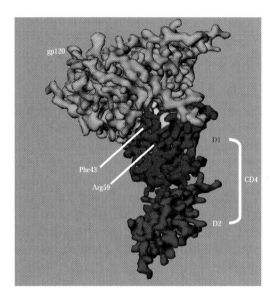

Figure 5.2.   Model of HIV-1gp120 (Purple) Binding to CD4

Space-filling model of CD4 domains D1 (red) and D2 (blue). The model demonstrates the extracellular component of the CD4 molecule with residues Phe 43 (cyan) and Arg 59 (green).

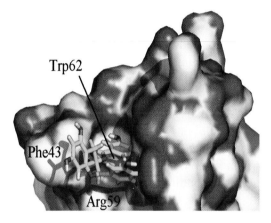

Figure 5.3.
A Model of EGCG Binding to the D1 Domain of CD4

Model drawn using PyMol, with the crystal structure coordinates 1CDJ. In the protein, carbon is yellow, oxygen is red, and nitrogen is purple. The view is approximately from the direction of binding of gp120.

Such a potential viral entry inhibitor is EGCG, a polyphenolic catechin that is one of the main active components of green tea. Recently, investigators have found that the antiviral effects can be targeted at HIV-1 infection (31, 46, 56, 57, 59).

Broadly neutralizing antibodies recognize discontinuous conserved epitopes on gp120, the most abundant of which are directed against the CD4 binding site and block gp120-CD4 interaction (60). In HIV-1 infection, interatomic contacts are made between 22 CD4 residues and 26 gp120 amino acid residues. The most critical of the CD4 residues are Phe 43 and Arg 59, with Phe 43 at the center of the cluster of residues involved in binding (Figure 5.2). Sixty-three percent of all interatomic contacts come from one span (40–48) in C'C" of CD4; Phe 43 alone accounts for 23% of the total (61). Molecular modeling utilizing the crystal structure coordinates, 1CDJ (61) (Figure 5.3), showed that there is an appropriate binding site for EGCG in the region of Phe 43, Arg 59, and Trp 62, which is the region of CD4 that interacts with gp120 (58, 61) and would therefore prevent docking of gp120 onto the D1 domain (56). EGCG is known to be particularly good at binding to arginine and aromatic residues, using mainly functions on rings D and B (62, 63). The model therefore agrees well with known affinities of EGCG. Modeling of interactions of CD4 with EGCG and gp120 has been carried out independently (64), and in agreement with this model, namely, stacking of the galloyl ring D against Trp 62, and interactions with Arg 59 and Phe 43. Therefore, the binding of EGCG to CD4 completely blocks binding of gp120 (59).

BINDING AFFINITY OF EGCG FOR CD4

Assessment of binding affinity was performed using nuclear magnetic resonance (NMR) spectroscopy. Saturation transfer difference (STD), an NMR technique, provides information on ligand binding to receptors and contact with the receptor (65, 66). As the receptor protein becomes progressively saturated with a radiofrequency pulse (interpreted right to left by increasing ppm), the portions of the ligand that is bound to the protein are recognized as strong signals or representative peaks as they become saturated by association (67).

Figure 5.4 shows NMR and STD experiments of 1.45 μM protein (5.8 μM binding site) and 310 μM EGCG, a ratio of EGCG to binding site of 53. Strong saturation was seen at the four signals arising from the aromatic rings of EGCG, indicating binding of EGCG to the protein at the polyphenolic rings (Figure 5.4A, 5.4B). STD experiments carried out at several different protein (CD4): ligand (EGCG) concentrations and ratios resulted in similar findings. STD experiments using a 1:1 ratio of EGCG to (−)-catechin (Figure 5.4C) produced

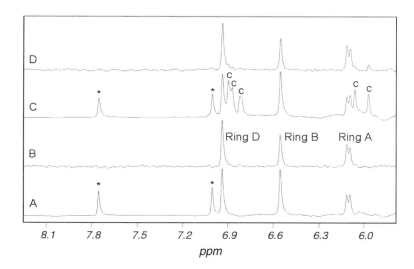

Figure 5.4.   Saturation Transfer Difference Spectra

A, NMR spectrum of 310 μmol/L EGCG in the presence of 1.45 μmol/L PRO 542 (5.8 μmol/L CD4). The signals marked with asterisks are from low-molecular-weight compounds present in the CD4 buffer. **B**, STD spectrum from this solution. The intensities of the STDs at rings D, B, and A are 10%, 7.4%, and 10%, respectively. **C**, NMR spectrum of 310 μmol/L EGCG plus 310 μmol/L (-)-catechin in the presence of 1.45 μmol/L PRO 542 (5.8 μmol/L CD4). The catechin signals are marked c. **D**, STD spectrum from this solution. The intensities of the STDs at rings D, B, and A of EGCG are 9%, 6%, and 9%, respectively, whereas the STDs from catechin are in the range of 1.5% to 3%. In B and D, there are no measurable STDs to the other signals marked with asterisks.

much larger effects on the EGCG than on catechin and only a slight reduction in the STD on EGCG (Figure 5.4D), suggesting that although there is some competition between (−)-catechin and EGCG, control (−)-catechin binds much more weakly than EGCG. Other low-molecular-weight components of the protein buffer (indicated by asterisks in Figure 5.4) produced no STDs (59). Thus the linear decrease of signal of free EGCG on titration with CD4, as well as the lack of exchange broadening by NMR, implied a dissociation constant stronger than $1\,\mu mol/L$. This combined with the STD effects resulted in a calculated approximate K_d of $10\,nmol/L$ (59).

INHIBITION OF HIV-1-GP120 BINDING TO HUMAN CD4[+] T-CELLS

Determination of an inhibitory effect of gp120 binding on human CD4[+] T-cells by EGCG was made in a cell-based system. Of critical importance was the determination of whether

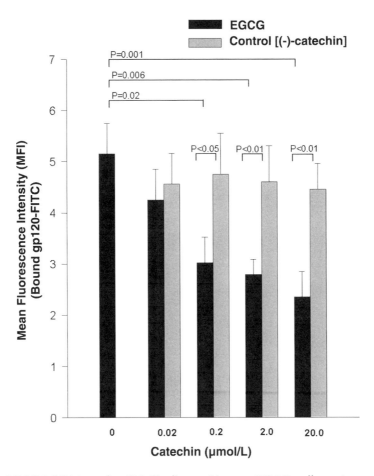

Figure 5.5. EGCG Inhibition of gp120 Binding to Human CD4 T-cells as Assessed by Flow Cytometry

The data are expressed as means ± SD of six independent experiments. Only significant differences are noted (59).

EGCG could inhibit binding of gp120 to CD4 at concentrations that could be achieved by drinking green tea or taking an oral tablet of EGCG. Previous investigations had shown that two cups of green tea would raise the blood level of EGCG to $0.2\,\mu M$ and EGCG tablets would yield a blood level of $1.7\mu M$. As shown in Figure 5.5, EGCG significantly inhibited the binding of gp120 to $CD4^+$ T-cells in a dose-dependent manner at 0.2 (42%), 2.0 (47%), and $20\mu M$ (55%) EGCG (p=0.02, 0.006, and 0.001, respectively). Thus, at physiologically relevant levels of EGCG (i.e., in this investigation, up to $2.0\mu M$), there was a statistically significant inhibitory effect, although complete inhibition of gp120 binding was not achieved. Incubation with control, (−)-catechin, did not alter the binding capacity of gp120 on $CD4^+$ T-cells (59).

This inhibition of HIV-1-gp120 binding to human $CD4^+$ T-cells by EGCG was also observed on HIV-1 infectivity as evaluated by measuring p24 antigen production. Three groups of HIV-1 have been described, labeled M, N, and O, based on genome differences. Most HIV-1 infections are caused by group M viruses, and these are divided into nine subtypes known as clades (A–D, F–H, J, and K). The DNA sequences of viruses in distinct clades can differ by 15% to 20% (68). The most common clade in the Americas, Europe, and Australia is clade B, whereas clade C predominates in the most heavily affected part of the world, southern Africa. Increasingly, recombinant HIV-1 (recombining different clades) are detected (68). Different clades might be transmitted with different levels of efficiency and might differ in their pathogenic potential (2). Human PBMC exposed to various strains and subtypes of HIV-1 exhibited detectable, intracellular, and extracellular p24 levels. Cultures exposed to increasing concentrations of EGCG resulted in the efficient suppression of p24 antigen production. EGCG exerted significant inhibitory activity on HIV-1 replication across subtype and tropisms with IC_{50} at a physiologically relevant level (Table 5.1).

Table 5.1. Inhibition of HIV-1 p24 Antigen by EGCG

| HIV-1 | | IC50 |
Subtype	Tropism[‡]	EGCG (mM)
B	R5	3
B	X4	6
B	R5/X4	6
C	R5	6
C	R5/X4	12
D	X4	12
D	R5	12
G	R5	12

Source: Table 1. HIV-1 p24 antigen measured in human PBMC by HIV-1 P24 ELISA. Taken from Nance, CL, Siwak E, Ram A, Willis V, Westerfield S, and Shearer WT. HIV-1 Infectivity inhibited by binding of the green tea catechin, epigallocatechin gallate, to CD4. *Clin Immunol* 2007;123:S13.
[‡]R5, CCR5 coreceptor; x4, CXCR5 coreceptor; Rt/X4, dual tropic coreceptor.

On the basis of the literature, the concentration of EGCG likely in the plasma after consuming the equivalent of two to three cups of green tea is within the range of 0.1 to 0.6 µmol/L and with greater consumption of green tea (seven to nine cups) at the level of 1 to 2 µmol/L (33, 47, 49, 69, 70). Therefore, interference of gp120 binding to CD4+ T-cells was assessed at the physiologically relevant levels of 0.2 to 2.0 µmol/L (59). These studies have demonstrated evidence of high-affinity binding of EGCG to the CD4 molecule with a K_d of 10 nM with subsequent inhibition of gp120 binding to human CD4+ T-cells. EGCG binds in the same molecular pocket on CD4 as does HIV-1-gp120. EGCG at concentrations equivalent to those obtained by the consumption of green tea is able to reduce the attachment of gp120 to CD4 (when present at physiological concentrations) by a factor of between 10-fold and 20-fold (59). Thus, the blockade of the binding of HIV-1-gp120 to CD4 by EGCG can efficiently inhibit HIV-1 infectivity of CD4+ cells. Therefore, EGCG at concentrations equivalent to those obtained by the consumption of green tea is able to significantly reduce the attachment of gp120 to CD4. Nevertheless, the results suggest that EGCG, possibly given as a therapeutic intervention such as in a capsular form as an alternative to drinking green tea, could be a useful way of reducing the risk of HIV-1 infection (26, 63).

TRANSLATIONAL MEDICINE: EGCG: BENCH TO BEDSIDE

ARV has decreased the number of AIDS cases dramatically (71). However, ARV is not able to eradicate HIV-1 from patients completely. On the other hand, the toxicity of currently available anti-HIV drugs makes it difficult to maintain patients' adherence to ARV therapy (72). The inevitable emergence of drug-resistant mutants, especially multidrug-resistant mutants, in response to ARV therapies makes the situation worse (73). The rates of success of ARV are predicted to decrease gradually with the increase in the emergence of drug-resistant strains. Therefore, continuous development of novel anti-HIV agents is necessary (18).

EGCG ANIMAL STUDIES

Absorption, distribution, metabolism, and excretion experiments in rodents and dogs have shown that EGCG is rapidly absorbed (74–79). The oral bioavailability of tea catechins has been found to be low in rodents. Results from the animal studies have shown the relative bioavailability to be 1.6% at a low dose (75 mg/kg body weight) and 13.9% at higher doses (250 mg/kg and 400 mg/kg). C_{max} and the AUC–time curve increased more than dose proportionally at lower doses of EGCG but leveled off at higher doses. T_{max} was reached after 60 to 115 minutes. The $t_{1/2}$ was approximately 2.2 hours after intravenous administration and 5 to 6 hours after oral administration. EGCG was characterized as having a high clearance (about 68 ml/min per kg), with a volume of distribution of approximately 2.2 l/kg. Animal studies have assessed the safety of EGCG consumption. No genotoxic effects were found in studies on mice and rats at EGCG concentrations comparable to those reported in human studies (80).

There was no indication of a teratogenic effect when EGCG was administered in the diets of rats during organogenesis at doses delivering up to a nominal 1000 mg EGCG/kg per day. The preliminary study in which EGCG was administered by subcutaneous injection provided supporting evidence of the absence of teratogenicity (81).

EGCG CLINICAL TRIALS

Safety, Toxicity, and Pharmacokinetics

Formulation of EGCG has become critical as purified EGCG is considered to be too costly for clinical use and is poorly absorbed, and tolerance has become an issue because of the caffeine content (47, 82, 83). Investigators have used supplemental or synthetic forms of EGCG and other tea catechins to help characterize dose-response kinetics and other biologic effects and to promote the design and development of chemopreventive drug candidates based on EGCG.

A decaffeinated supplemental preparation of tea catechins, Polyphenon® E, developed by the Division of Cancer Prevention (DCP) Chemoprevention Branch at the National Cancer Institute (NCI) and in conjunction with Mitsui Norin Co., Ltd., contains approximately 50% EGCG and 30% other catechins. In a phase I pharmacokinetic study of Polyphenon® E, 20 human subjects were given single-dose administration of 200, 400, 600, or 800 mg EGCG, with each capsule containing 200 mg of EGCG and 68 mg of other catechins. Peak plasma EGCG levels of 200 to 400 ng/ml ($0.4–0.8\,\mu$M) could be achieved after the administration of these formulations at doses equivalent to the EGCG content in 8 to 16 cups of green tea (depending on the cup size) (53).

A subsequent in-depth study of the safety and plasma kinetics of multiple-dose administration of purified EGCG and Polyphenon® E was performed. This study examined once-daily and twice-daily dosing regimens of EGCG and Polyphenon® E over a four-week period in 40 healthy volunteers (52). In this study, standardized, defined, and decaffeinated green tea polyphenol oral products in amounts similar to the EGCG content in 16 Japanese-style cups of green tea were consumed once daily or in divided doses twice daily (four capsules/day) for four weeks. EGCG intake at doses of 400 mg twice daily and 800 mg once daily established peak serum concentrations averaging 150 to 290 ng/mL. Peak concentrations were reached between 2.4 and 4.2 hours. Once-daily dosing of 800 mg resulted in approximately a 60% increase in the systemic exposure of free EGCG after chronic Polyphenon® E administration. Purified EGCG and Polyphenon® E were administered with food in these studies. All adverse events during the four-week period were rated as mild and overall were similar to placebo. Abdominal discomfort (19%) was the most frequent adverse event. Other side effects included headache (6%), excess gas (6%), and dizziness (6%) (52).

On the basis of the reported adverse events and clinical laboratory data in this trial, the study agents and dosing schedules have been found to be safe and well tolerated by the study subjects for at least one month. The reported adverse events were rated as mild events. The more common events include headache, stomachache, abdominal pain, and nausea, which have been reported in subjects receiving green tea polyphenol treatment as well as in subjects receiving placebo. There were no significant changes in blood counts and blood chemistry profiles after four weeks of green tea polyphenol treatment (52).

Fasting

As a significant fraction of the orally administered green tea catechin is either not absorbed or is eliminated presystemically, Chow et al. performed a randomized, single-dose, crossover pharmacokinetic study of Polyphenon® E in 30 healthy individuals comparing dosing with food and under fasting conditions (84). In this study, taking Polyphenon® E at 400, 800, or 1200 mg on an empty stomach after an overnight fast resulted in a dramatic increase in the blood levels of free EGCG. Fasting peak concentrations occurred between 1.0 and 2.0 hours. AUC and C_{max} were 2.3 to 3.5 times and 3.6 to 5.6 times higher, respectively, when taken on an empty stomach. Fasting doses were also generally well tolerated, with grade 1 or 2 nausea being the most frequent adverse effect, occurring in approximately 36% of subjects. Other side effects included abdominal discomfort (10%), headache (10%), dyspepsia (3%), diarrhea (7%), gas (3%), and rash (3%). Results showed that greater oral bioavailability of free catechins can be achieved by taking Polyphenon® E on an empty stomach after an overnight fast. Polyphenon® E up to a dose that contains 800 mg EGCG is well tolerated when taken under the fasting condition. This dosing condition is also expected to optimize the biological effects of tea catechins (84).

Metabolism

After oral intake, EGCG undergoes extensive hepatic first-pass metabolism including glucuronidation, sulfation, and methylation. In humans, EGCG is present mainly in the free form in plasma. EGCG is degallated to EGC. EGC is detected mainly as the glucuronidated form (57%–71%) or sulfated form (23%–36%), with only a small amount present as the free form (3%–13%) (69). In addition to these conjugation reactions, EGCG and EGC undergo gut metabolism to form ring fission products (69), which are then further broken down by gut flora to phenylacetic and phenylpropionoic acids (79). EGCG is not detected in the urine after ingestion (53, 69). These data suggest that EGCG is not excreted in the urine but transported to the liver for excretion into bile and feces.

In a study by Ullman et al., a complete set of plasma kinetic data for single oral doses of pure EGCG capsules (94% crystalline bulk EGCG, Roche Vitamins, Ltd.) in the dose range of 50 to 1600 mg was assessed under fasting conditions in 60 healthy volunteers (85). The plasma kinetic profile of Roche bulk EGCG revealed a rapid absorption with a one-peak plasma concentration versus time course, followed by a distribution phase and an elimination phase. A dose linearity can be assumed for rate and extent. Single oral doses of Roche bulk EGCG up to 1600 mg were very well tolerated in this study, and no clinical or biological adverse events occurred (85). Other clinical studies have assessed the drug interactions of EGCG with cytochrome P450 activity or long-term EGCG dosing. Two studies showed no significant alteration in the disposition of medications primarily dependent on the CYP2D6 or CYP3A4 pathways of metabolism (86, 87).

Drug interactions may result from either pharmacokinetic or pharmacodynamic sources. Pharmacokinetic interactions can affect absorption, transport, distribution, metabolism, or elimination of a drug. Pharmacodynamic interactions alter the pharmacologic response to a drug but may not affect the drug's body concentrations. Risk of drug interactions of EGCG may be decreased due to minimal interaction with major cytochrome P450 (CYP) isozymes. Four weeks of Polyphenon® E 800 mg once daily did not change the activities of CYP1A2, CYP2D6, and CYP2C9 but inhibited CYP3A4 activity by approximately 20% compared to baseline (p = 0.01) (84). This is not likely to be clinically relevant. Lack of significant effect on CYP isozymes is beneficial, because of the 22 currently FDA-approved agents for HIV treatment, 14 are substrates, inducers, or inhibitors of CYP enzymes. These results suggest that EGCG administration may be less likely to affect the pharmacokinetics of commonly used pharmaceutical drugs, in particular many of the available ARV agents; however, it could enhance the detoxification of compounds that are significantly glucuronidated. Of the available ARVs, at least five are either primary substrates for UDP glucuronosyltransferases (UGT) or increase/inhibit UGT activity and thus may be a potential source for drug interactions. Effects of EGCG on drug transporters are currently unknown.

Cancer Studies

A phase I clinical trial of EGCG dosing of 600 mg daily for one year resulted in a 90% reduction in the rate of high-grade prostate intraepithelial neoplasia-positive men developing prostate cancer. No significant side effects were observed (88).

Doses of green tea extract (GTE) containing 13.2% EGCG, 6.8% caffeine, up to 5.05 g/m² per day GTE for up to six months have been evaluated in adults with solid tumors (54). Single doses of up to 1600 mg were generally well tolerated (89). In this study of 49 adult cancer patients, the maximum-tolerated dose was 4.2 g/m² once daily (6.1–9.9 g/day GTE) or 1.0 gm/m² three times daily (4.8–6.7 g/day GTE). At 4.2 gm/m² once daily, no notable increase in toxicity occurred compared to the 3.37 gm/m² once daily cohort. At 4.2 gm/m² once daily, the following adverse effects occurred in one out of six patients: polyphagia, vomiting, paresthesia, restlessness, and headache (all grade 1); fatigue and nausea (grade 2). Three out of six patients at 4.2 gm/m² once daily experienced grade 1 nausea. Dosing at 1.0 gm/m² three times daily was associated with similar adverse effects: grade 2 fatigue (1/8), grade 1 flatulence (1/8), grade 1 nausea (1/8), grade 1 agitation (2/8), grade 1 insomnia (2/8), and grade 1 headache (1/8). No hematologic toxicities were observed in this study. In follow-up laboratory examinations, no significant changes were found in serum chemistries, coagulation, electrocardiographs, or urinalysis. Many of the side effects seen in this study were attributed to the caffeine contained in the studied formulation.

Several case reports have implicated concentrated extracts of Chinese green tea (*Camellia sinesis*) in causing hepatotoxicity, usually with a mixed hepatocellular-cholestatic picture (90, 91). Cumulative amount of extract consumed ranged from 5.9 to 240 g. Most patients were younger than 40 years of age (8 of 11 cases) and women (9 of 11). Ten of 11 patients recovered after discontinuing the implicated substance. One patient required liver transplantation.

CONCLUSIONS

Overall, EGCG is the most prevalent compound found in GTEs. It has been shown to have significant in vitro anti-HIV-1 activity at physiologically achieved plasma concentrations.

A major drawback of present conventional ARV drugs is their high cost and unavailability in the Third World. A cheap, readily available, and safe treatment, such as could be provided by this complementary and alternative medicine, component of green tea, would have an enormous impact on public health. Proteins, monoclonal antibodies, and synthetic peptide formulations may be prohibitively expensive in the millimolar amounts likely to be needed per application, while the cost of making conventional small molecule inhibitors, such as EGCG, might not be unreasonable.

Until now, most of the FDA-approved anti-HIV drugs are HIV reverse transcriptase inhibitors (RTIs), including the nucleotide RTIs (NRTIs) and nonnucleotide RTIs (NNRTIs), and protease inhibitors (PIs), except for the first member of a new kind of anti-HIV drug, HIV entry inhibitors T-20 (92, 93). Clinical applications of these drugs in various combinations, known as ARV, have dramatically reduced the morbidity and mortality of AIDS and have significantly improved life expectancy for HIV-positive patients. However, substantial numbers of HIV-infected patients on ARV regimens cannot use the RTIs or PIs because of the emergence of drug-resistant HIV mutants and serious adverse effects. Thus, the development of new classes of anti-HIV drugs targeting different stages of HIV replication, such as HIV entry, integration, and maturation, is urgently needed (31).

Novel therapeutic complementary and alternative medicine has been found in natural products. One such candidate for complementary and alternative medicine is the green tea catechin, EGCG. EGCG, a naturally derived anti-HIV agent, has been shown to bind to the HIV-1-gp120 binding site on the CD4 molecule with sufficient affinity to prevent the HIV-1 virion from attaching to the target cell, CD4, thus inhibiting infection. The outcome of phase I clinical trials has established EGCG to be safe and well tolerated in healthy participants.

No studies to date have evaluated the safety, efficacy, and pharmacokinetic characteristics of EGCG in HIV-1-infected individuals. EGCG in the formulation Polyphenon® E is standardized and has the most clinical data to date in humans, especially regarding safety and pharmacokinetics. Based on these data, several potential doses of EGCG administered as Polyphenon® E have been selected as likely to achieve the concentrations previously shown in vitro to be necessary for anti-HIV-1 activity (0.2 to 5 mM = 92 to 2292 ng/mL), and Polyphenon® E has been selected as the formulation to be used in our phase I clinical study.

We are now poised to begin the next phase of the translational process to develop the green tea catechin, EGCG, as a complementary and alternative medicine in the management of HIV/AIDS. A phase I, dose-blinded, randomized, placebo-controlled clinical trial will be initiated to determine the safety, toxicity, dosing, and antiviral effects of EGCG in capsule form (Polyphenon® E), administered orally once or twice daily at three different doses in HIV-1-infected, clinically stable, treatment-naïve, and treatment-experienced adults not on concomitant ARV therapy. The results from this preliminary research in humans will lay a foundation for justification of larger clinical trials and the development and advancement of EGCG as a complementary and alternative medicine in the management of HIV/AIDS.

ACKNOWLEDGMENTS

The author wishes to thank Michael P. Williamson, Edward B. Siwak, Melinda P. D'Souza, and Rebecca A. Davis, all of whom were involved in various aspects of these studies. The original work reported was supported by Grant AT003084 from the National Center for Complementary and Alternative Medicine and AI 1036211 from the Center for AIDS Research, National Institute of Allergy and Infectious Diseases.

REFERENCES

[1]UNAIDS. AIDS epidemic update: December 2005. UNAIDS and WHO wwwunaidsorg/epi/2005/doc/ EPIupdate2005_pdf_en/epi- update2005_enpdf. 2005.

[2]Cohen M, Hellmann N, Levy J, DeCock K, Lange J. The spread, treatment, and prevention of HIV-1: evolution of a global pandemic. *J Clin Invest*. 2008;118(4):1244–1254.

[3]Walker B, Burton D. Toward an AIDS vaccine. *Science*. 2008;320:760–764.

[4]NIAID Fact Sheet: HIV infection in women, May 2003 and HIV/AIDS statistics, December 2002. (www .niadnih.gov/factsheets/womenhivhtm) (http://biodefenseniaidnihgov/factsheets/aid sstathtm). 2002.

[5]Doncel G, Mauck C. Vaginal microbicides: a novel approach to preventing sexual transmission of HIV. *Current HIV/AIDS Reports*. 2004;1:25–32.

[6]Kwong P, Wyatt R, Robinson J, Sweet R, Sodroski J, Hendrickson W. Structure of an HIV gp120 envelope glycoprotein in complex with the CD4 receptor and a neutralizing human antibody. *Nature*. 1998;393: 648–659.

[7]Berger E, Murphy P, Farber J. Chemokine receptors as HIV-1 coreceptors: roles in viral entry, tropism, and disease. *Annu Rev Immunol*. 1999;17:657–700.

[8]Levy J. Infection by human immunodeficiency virus-CD4 is not enough. *N Engl J Med*. 1996;335: 1528–1530.

[9]Campbell G, Spector S. CCL2 increases X4-tropic HIV-1 entry into resting CD4$^+$ T cells. *J Biol Chem*. In press 2008. p. 18.

[10]Sleasman JW, Goodenow MM. HIV-1 infection. *J Allergy Clin Immunol*. 2003 Feb;111(2 Suppl): S582–S592.

[11]Wei X, Decker JM, Wang S, Hui H, Kappes JC, Wu X, Salazar-Gonzalez JF, Salazar MG, Kilby JM, Saag MS, Komarova NL, Nowak MA, Hahn BH, Kwong PD, Shaw GM. Antibody neutralization and escape by HIV-1. *Nature*. 2003 Mar 20;422(6929):307–312.

[12]Chinen J, Shearer W. Molecular virology and immunology of HIV infection. *J Allergy Clin Immunol*. 2002;110:189–198.

[13]Chinen J, Shearer W. *Immune-Based Therapies for HIV Infection*. Shearer W, Hanson I, eds. Philadelphia, PA: Saunders/Elsevier Science; 2003.

[14]Lee J, Kim H, Lee Y. A new anti-HIV flavonoid glucuronide from Chrysanthemum morifolium. *Planta Med*. 2003;69:859–861.

[15]Wu J, Wang X, Yi Y, Lee K. Anti-AIDS agents 54. A potent anti-HIV chalcone and flavonoids from genus Desmos. *Bioorg Med Chem Lett*. 2003a;13:1813–1815.

[16]Cos P, Maes L, Vanden Berghe D, Hermans N, Pieters L, Vlietinck A. Plant substances as anti-HIV agents selected according to their putative mechanism of action. *J Nat Prod*. 2004;67:284–293.

[17]De Clercq E. Current lead natural products for the chemotherapy of human immunodeficiency virus (HIV) infection. *Med Res Rev*. 2000 Sep;20(5):323–349.

[18]Wang R, Gu Q, Wang Y, Zhang X, Yang L, Zhou J, Chen J, Zheng Y. Anti-HIV-1 activities of compounds isolated from the medicinal plant *Rhus chinensis*. *J Ethnopharmacol*. 2008;117(2):249–256.

[19]Patwardham B, Gautam M. Botanical immunodrugs: scope and opportunities. *Drug Discovery Today*. 2005;10:495–502.

[20]Asres K, Seyoum A, Veersham C, Bucar F, Gibbons S. Naturally derived anti-HIV agents. *Phytother Res*. 2005;19:557–581.

[21]NCI, DCPC Chemoprevention Branch and Agent Development Committee. Clinical development plant: tea extracts, green tea polyphenols, epigallocatechin gallate. *J Cell Biochem*. 1996;26:S236–S257.

[22]Dufresne C, Farnworth E. A review of latest reserach findings on the health promotion properties of tea. *J Nutr Biochem*. 2001;12:404–421.

[23]Deana R, Turetta L, Donella-Deana A, Dona M, Brunati AM, De Michiel L, Garbisa S. Green tea epigallocatechin-3-gallate inhibits platelet signalling pathways triggered by both proteolytic and non-proteolytic agonists. *Thromb Haemost*. 2003 May;89(5):866–874.

[24]Ludwig A, Lorenz M, Grimbo N, Steinle F, Meiners S, Bartsch C, Stangl K, Baumann G, Stangl V. The tea flavonoid epigallocatechin-3-gallate reduces cytokine-induced VCAM-1 expression and monocyte adhesion to endothelial cells. *Biochem Biophys Res Commun*. 2004 Apr 9;316(3):659–665.

[25]Sakata R, Ueno T, Nakamura T, Sakamoto M, Torimura T, Sata M. Green tea polyphenol epigallocatechin-3-gallate inhibits platelet-derived growth factor-induced proliferation of human hepatic stellate cell line LI90. *J Hepatol*. 2004 Jan;40(1):52–59.

[26]Nakachi K, Matsuyama S, Miyake S, Suganuma M, Imai K. Preventive effects of drinking green tea on cancer and cardiovascular disease: epidemiological evidence for multiple targeting prevention. *Biofactors*. 2000;13(1–4):49–54.

[27]Yang C, Landau J. Effects of tea consumption on nutrition and health. *J Nutr.* 2000;130:2409–2412.

[28]Havsteen B. The biochemistry and medical significance of the flavonoids. *Pharmacol Ther.* 2002;96: 67–202.

[29]Nair M, Kandaswami C, Mahajan S, Nair H, Chawda R, Shanahan T, Schwartz S. Grape seed extract proanthocyanidins downregulate HIV-1 entry coreceptors, CCR2b, CCR3 and CCR5 gene expression by normal peripheral blood mononuclear cells. *Biol Res.* 2002;35:421–431.

[30]Leung L, Su Y, Chen R, Zhang Z, Huang Y, Chen Z. Theaflavins in black tea and catechins in green tea are equally effective antioxidants. *J Nutr.* 2001;131:2248–2251.

[31]Liu S, Lu H, Zhao Q, He Y, Niu J, Debnath AK, Wu S, Jiang S. Theaflavin derivatives in black tea and catechin derivatives in green tea inhibit HIV-1 entry by targeting gp41. *Biochimica et Biophysica Acta.* 2005; 1723:270–281.

[32]Sartippour M, Heber D, Ma J, Lu Q, Go V, Nguyen M. Green tea and its catechins inhibit breast cancer xenografts. *Nutr Cancer.* 2001;40:149–156.

[33]NCI. Clinical development plan: tea extracts. Green tea polyphenols. Epigallocatechin gallate. *J Cell Biochem Suppl.* 1996;26:236–257.

[34]Kemberling J, Hampton J, Keck R, Gomez M, Selman S. Inhibition of bladder tumor growth by the green tea derivative epigallocatechin-3-gallate. *J Urol.* 2003;170:773–776.

[35]Adhami V, Ahmad N, Mukhtar H. Molecular targets for green tea in prostate cancer prevention. *J Nutr.* 2003;133:2417S–2424S.

[36]Landau J, Wang Z, Yang G, Ding W, Yang C. Inhibition of spontaneous formation of lung tumors and rhabdomyosarcomas in A/J mice by black and green tea. *Carcinogenesis.* 1998;19:501–507.

[37]Liao J, Yang G, Park E, Meng X, Sun Y, Jia D, Seril D, Yang C. Inhibition of lung carcinogenesis and effects on angiogenesis and apoptosis in A/J mice by oral administration of green tea. *Nutr Cancer.* 2004;48: 44–53.

[38]Mittal A, Piyathilkae C, Hara Y, Katiyar S. Exceptionally high protection of photocarcinogenesis by topical application of (–)-epigallocatechin-3-gallate in hydrophilic cream in SKH-1 hairless mouse model: relationship to inhibition of UVB-induced global DNA hypomethylation. *Neoplasia.* 2003;5:555–565.

[39]Zhang G, Miura Y, Yagasaki K. Effects of dietary powdered green tea and theanine on tumor growth and endogenous hyperlipidemia in hepatoma-bearing rats. *Biosci Biotechnol Biochem.* 2002;66:711–716.

[40]Umemura T, Kai S, Hasegawa R, Kanki K, Kitamura Y, Nishikawa A, Hirose M. Prevention of dual promoting effects of pentachlorophenol, an environmental pollutant, on diethylnitrosamine-induced hepato-and cholangiocarcinogenesis in mice by green tea infusion. *Carcinogenesis.* 2003;24:1105–1109.

[41]Kohlmeier L, Weterings KG, Steck S, Kok FJ. Tea and cancer prevention: an evaluation of the epidemiologic literature. *Nutr Cancer.* 1997;27(1):1–13.

[42]Mukhtar H, Ahmad N. Tea polyphenols: prevention of cancer and optimizing health. *Am J Clin Nutr.* 2000;71:1698s–1702s.

[43]Higdon J, Frei B. Tea catechins and polyphenols: health effects, metabolism, and antioxidant functions. *Crit Rev Food Sci Nutr.* 2003;43(1):89–143.

[44]Okubo S, Sasaki T, Hara Y, Mori F, Shimamura T. Bactericidal and anti-toxin activities of catechin on enterohemorrhagic *Escherichia coli. J Jpn Assoc Infect Dis.* 1997;72(3):211–217.

[45]Fassina G, Buffa A, Benelli R, Varnier OE, Noonan DM, Albini A. Polyphenolic antioxidant (–)-epigallocatechin-3-gallate from green tea as a candidate anti-HIV agent. *AIDS.* 2002 Apr 12;16(6): 939–941.

[46]Yamaguchi K, Honda M, Ikigai H, Hara Y, Shimamura T. Inhibitory immunodeficiency virus type 1 (HIV-1). *Antiviral Res.* 2002 Jan;53(1):19–34.

[47]Lambert JD, Yang CS. Mechanisms of cancer prevention by tea constituents. *J Nutr.* 2003 Oct;133(10): 3262S–3267S.

[48]Zaveri NT. Synthesis of a 3,4,5-trimethoxybenzoyl ester analogue of epigallocatechin-3-gallate (EGCG): a potential route to the natural product green tea catechin, EGCG. *Org Lett.* 2001 Mar 22;3(6):843– 846.

[49]Lee MJ, Maliakal P, Chen L, Meng X, Bondoc FY, Prabhu S, Lambert G, Mohr S, Yang CS. Pharmacokinetics of tea catechins after ingestion of green tea and (–)-epigallocatechin-3-gallate by humans: formation of different metabolites and individual variability. *Cancer Epidemiol Biomarkers Prev.* 2002 Oct;11: 1025–1032.

[50]Sartippour MR, Shao ZM, Heber D, Beatty P, Zhang L, Liu C, Ellis L, Liu W, Go VL, Brooks MN. Green tea inhibits vascular endothelial growth factor (VEGF) induction in human breast cancer cells. *J Nutr.* 2002 Aug;132(8):2307–2311.

[51]Maeda-Yamamoto M, Kawahara H, Tahara N, Tsuji K, Hara Y, Isemura M. Effects of tea polyphenols on the invasion and matrix metalloproteinases activities of human fibrosarcoma HT1080 cells. *J Agric Food Chem.* 1999 Jun;47(6):2350–2354.

[52]Chow HH, Cai Y, Hakim IA, Crowell JA, Shahi F, Brooks CA, Dorr RT, Hara Y, Alberts DS. Pharmacokinetics and safety of green tea polyphenols after multiple-dose administration of epigallocatechin gallate and polyphenon E in healthy individuals. *Clin Cancer Res.* 2003 Aug 15;9(9):3312–3319.

[53]Chow H, Cai Y, Alberts D, Hakim I, Dorrl R, Shahi F, Crowell J, Yang C, Hara Y. Phase I pharmacokinetic study of tea polyphenols following single-dose administration of epigallocatechin gallate and polyphenon E. *Cancer Epidemiol Biomarkers Prev.* 2001;10:53–58.

[54]Pisters K, Newman R, Coldman B, Shin D, Khuri F, Hong W, Glisson B, Lee J. Phase I trial of oral green tea extract in adult patients with solid tumors. *J Clin Oncol.* 2001;19:1830–1838.

[55]Sugaya M, Lore K, Koup R, Douek DC, Blauvelt A. HIV-infected Langerhans cells preferentially transmit virus to proliferating autologous CD4+ memory T cells located within Langerhans cell-T cell clusters. *J Immunol.* 2004;172:2219–2224.

[56]Nance C, Shearer W. Is green tea good for HIV-1 infection? *J Allergy Clin Immunol.* 2003;112(5):851–853.

[57]Kawai K, Tsuno NH, Kitayama J, Okaji Y, Yazawa K, Asakage M, Hori N, Watanabe T, Takahashi K, Nagawa H. Epigallocatechin gallate, the main component of tea polyphenol, binds to CD4 and interferes with gp120 binding. *J Allergy Clin Immunol.* 2003 Nov;112(5):951–957.

[58]Arthos J, Deen KC, Chaikin MA, Fornwald JA, Sathe G, Sattentau QJ, Clapham PR, Weiss RA, McDougal JS, Pietropaolo C, et al. Identification of the residues in human CD4 critical for the binding of HIV. *Cell.* 1989 May 5;57(3):469–481.

[59]Williamson MP, McCormick TG, Nance CL, Shearer WT. Epigallocatechin gallate, the main polyphenol in green tea, binds to the T-cell receptor, CD4: Potential for HIV-1 therapy. *J Allergy Clin Immunol.* 2006;118:1369–1374.

[60]Ho DD, McKeating JA, Li XL, Moudgil T, Daar ES, Sun NC, Robinson JE. Conformational epitope on gp120 important in CD4 binding and human immunodeficiency virus type 1 neutralization identified by a human monoclonal antibody. *J Virol.* 1991 Jan;65(1):489–493.

[61]Wu H, Myszka DG, Tendian SW, Brouillette CG, Sweet RW, Chaiken IM, Hendrickson WA. Kinetic and structural analysis of mutant CD4 receptors that are defective in HIV gp120 binding. *Proc Natl Acad Sci USA.* 1996 Dec 24;93(26):15030–15035.

[62]Charlton AJ, Baxter NJ, Khan ML, Moir AJ, Haslam E, Davies AP, Williamson MP. Polyphenol/peptide binding and precipitation. *J Agric Food Chem.* 2002 Mar 13;50(6):1593–1601.

[63]Charlton AJ, Haslam E, Williamson MP. Multiple conformations of the proline-rich protein/epigallocatechin gallate complex determined by time-averaged nuclear Overhauser effects. *J Am Chem Soc.* 2002 Aug 21;124(33):9899–9905.

[64]Hamza A, Zhan CG. How can (–)-epigallocatechin gallate from green tea prevent HIV-1 infection? mechanistic insights from computational modeling and the implication for rational design of anti-HIV-1 entry inhibitors. *J Phys Chem B.* 2005;110:2910–2917.

[65]Benie AJ, Moser B, Bauml E, Blaas D, Peters T. Virus-ligand interactions: identification and characterization of ligand binding by NMR spectroscopy. *J Am Chem Soc.* 2003;125(1):14–15.

[66]Mayer M, Meyer B. Group epitope mapping by saturation transfer difference NMR to identify segments of a ligand in direct contact with a protein receptor. *J Am Chem Soc.* 2001 Jun 27;123(25):6108–6117.

[67]Meyer B, Peters T. NMR spectroscopy techniques for screening and identifying ligand binding to protein receptors. *Angew Chem Int Ed Engl.* 2003 Feb 24;42(8):864–890.

[68]McCutchan F. Understanding the genetic diversity of HIV-1. *AIDS.* 2000;14(Suppl3):S31–S44.

[69]Lee M, Wang Z, Li H, Chen L, Sun Y, Gobbo S, Balentine D, Yang C. Analysis of plasma and urinary tea polyphenols in human subjects. *Cancer Epidemiology, Biomarkers and Prevention.* 1995;4:393–399.

[70]Behr M, Small P. Inhibition of carcinogenesis by tea. *Nature.* 1997;389:134–135.

[71]Palella Jr. F, Delaney K, Moorman A, Loveless M, Fuhrer J, Satten G, Aschman D, Holmberg S. Declining morbidity and mortality among patients with advanced human immunodeficiency virus infection. *N Engl J Med.* 1998;338:853–860.

[72]Siliciano J, Kajdas J, Finzi D, Quinn T, Chadwick K, Margolick J, Kovacs C, Gange S, Siliciano R. Long-term follow-up studies confirm the stability of the latent reservoir for HIV-1 in resting CD4 T cells. *Nat Med.* 2003;9:727–728.

[73]Grant R, Hecht F, Warmerdam M, Liu L, Liegler T, Petropoulos C, Hellmannn N, Chesney M, Busch M, Kahn J. Time trends in primary HIV-1 drug resistance among recently infected persons. *JAMA.* 2002;288: 181–188.

[74]Swezey R, Aldridge D, LeValley S, Crowell, JA, Hara Y, Green CE. Absorption, tissue distribution and elimination of 4-[(3)h]-epigallocatechin gallate in beagle dogs. *Int J Toxicol.* 2003;22:1887–1893.

[75]Unno T, Takeo T. Absorption of (–)-epigallocatechin gallate into the circulation system of rats. *Biosci Biotechnol Biochem.* 1995;59:1558–1559.

[76]Nackagawa K, Miyazawa T. Absorption and distribution of tea catechin (–)-epigallocatechin-3-gallate in the rat. *J Nutr Sci Vitaminol.* 1997;43:679–684.

[77]Zuhu M, Chen Y, Li R. Oral absorption and bio-availability of tea catechins. *Planta Med.* 2000;66: 444–447.

[78]Kim D, Lim J. Pharmacokinetic study of epigallocatechin gallate in rats. *J Kor Pharm Sci.* 1999;29: 179–184.

[79]Chen L, Lee M, Li H, Yang C. Absorption, distribution and elimination of tea polyphenols in rats. *Drug Metab Dispos.* 1997;25:1045–1050.

[80]Isbrucker RA, Bausch J, Edwards JA, Wolz E. Safety studies on epigallocatechin gallate (EGCG) preparations. Part 1: genotoxicity. *Food and Chem Toxicology.* 2006;44:626–635.

[81]Isbrucker RA, Edwards JA, Wolz E, Davidovich A, Bausch J. Safety studies on epigallocatechin gallate (EGCG) preparations. Part 3: teratogenicity and reproductive toxicity studies in rats. *Food Chem Toxicol.* 2006;44:651–661.

[82]Fujiki H, Suganuma M, Imai K, Nakachi K. Green tea: cancer preventive beverage and/or drug. *Cancer Lett.* 2002 Dec 15;188(1–2):9–13.

[83]Fujiki H, Suganuma M, Okabe S, Sueoka E, Sueoka N, Fujimoto N, Goto Y, Matsuyama S, Imai K, Nakachi K. Cancer prevention with green tea and monitoring by a new biomarker, hnRNP B1. *Mutat Res.* 2001 Sep 1;480–81:299–304.

[84]Chow HH, Hakim I, Vining DR, Crowell JA, Ranger-Moore J, Chew WM, Celaya CA, Rodney SR, Hara Y, Alberts DS. Effects of dosing condition on the oral bioavailability of green tea catechins after single- dose administration of polyphenon E in healthy individuals. *Clin Cancer Res.* 2005;11(12):4627–4633.

[85]Ullman U, Haller J, Decourt J, Girault N, Girault J, Richard-Caudron A, Pineua B, Weber P. A single ascending dose study of epigallocatechin gallate in healthy volunteers. *J Int Med Res.* 2003;31:88–101.

[86]Chow HH, Hakim I, Vining DR, Crowell J, Cordova CA, Chew WM, Xu M, Hsu C, Ranger-Moore J, Alberts D. Effects of repeated green tea catechin administration on human cytochrome P450 activity. *Cancer Epidemiol Biomarkers Prev.* 2006;15(12):2473–2476.

[87]Donovan J, Chavin K, DeVane C, Taylor R, Wang J, Ruan Y, Markowitz J. Green tea (Camellia sinensis) extract does not alter cytochrome P45o 3A4 or 2D6 activity in healthy volunteers. *DMD.* 2004;32(9):906–908.

[88]Bettuzzi S, Brausi M, Rizzi F, Castagnetti G, Peracchia G, Corti A. Chemoprevention of human prostate cancer by oral administration of green tea catechins in volunteers with high-grade prostate intraepithelial neoplasia: a preliminary report from a one-year proof-of-principle study. *Cancer Res.* 2006;66(2):1234–1240.

[89]Sleasman JW, Goodenow MM. HIV-1 infection. *J Allergy Clin Immunol.* 2003;111(2):S582–S592.

[90]Gloro R, Hourmand-Ollivier I, Mosquet B, Mosquet L, Rousselot R, Salame E, Piquet M, Dao T. Fulminant hepatitis during self-medication with hydroalcoholic extract of green tea. *Eur J Gastroenterol Hepatol.* 2005;17(10):1135–1137.

[91]Bonkovsky HL. Hepatotoxicity associated with supplements containing Chinese green tea (Camellia sinensis). *Ann Intern Med.* 2006;144(1):68–71.

[92]De Clercq E. Antiviral drugs in current clinical use. *J Clin Virol.* 2004;30:115–133.

[93]Moore JP, Doms RW. The entry of entry inhibitors: a fusion of science and medicine. *PNAS.* 2003 Sept 16, 2003;100(19):10598–10602.

Chapter 6

Curcuminoids from *Curcuma longa* in Disease Prevention and Treatment

Vladimir Badmaev

CHRONIC INFLAMMATION

Inflammation as a lingering rather than an acute process is increasingly important for researchers and clinicians from diversified fields of medicine. Chronic inflammation is considered an underlying pathology of many diseases that remain poorly understood or treated. Cardiovascular disease, a leading cause of mortality in the world, is no longer considered as only a disorder of lipid accumulation but also as a disease process characterized by low-grade inflammation of the endothelial cells and an inappropriate healing response of the vascular lining (1). Cancer is another chronic degenerative disease that is initiated and promoted by lingering inflammation, often triggered by environmental or nutritional factors (2). Similarly, the neurodegenerative conditions, for example, Alzheimer's disease, are hypothesized as being caused by dysfunction of the immune system reacting to chronic inflammation of the central nervous system (3).

Several epidemiological and laboratory studies have demonstrated that patients with clinically different diseases may have a similar pattern of elevated serum levels of inflammatory biomarkers including nuclear factor kappa beta (NF-κB), interleukin-6 (IL-6), cyclooxygenase enzymes (COX-1 and COX-2), tumor necrosis factor-alpha (TNF-alpha), cell adhesion molecules, for example, intercellular adhesion molecule-1 and P-selectin, and acute-phase proteins including C-reactive protein (CRP), fibrinogen, and amyloid (1, 2, 3). Dysregulation of tumor necrosis factor, or TNF, has been implicated in a wide variety of inflammatory diseases including rheumatoid arthritis, Crohn's disease, multiple sclerosis, psoriasis, scleroderma, atopic dermatitis, systemic lupus erythematosus, type 2 diabetes, atherosclerosis, myocardial infarction, osteoporosis, and autoimmune deficiency disease. TNF upregulates nuclear factor kappa beta (NF-κB is critically important as a transcription factor for the expression of TNF), and it also mediates its biological effects through activation of caspases,

Sabinsa Corporation, Piscataway, New Jersey 08854; vebadmaev@attglobal.net
Dedicated to the pioneering work of Dr. Muhammed Majeed and Sami Labs and the Sabinsa team in introducing Ayurvedic standardized botanicals to the West.

activator protein 1 (AP-1, a transcription factor needed for expression of TNF), c-jun N-terminal kinase (JNK, which belongs to mitogen-activated protein kinases [MAPK]), p38 mitogen-activated protein kinases (p38 MAPK), and p44/p42 MAPK. These changes in levels and activity of biomarkers may signal a chronic inflammatory process in a high-risk group of patients predisposed to or suffering from a degenerative disease and cancer.

Although synthetic drugs effectively reduce inflammation and pain in both acute and chronic inflammatory conditions, they work in a very selective way that may be counterproductive to the purpose of treatment. Recent research reveals that selective COX-2 inhibitor drugs may induce metabolic imbalances that can result in the overproduction of toxic cytokines, TNF-alpha, and certain interleukins that are involved in the inflammatory process (4).

In the emerging trend to search for natural therapies, turmeric root, ginger root, rosemary leaves, green tea leaves, and their respective active phytochemical constituents are reported to be effective COX-2 inhibitors that also may inhibit the formation of inflammatory leukotrienes and toxic cytokines. These botanicals, unlike synthetic COX-2 enzyme inhibitors, do not irritate the gastrointestinal lining and generally have a safe record of traditional use spanning centuries. Furthermore, no adverse effects have been reported with these botanical preparations in clinical studies performed to validate their therapeutic properties. In fact,

Table 6.1. Comparison of Cancer Incidence in U.S. (Curcumin Non-Users) and India (Curcumin Users)

	U.S.		India	
Cancer	Cases	Deaths	Cases	Deaths
Breast	660	160	79	41
Prostate	690	130	20	9
Colon/rectum	530	220	30	18
Lung	660	580	38	37
Head and neck SCC	140	44	153	103
Liver	41	44	12	13
Pancreas	108	103	8	8
Stomach	81	50	33	30
Melanoma	145	27	1.8	1
Testis	21	1	3	1
Bladder	202	43	15	11
Kidney	115	44	6	4
Brain, nervous system	65	47	19	14
Thyroid	55	5	12	3
Endometrial cancers	163	41	132	72
Ovary	76	50	20	12
Multiple myeloma	50	40	6	5
Leukemia	100	70	19	17
Non-Hodgkin's lymphoma	180	90	17	15
Hodgkin's disease	20	5	7	4

Showing cases per 1 million persons calculated on the basis of current consensus: endometrial cancers include Cervix uteri and Corpus uteri.

Source: GLOBOCAN 2000: Cancer Incidence, Mortality and Prevalence Worldwide, Version 1.0. IARC Cancer Base No. 5. Lyon, IARC Press, 2001.

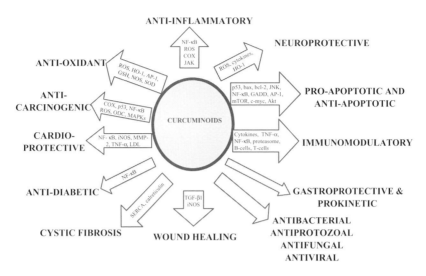

Figure 6.1. Mode of Action of Curcuminoids

Acknowledgment: Gescher Andy, University of Leicester, UK

many of the compounds found in the extracts are on the U.S. Food and Drug Administration (FDA) GRAS (generally recognized as safe) list of compounds that are safe to use in daily nutrition. In this regard, based on the current body of scientific evidence, turmeric's (curry) curcuminoids are considered the most promising food-derived compounds to fight inflammation and related diseases (5, 6) (Table 6.1).

There is a significant amount of research conducted on the health benefits of curcuminoids summarized in Figure 6.1. In this chapter the potential for curcuminoids in inflammatory processes will be discussed. In view of the efficacy and apparently low toxicity of curcuminoids, securing a predictable delivery of curcuminoids to the target tissue(s) will be essential to fulfill their promise for medicinal food or novel drug applications in prevention and treatment of inflammatory and neoplastic diseases.

STANDARDIZATION OF TURMERIC'S CURCUMINOIDS

Curcumin (chemically diferuloylmethane) and its derivatives demethoxycurcumin and bisdemethoxycurcumin, collectively known as curcuminoids, are responsible for the yellow pigment derived from the roots of the perennial herb turmeric (*Curcuma longa* L. Family *Zingiberaceae*) (Figure 6.2). The same ground, dried roots of turmeric, which have been used for centuries as a spice (curry), a food preservative, and a coloring agent, have been found to be a rich source of phenolic compounds (curcuminoids) with versatile biological mechanisms (6) and (6a). In dietary supplement practice and in a growing body of scientific research, an extract of turmeric roots is now being utilized that is standardized for a high purity of curcuminoids, for example, 95% curcuminoids, devoid of environmental contaminants (7–22). The standardization is achieved on the basis of the content of a group of bioactives, that is, curcuminoids, by a high-pressure liquid chromatography (HPLC) method, resulting in the following combination:

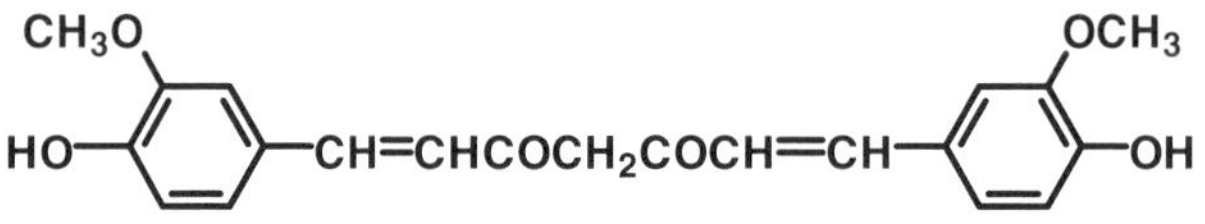

CURCUMIN *Diferuloyl methane*

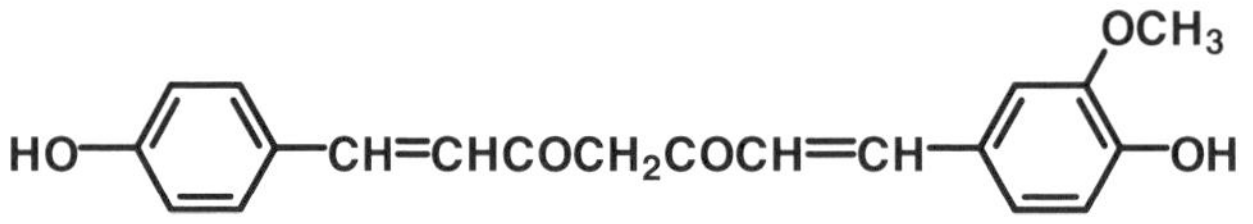

DEMETHOXY CURCUMIN *p-Hydroxy-cinnamoyl-feruloyl-methane*

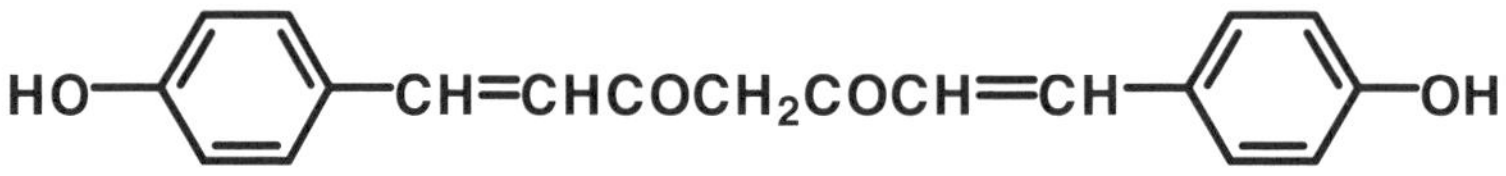

BISDEMETHOXY CURCUMIN *pp'-Dihydroxy-dicinnamoyl-methane*

Figure 6.2. Chemical Structures of Curcuminoids

(total curcuminoids not less than 95.0% calculated on dried basis)
(bisdemethoxy curcumin not less than 2.5% and not more than 6.5%)
(demethoxycurcumin not less than 15.0% and not more than 25.0%)
(curcumin not less than 70.0% and more than 80.0%)

but also based on limits for various quality parameters such as the ash content (no more than 1.0%), melting range (172–178°C), bulk density (0.5 g/ml), sieve values (standard size of the particles of the extract), solubility in water (insoluble in water) and organic solvents (slightly soluble in alcohol, soluble in acetone and glacial acetic acid), microbial (total microbial count < 100 cfu/g and absence of pathogenic bacteria) and mold and yeast (< 10 cfu/g) loads, residual solvents from the extraction process, and pesticide (e.g., in Japan there is a list of 183 pesticides for which curcuminoids have to test negative) and aflatoxin levels (have to be < 20 ppb).

The limits for heavy metals (total heavy metals under 10 ppm, arsenic < 1 ppm, lead < 0.5 ppm) are an important quality control and standardization parameter. There are two possible sources of heavy metals in the turmeric extract. The first one is the plant's ability to absorb from the soil, that is, "naturally occurring." The second is contamination from the process (equipment, process water, and the solvents and chemicals used in the manufacture).

CURCUMINOIDS IN TREATMENT OF CANCER

Potential Mechanisms of Action

In the last three years alone, several pioneering IND (Investigational New Drug) studies have been granted by the FDA and other studies funded by the National Institutes of Health to investigate curcumin and its derivatives in the treatment of patients with cancer (16, 17, 18). Some of the leading clinical research centers in the United States, including MD

Anderson Hospital in Houston, Texas, are involved in preclinical and clinical research of the anticancer mechanism and application of curcuminoids in conditions including multiple myeloma and colon, pancreatic, breast, prostate, head and neck, and respiratory tract cancers. These cancer conditions are either currently being studied in clinical experiments or considered next in line for systematic evaluation with curcuminoid therapy.

Curcuminoids act by inhibiting several processes that contribute to the survival, proliferation, invasion, and metastasis of tumor cells (23). Curcuminoids act by interfering with signaling mechanisms (critical for tumor growth), regulation of apoptosis, and tumor angiogenesis. Current research is designed to determine which of these fundamental processes in cancer development account for the clinical effects of curcumin and its derivatives.

Curcuminoids have significant immunomodulating and anti-inflammatory effects, in part caused by the inhibition of cyclooxygenase type 2 enzyme (COX-2) and its subsequent arachidonic acid metabolism (24, 25). Curcuminoids, like several other immunomodulators, inhibit the activation of the nuclear factor kappa-B (NF-κB) family of transcription factors that are known to be activated in a wide variety of solid tumors, lymphomas, and leukemias (26, 27, 28) (Graph 6.1, Table 6.2). The activation of NF-κB may shield tumor cells from apoptosis, or programmed cell death, and promote tumor growth factors and those factors that facilitate invasion and metastasis of tumors. Curcuminoids block the NF-κB–mediated gene expression responsible for the chain of events leading to tumor development, progression, and expansion. A probable mechanism of curcuminoids appears to be blocking the degradation of the inhibitors of NF-κB (Graph 6.1; 26). In vitro, curcuminoids induce apoptosis and thus inhibit tumor growth in a broad range of tumor cells, including cell lines from colon, breast, prostate, squamous cell, renal cell, and hepatocellular carcinomas; B- and T-cell lymphomas; leukemias; melanoma; and sarcoma cells (29).

Curcuminoids also affect a signaling mechanism that involves expression and activation of certain growth factor receptors that promote tumor growth. For example, HER-2/neu is

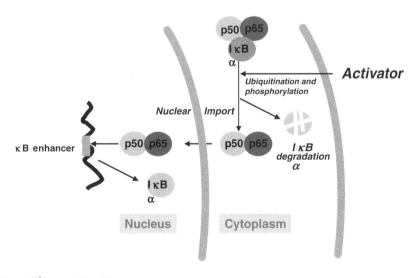

Graph 6.1. What Is NF-κB?

Source: *Leukemia*. 2002 Jun;16(6):1053–1068

Table 6.2. Tumors Linked to NF-κB Expression

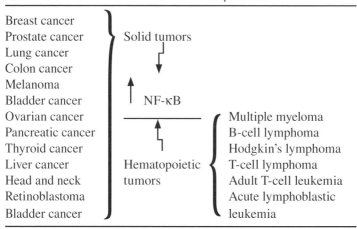

Source: *Curr. Opin. Oncol.* 2003; 15(6): 405–411.

a member of the Epidermal Growth Factor Receptor family, which is overexpressed in approximately 30% of breast cancer patients. HER-2/neu–positive breast cancer cells, when exposed to curcumin, were found to have decreased expression of the HER-2 receptor (29, 30, 31).

This ability makes curcumin a promising agent for combination with paclitaxel (Taxol) (29). The drug Taxol is derived from the Pacific yew tree and is produced semisynthetically using a combination of fermentation and synthesis. It is used as first-line chemotherapy in breast cancer. It induces the apoptosis of breast tumor cell lines, but overexpression of HER-2/neu may block these apoptotic effects and induce resistance to Taxol. Further, HER-2/neu and Taxol can activate antiapoptotic pathways through activation of NF-κB. Thus, agents such as curcuminoids that can down-regulate activation of NF-κB and decrease HER-2/neu overexpression and other markers of tumorigenesis may augment the therapeutic effects of Taxol against breast cancer (Figure 6.3).

Interestingly, curcuminoids may have a comparable mechanism of action to the drug therapy involving Herceptin for breast cancer patients with HER-2 receptor–positive cancer cells. Herceptin is an antibody against HER-2 receptors, binding, blocking, and inactivating those receptors. In vitro, the growth of breast cancer cells with multidrug resistance (MDR) characteristics is inhibited by these turmeric phenolics; the stimulation of estrogen receptor (ER)–positive cell lines by estrogenic pesticides is also inhibited by curcuminoids (31, 32). Curcuminoids have also been found to inhibit epidermal growth factor receptor expression or activation in skin cancer cell lines as well as in androgen-sensitive and androgen-insensitive prostate cancer cell lines (33).

An important anticancer mechanism of curcuminoids is restriction of vital blood supply to the rapidly growing tumor (34, 35). In vitro, these compounds inhibit the blood vessel endothelial and smooth muscle cell growth and proliferation, which is the basis for inhibition of angiogenesis (new blood vessel formation). Curcuminoids also inhibit new vessel formation induced by growth factors, such as fibroblast growth factor-2 (FGF-2) (34). Furthermore, curcuminoids inhibit the production of vascular endothelial growth factor (VEGF) in human melanoma cells (36). The antiangiogenic effect of turmeric compounds

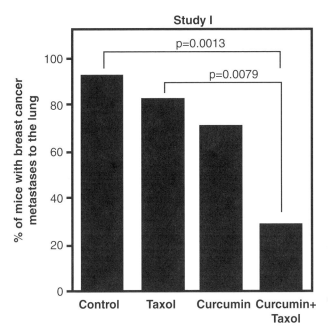

Figure 6.3. Effect of Curcumin, Taxol, or Their Combination on Breast Cancer Metastasis to the Lung

Source: *Clin Cancer Res.* 2005 Oct 15;11(20):7490–7498.

can be explained by the aforementioned selective COX-2 inhibition with curcuminoids. COX-2 enzyme activity may contribute to tumor growth (inhibition of apoptosis) along with increased production of the new vessel growth factors (VEGF, FGF) and the formation of new blood vessels. In in vitro experiments, COX inhibitors inhibited the growth of human colon, prostate, gastric, lung, head and neck, pancreatic, liver, and breast cancer cell lines (37, 38).

CLINICAL TRIALS IN CANCER

Human clinical trials with curcuminoids have been undertaken in several cancers in view of evidence of safety and efficacy in preclinical studies of these compounds in prevention and treatment of several forms of cancer. Several examples of clinical trials against various cancers are discussed. The data include design, use of biomarker measurements, adverse events, and a discussion of dosing and clinical outcome.

Clinical Trials in Patients with Colon Cancer

Gastrointestinal cancer has been of particular interest because of its epidemiological significance. Curcuminoids were evaluated in the Department of Oncology, University of Leicester, United Kingdom, in a dose-escalation study in patients with advanced colorectal cancer refractory to standard chemotherapy (7). The primary objective of this four-month study was to evaluate markers of efficacy of the novel chemopreventive agent. Three biomarkers of the potential activity of curcuminoids were measured in the peripheral blood leukocytes: glutathione *S*-transferase activity (GST), levels of M1G (DNA adduct [M1G] formation), and prostaglandin E2 (PGE2) production induced ex vivo.

Design of the Trial

Fifteen patients with histologically proven adenocarcinoma of the colon or rectum for which no additional conventional therapies were available were selected for the study based on the following criteria: measurable or evaluable disease; age > 18 years; World Health Organization (WHO) performance status of 0 to 2 and life expectancy > 12 weeks; absolute neutrophil count > 1.5×109/L; hemoglobinn > 10 g/dL; platelets > 100×109/L; aspartate aminotransferase and alanine aminotransferase < 2.5 times the upper limit of normal; serum bilirubin and creatinine < 1.5 times the upper limit of normal; and no previous investigational or chemotherapeutic drugs within 28 days before enrollment. Patients were asked to abstain from nonsteroidal anti-inflammatory drug use and the consumption of foods containing the spice turmeric during the study period, and their general practitioners were asked not to prescribe nonsteroidal anti-inflammatory drugs. Written informed consent was obtained from each patient before enrollment. All of the patients were Caucasians except for one patient who was Indian. The trial and formulation were approved by the local ethics committee and the United Kingdom Medicines Control Agency.

Each patient was assigned to the dose level (DL), and depending on dose level, patients consumed one, two, four, or eight capsules, providing 450 (DL1), 900 (DL2), 1800 (DL3), or 3600 (DL4) mg of curcuminoids, respectively, once daily. The capsules of a daily dose of curcuminoids were consumed together with water in the morning after at least two hours of fasting. Treatment was continued until disease progression was established or consent was withdrawn. The three indices of the potential pharmacological activity of curcumin measured in patient blood leukocytes were GST activity, levels of a deoxyguanosine adduct (M1G) formed via oxidative DNA damage, and inducible prostaglandin E2 (PGE2) levels as an indicator of COX-2 activity induced ex vivo by lipopolysaccharide (LPS). Serum levels of total cholesterol and the tumor markers carcinoembryonic antigen CA19.9 and CA125 were measured before treatment and every month of treatment. Blood samples for analysis of GST activity and M1G levels were collected one week before and on days 1, 2, 8, and 29 of treatment, immediately before dosing for M1G or immediately before and one hour after each dose for GST. Blood was also taken for assessment of plasma PGE2 concentration induced ex vivo.

Patients were evaluated for tumor response every eight weeks, using computed tomography or magnetic resonance imaging scanning, in addition to monthly chest X-rays. Measurements were made using the WHO Solid Tumor Response Criteria. Partial response was defined as at least a 50% decrease in measurable lesions from baseline and with no development of new lesions. Progressive disease was defined as at least a 25% increase, clear worsening from previous assessment of any evaluable disease, reappearance of any lesion that had disappeared, or appearance of any new lesion or site. Stable disease was defined as the scenario in which the disease status had neither responded to meet the partial response criterion nor progressed to meet the progressive disease criteria.

Tolerance and Side Effects

Curcuminoids were well tolerated at all of the dose levels. Two types of gastrointestinal adverse events were reported by patients, which were probably related to curcuminoids' consumption. One patient consuming 0.45 g curcuminoids daily and one patient consuming

3.6 g curcuminoids daily developed diarrhea (National Cancer Institute grades 1 and 2) one month and four months into treatment, respectively. In the first case, diarrhea was controlled with an antidiarrheal drug. The other patient withdrew consent from the study, and the diarrhea resolved after cessation of treatment. One patient consuming 0.9 g curcumin daily experienced nausea (National Cancer Institute toxicity grade 2), which resolved spontaneously despite continuation of treatment. Two abnormalities were detected in blood tests, both possibly related to treatment: a rise in serum alkaline phosphatase level was observed in four patients, consistent with National Cancer Institute grade 1 toxicity in two patients and grade 2 toxicity in two patients; serum lactate dehydrogenase levels rose to > 150% of pretreatment values in three patients.

Clinical Status

All of the patients enrolled exhibited radiologic evidence of progressive disease before recruitment. No partial responses to treatment were observed. Two patients exhibited stable disease by radiologic criteria after two months of treatment, and they remained on treatment for a total of four months. The first of these two patients (DL2) developed progressive disease on her second computed tomography scan. The other patient (DL3) demonstrated continued stable disease on a computed tomography scan after four months, but she withdrew consent on account of diarrhea, which she thought was treatment related. Decreases in tumor markers were not observed as a result of treatment in any of the patients. Three significant changes in quality of life scores were recorded: one patient noticed a significant improvement after one month of treatment, and two patients deteriorated after two months of treatment, both of whom were found to have radiologic progressive disease.

Biomarkers of the Trial

Oral administration of curcuminoids did not impact on basal PGE2 levels in leukocytes, nor did doses of 0.45 to 1.8 g daily alter LPS-induced PGE2. However, consumption of 3.6 g of curcumin daily affected LPS-induced PGE2 levels. When values obtained immediately predose or one hour postdose on days 1, 2, 8, and 29 were pooled for the six patients consuming this dose, PGE2 levels observed postdose were significantly lower, 46%, than those measured immediately predosing (p = 0.028). There was no time-dependent trend in basal or LPS-stimulated PGE2. A subset analysis revealed no difference between inducible PGE2 levels in samples from the three patients in which curcumin was detected compared with those in which curcumin was not detected. These results suggest that consumption of 3.6 g of curcumin daily is linked with inhibition of PGE2 induction in blood taken postdose compared with blood taken predose. Oral curcuminoids at any dose level showed no effect on GST and M1G formation.

Levels of Curcumin and Derivatives in Plasma, Urine, and Feces

Curcumin was detected in plasma samples taken 0.5 and 1 hour postdose from patients consuming 3.6 g of curcumin daily. Glucuronides and sulfates of curcumin and desmethoxycurcumin were found in the plasma from all patients consuming 3.6 g of curcumin daily at all of the time points studied. Curcumin and its glucuronide and sulfate metabolites were detected in plasma in the 10 nmol/L range. Analysis of urine suggested the presence of curcumin and the conjugates in all of the samples from patients consuming 3.6 g of curcumin daily. Using HPLC, such chromatographic peaks were not seen in any extracts of urine samples from patients on the lower doses. The HPLC techniques demonstrated the presence of curcumin and curcumin glucuronide, desmethoxycurcumin and desmethoxy-curcumin glucuronide, and curcumin sulfate in urine. Abundant amounts of curcumin were recovered from the feces at all of the dose levels. Trace amounts of curcumin sulfate were detected in feces from three patients consuming 3.6 g of curcumin daily.

The study presented herein provides the first report of the systemic parameters of pharmacokinetics and activity of curcuminoids that may facilitate the phase II chemoprevention or anticancer trials. The results allow the following conclusions regarding oral curcuminoids in humans: (a) administration of 0.5 to 3.6 g daily for up to four months is associated with mild diarrhea in colon cancer patients as the only reported side effect of the treatment; (b) consumption of 3.6 g of curcuminoids daily generates detectable levels of parent compound and conjugates in plasma, urine, and feces; and (c) consumption of 3.6 g of curcumin daily causes inhibition of PGE2 production in blood leukocytes measured ex vivo.

In conclusion, a daily oral dose of 3.6 g of curcuminoids is advocated for phase II evaluation in the prevention or treatment of colorectal cancer. PGE2 blood levels may indicate the biological activity; however, the possibility of induction of GST enzymes and suppression of oxidative genetic material damage (DNA adduct [M1G] formation) with curcuminoids should not be discounted.

Clinical Trial in Patients with Pancreatic Cancer

In a clinical trial conducted at MD Anderson Medical Center, Houston, Texas, curcuminoids were evaluated in treatment of patients with pancreatic cancer. Pancreatic cancer is one of the most lethal cancers, with an overall five-year survival rate of < 5%, with most patients dying of the disease within one year. The poor prognosis of pancreatic cancer is due to its tendency for late presentation; aggressive, local invasion; early metastases; and poor response to chemotherapy. The only drugs approved by the FDA for treatment of pancreatic cancer are gemcitabine and erlotinib. Both of these drugs elicit responses in only a small percentage of patients (fewer than 10%), their effect on survival is measured in weeks, and treatment is associated with multiple adverse effects and drug resistance. There is a need for novel strategies involving less toxic agents that can sensitize pancreatic cancer cells to chemotherapy.

Several in vitro and in vivo studies have shown that nuclear transcription factor-κB (NF-κB) is activated in an experimental model of pancreatic cancer. The transcription factor has been linked with cell proliferation, invasion, angiogenesis, metastasis, suppression of apoptosis, and chemoresistance in multiple tumors including pancreatic cancer. The preclinical studies have shown that curcuminoids suppress NF-κB activation and the growth of human pancreatic cancer xenografts in mice. Phase I human clinical trials of curcuminoids have shown that curcuminoids are safe at doses of up to 8 g per day (39). Subsequently, the phase II clinical trial described below was undertaken to determine whether orally administered curcuminoids have biological activity in patients with advanced pancreatic cancer (40).

Design of the Trial

This trial was a nonrandomized, open-label, phase II clinical study. Twenty-five patients (13 men, 12 women; aged 43–77) with histologically confirmed pancreatic cancer and a Karnofsky performance score greater than 60 but preserved hepatic function and renal function were enrolled in the phase II trial. Patients took 8 g of curcuminoids in capsule form daily for up to 18 months. The patients could not receive any concomitant chemotherapy and radiotherapy. Patients who were diagnosed as at least with stable disease after eight weeks received continued therapy with curcuminoids at 8 g per day.

A physical examination, an electrocardiogram, a chest X-ray, diagnostic imaging, and disease staging were performed at baseline, repeated every four weeks and at the end of therapy for all patients enrolled in the study; diagnostic imaging was repeated every eight weeks during the course of treatment. Blood samples were used to measure the following values: cytokine concentrations (interleukin-6, -8, and -10 and interleukin-1 receptor antagonist [IL-1RA]), tumor markers (CA 19-9, CA 27.29, CA 125, and carcinoembryonic antigen) concentrations, and peripheral blood mononuclear cell expression of NF-κB, COX-2, and signal transducer and activator of transcription 3 (pSTAT3). Blood samples were collected pretherapy at 24 hours, 8 days, 4 weeks, and 8 weeks and analyzed using enzyme-linked immunosorbent assay (ELISA) and electrophoretic mobility shift assay (EMSA), assessed for pharmacokinetics of curcuminoids. The adverse events were assessed on the basis of the National Cancer Institute Expanded Common Toxicity Criteria, and tumor response was evaluated on the basis of the Response Evaluation Criteria in Solid Tumors.

Clinical Status

Twenty-four patients were available for the toxicity evaluation, and 21 patients were available for evaluation of the response to treatment with curcuminoids. The breakdown of non-evaluable patients was as follows: one patient developed gastric obstruction on day 1, one patient was noncompliant, and two patients were lost because of inadequate follow-up.

There were no treatment-related adverse effects. Two of the 21 patients exhibited a favorable response to curcuminoids. In addition, a third patient remained on the study for approximately eight months with stable weight and a feeling of well-being—however, with progression of the lesions. Pancreatic cancer remained stable in one of the aforementioned patients for longer than 18 months. This patient was previously treated with failed Whipple's surgery followed by gemcitabine and radiation therapy. The patient had an elevated CA 125 but not CA 19.9 level. With the treatment of curcuminoids, the CA 125 antigen levels decreased gradually over the course of 12 months (Graph 6.2).

The first patient remained in relatively good physical condition, maintained his body weight, and did not develop ascites or edema. His neoplastic lesions remained stable in size as evaluated by serial positron emission tomography or computer tomography scans. The second patient had a marked response that lasted one month and was manifested by 73% reduction in the tumor size. Curiously, once the tumor progression started again, the lesions that had regressed remained small, but other lesions grew larger.

Biomarkers of the Trial

The baseline serum cytokines were elevated in the majority of the patients. In contrast, the majority of healthy volunteers had undetectable serum levels of IL-6, IL-8, and IL-10, with all having detectable serum levels of IL-IRA. Interestingly, the two patients who had a positive response to curcuminoids had their baseline IL-6 below the median levels and the IL-1RA above the median levels; the patient who benefited most, that is, had over 18 months of gradual improvement, had the highest initial IL-1RA level among all participants of the study. Treatment resulted in variable changes in cytokine levels. Of particular interest was

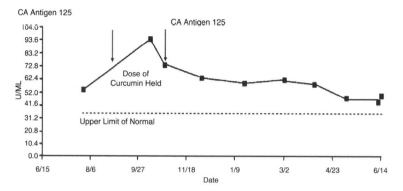

Graph 6.2. Pancreatic Cancer Trial: CA125 [Cancer Antigen 125] Levels in a Patient

Serum levels of CA125 increased before dropping again when curcuminoids were administered. CA 19-9 was not elevated.

Source: *Clin Cancer Res.* 2008 Jul 15;14(14); 4491–4499.

the patient with brief and dramatic regression of tumor who now had a significant increase in serum levels of all measured cytokines, for example, the in-treatment IL-6 level that reached 35-fold of the baseline level for this patient. One way to explain the surge in cytokines is release of cytokines from the tumor associated with shrinkage of the tumor mass. Of potential importance in this patient is the observation that the tumors that originally had regressed continued to show regression in follow-up, whereas the tumors that grew previously had been dormant. This finding suggests that there was a malignant clone that responded to curcuminoids, while another resistant clone emerged. The patient who had the stable disease condition for more than 18 months experienced gradual decrease in all cytokine levels over time. As previously mentioned, this patient had the highest baseline levels of IL-1RA of the tested patients. This finding may be biologically relevant because IL-1RA opposes IL-1, which can stimulate growth of pancreatic cell lines in vitro.

The NF-κB and the activated-by-NF-κB COX-2 play critical roles in the growth and angiogenesis of pancreatic cancer. Immunocytochemistry of peripheral blood mononuclear cells (PBMC) showed constitutively active NF-κB in all patients who consented to optional tests (19 out of 25 patients), whereas activation of the transcription factor was not detected in healthy volunteers. On treatment with curcuminoids, immunocytochemistry values showed a decline (without reaching statistical significance p=0.1) in cellular expression of NF-κB compared with that in normal volunteers. PMBC in all 19 patients examined expressed COX-2, which declined significantly (p<0.03) in the course of treatment with curcuminoids. The expression of NF-κB correlated well with the expression of COX-2, and the majority of the patients showed down-regulation of NF-κB and COX-2 after treatment with curcuminoids. This is the first study to show that curcuminoids can down-regulate the expression of NF-κB and COX-2 in humans. Nevertheless, the down-regulation was not associated with clinical response in many patients, possibly because the down-regulation in PBMC does not reflect the changes in the tumor itself.

The expression of activated pSTAT3 in PBMC was also evaluated, because this compound is regulated by growth factors, for example, epidermal growth factor, and it is implicated in tumorgenesis and chemoresistance. All tested patients had activated STAT3 at baseline, and there was a statistically significant decline (p=0.009) in the percentage of pSTAT3-positive PBMCs in course of treatment with curcuminoids.

Clinical Trial in Patients with Pancreatic Cancer

Another study performed at the Department of Oncology, Rambam Medical Center, Haifa, Israel, was undertaken to evaluate feasibility and efficacy of gemcitabine in combination with curcuminoids in patients with advanced pancreatic cancer (41). Patients received 8 g of curcuminoids by mouth daily, concurrently with gemcitabine 1000 mg/m2 IV weekly times three out of four weeks. Time to tumor progression was the primary end point and the toxicity profile the main secondary end point. Seventeen patients (ten male, seven female, aged 54–78) were enrolled for the study. Six patients had locally advanced tumors and 11 patients had metastatic disease, all in the liver. Patients received a median of two cycles of gemcitabine. Five patients discontinued curcuminoids after a few days to two weeks because of intractable abdominal fullness or pain. One patient died unrelated to the treatment event. In the 11 patients, curcuminoids and gemcitabine were delivered concomitantly for a period of 1 to 12 months. The dose of curcuminoids was reduced to 4 g per day in three of the patients because of abdominal discomfort. One patient out of the 11 evaluable patients had partial response (7 months), four had a stable disease condition (2, 3, 6, and 12 months), and six had tumor progression. Time to tumor progression was 1 to 12 months (median 2) and overall survival 1 to 24 months (median 6). These preliminary results suggest that a combination of gemcitabine and curcuminoids for patients with advanced pancreatic cancer is feasible. Based on the outcome of this study, a clinically acceptable daily oral dose of curcuminoids in pancreatic cancer patients on chemotherapy should be less than 8 g per day.

Clinical Trials in Cancer-Predisposing Plasma Cell Dyscrasias

The hypothetical role of curcuminoids as chemopreventive agents in management of plasma cell dyscrasias has been studied in a clinical trial at St. George Hospital, Sydney, Australia. The trial assessed a potential therapeutic effect of curcuminoids in patients diagnosed with monoclonal gammopathy of undefined significance (MGUS) (19).

Plasma cell dyscrasias, most commonly associated with paraproteinaemia, are a diverse group of disorders that includes multiple myeloma, Waldenstrom's macroglobulinaemia, heavy chain disease, MGUS, and immunocytic amyloidosis. The incidence of plasma cell dyscrasias is age related. It occurs in 1% of the population over age 25 and 4% of those over age 70.

MGUS is the most common of the monoclonal gammopathies. While this condition occurs in association with a variety of diseases, it can also precede the onset of multiple myeloma. MGUS patients have a serum M-protein value of<30 g/L, fewer than 10% plasma cells in the bone marrow, no or a small amount of M protein in the urine, and absence of lytic bone lesions, anemia, hypercalcemia, or renal insufficiency related to the plasma-cell proliferative process. MGUS is largely considered a benign condition; however, a number of studies show that patients with MGUS are at increased risk of developing fractures even before progression to multiple myeloma. Multiple myeloma is a progressive neoplastic disease and is characterized by high bone turnover, significant bone loss, and pathological fractures resulting in significant morbidity and a high mortality. It is also associated with hypercalcemia, anemia, renal damage, and increased susceptibility to bacterial infections.

Current management of MGUS patients includes the regular clinical observation for changes in clinical and immunochemical status at four- to six-month intervals. Overall, the risk of progression of MGUS to myeloma or related disorder is 1% per year. Younger patients are more likely to have progression to cancer during their lifetime because they are at risk longer. It is currently not possible to predict the course in any individual patient, and clinically, symptomatic myeloma may not evolve for as long as 20 years.

Because disease progression with MGUS is uncertain, early intervention to reduce the paraprotein load and the potential negative effects on the skeleton would provide an innovative therapeutic tool. Curcuminoids were selected for the trial with MGUS patients because numerous reports suggest that curcumin and its derivative curcuminoids have chemopreventive and chemotherapeutic effects. Curcumin has been shown to inhibit the proliferation of multiple myeloma cells through the down-regulation of IL-6 as well as to induce apoptosis in multiple myeloma cells. Curcumin has also been shown to inhibit osteoclastogenesis through the suppression of the receptor activator of nuclear factor kappa B ligand (RANKL is the primary mediator of osteoclast formation, function, and survival) signaling and subsequently to reduce bone turnover.

Design of the Trial

In a single-blind, randomized control pilot study, curcuminoid formula or placebo was administered orally, 2 g (2 caplets each 1000 mg curcuminoids) twice daily to a cohort of 26 MGUS patients. Patients were asked to abstain from drugs affecting bone metabolism for at least three months prior to and during the study. No patients had evidence of metabolic bone disorder. All the patients were Caucasian, aged over 45 years. The study design was approved by the local ethics committee. Written informed consent was obtained from each patient before enrollment.

Blood and urine samples were collected at baseline (V1), one week (V2), one month (V3), and three months (V4) after initiating the therapy. Full blood count, B2 microglobulin, serum paraprotein, and immunoglobulin electrophoresis (IEPG and EPG) were determined for all patients at each visit. Serum calcium, 25 hydroxyvitamin D3, and bone-specific alkaline phosphatase (bsALP) were determined at baseline only. Urine, as a morning second-void sample, was collected at each visit for uNTx (urinary N-telopeptide of type I collagen) measurements.

Clinical Status: Paraprotein Levels

Of the 26 patients randomized into the study—16 men and 10 women with average age of 68 years—24 patients completed the study. Seven (of the 17) patients were administered curcuminoids only during the course of the study. Two patients withdrew from the study before crossover, as they developed diarrhea, which resolved after cessation of treatment. The other five patients elected to remain on curcuminoids and refused crossover.

Baseline clinical data and serum biochemistry of the patients who completed the study are summarized below. Serum paraprotein concentration ranged from 8 to 36 g/L, with a median value of 20 g/L. Nine of the 26 patients randomized into the study had IgGk (35%), nine had IgGl (35%), four had IgMk (15%), three had IgAk (11%), and one had IgAl

(4%) paraproteins. All patients had a normal serum calcium level (mean = 2.62 mmol/L). There were nine patients with vitamin D deficiency (< 50 nmol/L). Two patients had elevated baseline serum bone-specific alkaline phosphatase measurements. All patients had elevated baseline B2 microglobulin levels (mean = 2.9 ± 1 mg/L), which remained unchanged throughout the study. All patients had normal baseline uNTx levels (mean of 27 ± 16 nmol/mmol creatinine), with no patient having a baseline value greater than 100 nmol/mmol creatinine.

Of the 17 patients who were started on curcuminoids, 10 had a baseline serum paraprotein level greater than or equal to 20 g/L (mean = 20.2 g/L) and 7 less than 20 g/L. In patients with a serum paraprotein ≥ 20 g/L, 50% of these (i.e., five patients) had a 5% to 30% decrease in serum paraprotein levels in response to curcumin. The most significant decrease was seen at V2 (p < 0.05 for group comparison between V1 and V2) (Figure 6.4). This decrease remained stable in most patients until they were crossed over to placebo. Two patients then demonstrated a rebound in their serum paraprotein levels. Patients with a baseline serum paraprotein less than 20 g/L did not show a response to curcuminoids, but their serum paraprotein levels remained stable throughout the study period.

Nine patients were randomly assigned to receive placebo at baseline. In contrast to a decrease in serum paraprotein seen in patients initiating curcuminoid therapy, patients receiving placebo demonstrated stable or increased serum paraprotein levels at V2 (Figure 6.5). At V4 (i.e., crossover), two patients demonstrated a decrease in their serum paraprotein.

Clinical Status: uNTx Levels

While 73% of patients did not show a change in their uNTx levels while taking curcuminoids or placebo, 27% of patients showed a decrease in their uNTx levels when taking curcuminoids. This response was most marked in two patients at crossover. Although the difference between the groups (i.e., curcuminoids vs. placebo) does not reach statistical significance, the results do indicate that certain patients may show a decrease in bone resorption in response to curcuminoids.

The present study demonstrates that oral curcuminoids are able to decrease paraprotein load and bone resorption in a select group of patients with MGUS. Fifty percent of patients

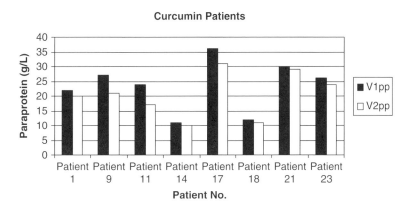

Figure 6.4.   MGUS Trial: Paraprotein Levels in Patients Receiving Curcuminoids

Source: *Clin Cancer Res.* 2008. In press.

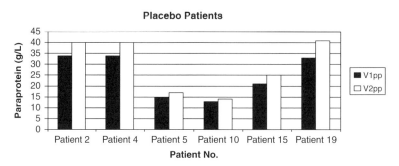

Figure 6.5. MGUS Trial: Paraprotein Levels in Patients on Placebo

Source: *Clin Cancer Res.* 2008. In press.

with a paraprotein $\geq 20\,\mathrm{g/L}$ responded with a 5% to 30% decrease in their paraprotein levels when taking $4\,\mathrm{g}$ per day curcuminoids orally. This response occurred already after seven days of curcuminoid therapy. Patients taking placebo had no such decrease in their paraprotein levels.

Bone resorption was determined by urinary N-telopeptide of type 1 collagen (uNTx) excretion rates. The 26 MGUS patients in this study had a mean uNTx level of 27.3 nmol/mmol creatinine at baseline with no patient having a baseline value above the upper range of normal. Nonetheless, a reduction in uNTx was noted in 7 out of 26 patients when given curcuminoids. This response coincided with the decrease in serum paraprotein and occurred after only one week of therapy.

The presented pilot study suggests that curcuminoids may decrease both serum paraprotein (in patients with levels $\geq 20\,\mathrm{g/L}$) and uNTx in patients with MGUS. The potential role of curcuminoids as a therapeutic intervention for MGUS patients warrants further investigation. A double-blind, randomized control trial using higher dosages of curcuminoids in a larger cohort of MGUS patients with significant paraproteinaemia is planned next. Also, a more detailed study is required to assess the therapeutic role of curcuminoids in MGUS patients with elevated uNTx values.

Clinical Trials in Leukemia Predisposing Myelodysplastic Syndrome

The myelodysplastic syndrome (MDS), sometimes referred to as preleukemia, is a hematological condition characterized by ineffective production, or dysplasia, of myeloid blood cells and risk of transformation to acute myelogenous leukemia (AML). The anemia of MDS requires blood transfusions.

Potential of curcuminoids and ginger therapy in MDS patients was evaluated in 2006 at Saint Vincent's Comprehensive Cancer Center, New York, and University of Massachusetts Medical Center, Worcester (18). Management of lower-risk MDS patients who are still transfusion independent has not been extensively examined, being typically withheld until patients either become transfusion dependent or show signs of disease progression. Low-intensity therapies could be tried in these patients for two potential benefits: to improve the cytopenias and to determine whether intervention at this early stage could arrest or reverse the expansion of the abnormal cell clone. In the clinical trial reported here, curcuminoids were combined with extract of ginger root (*Zingiber officinale* Roscoe, Fam. *Zingiberaceae*) standardized for gingerol (5% gingerol), the active constituent of ginger, to treat nine patients with low risk of myelodysplasia. Curcuminoids were administered in an incremental dosing schedule starting with 2.0 g in four divided doses per day increasing to 8 g per day, ginger extract 350 mg bid increasing to 1.4 g per day. The high dose of curcuminoids and ginger extract has been well tolerated with few or no side effects. The preliminary results have been very encouraging. Patients have been followed for 4 to 18 months and included seven males and two females: six presenting with refractory anemia (RA), two with refractory anemia with ringed sideroblasts (RARS), and one unclassified. Of the six evaluable patients, four have shown overall hematologic improvement. Two patients had stable disease. In conclusion, the curcuminoid and ginger extract combined therapy is well tolerated and potentially beneficial for early-stage MDS patients who are not transfusion dependent.

Clinical Trial in psoriasis vulgaris

Based on the physiological effects of curcumin and the positive anecdotal reports of its benefit for psoriasis, an open-label clinical trial to assess the safety and efficacy of oral curcuminoids in the treatment of chronic *psoriasis vulgaris* was conducted in the Department of Dermatology at the University of Pennsylvania School of Medicine and the Department of Dermatology at the University of Rochester, Rochester, New York (42).

Psoriasis is a chronic inflammatory skin condition classified as an autoimmune disorder which affects approximately 1% to 3% of the population worldwide and about 5.5 million people in the United States. There is a need for safe, inexpensive, and effective psoriasis therapies, especially because 95% of patients are willing to try new treatments. Curcuminoids have been used successfully to treat psoriasis based on anecdotal reports. A strong scientific rationale suggests that curcuminoids may in fact be promising for the treatment of psoriasis. In vitro and animal studies have demonstrated the inhibitory effect of curcuminoids on immune pathways critical to the pathology of psoriasis such as NFκB and downstream, inflammatory gene products such as Th-1–type cytokines (i.e., TNF-α, IFN γ,).

Design of the Trial

Patients were eligible if they were at least 18 years of age and had active but clinically stable plaque psoriasis that involved at least 6% of the body surface area and was of moderate plaque thickness as defined by a thickness score of 2 on the Psoriasis Area Severity Index (PASI). Patients were included if they were using a medically acceptable method of contraception throughout the entire study period. Patients with guttae, erythrodermic, or pustular psoriasis were excluded, as were patients who used systemic treatments for psoriasis (including methotrexate, cyclosporine, alefacept, adalimumab, efalizumab, infliximab, etanercept, etretinate, systemic steroids, and PUVA) within three months prior to day 0 or at any time during the study. Patients were excluded if they had used topical treatments or phototherapy for their psoriasis within 14 days prior to day 0 or at any time during the study. Patients who were pregnant or nursing a child, had clinically significant laboratory abnormalities at screening, or had significant uncontrolled comorbidities were excluded from the study. Subjects for whom the dose of clonidine, digoxin, beta-blockers, lithium, or antimalarials had changed in the past month prior to enrollment were excluded from the study. Enrolled subjects were required to avoid prolonged exposure to sun or UV light and to discontinue nonmedicated emollients and medicated psoriasis shampoos 24 hours before each study visit.

The study was designed to determine the safety and efficacy of oral curcuminoids in patients with plaque psoriasis receiving 4.5 g per day of oral curcuminoids for the first 12 weeks followed by a 4-week observation period after discontinuing the study drug. End points included improvement in Physicians Global Assessment (PGA) score, PASI score, and safety end points throughout the study.

The primary measure of efficacy was the proportion of patients who were classified as a responder using the PGA of Change at week 12. A responder was defined as achieving a rating of good (50%–74% improvement), excellent (75%–99% improvement), or cleared (100% improvement) on the PGA compared to baseline. Secondary end points included PASI scores and health-related quality of life as measured by the Skindex-29. Other outcome measures include PASI 75 and PASI 50, which correspond to 75% and 50% improvements in PASI scores from baseline, respectively, and have been shown to represent a meaningful end point in psoriasis clinical trials. Subjects were classified as responders based on week 12 PGA scores and a response rate was calculated with 95% exact confidence intervals.

Median PASI and Skindex-29 scores were calculated at baseline and week 12. The 12 subjects were enrolled and received the investigational drug at day 0. Of the five subjects who did not receive the drug, three were excluded because they did not have ≥6% of their body surface area covered with psoriasis and another subject was excluded because of anemia. Subjects were instructed to take three capsules (each capsule containing 500 mg curcuminoids) three times per day. All subjects who completed the trial were at least 85% compliant with the treatment regimen as determined by patient diaries, patient interviews, and pill counts.

Tolerance and Side Effects

There were no study-related adverse events that necessitated participant withdrawal. The 4.5 g per day for 12 weeks of oral curcuminoids was well tolerated and safe in subjects with psoriasis. All adverse events possibly related to the study drug were mild and limited to gastrointestinal upset and heat intolerance or hot flashes. One subject who was eligible for the study was lost to follow-up before receiving any study drug. Eight subjects completed the trial up to week 16. Four of the 12 enrolled subjects did not complete the trial; one was withdrawn by the investigators due to worsening of her psoriasis and three withdrew prior to week 12 because of lack of efficacy. Subjects who failed to complete the trial had similar degrees of psoriasis severity as measured by PASI compared to patients who completed the trial, but noncompleters had more impairment in health-related quality of life at baseline as measured by Skindex-29 (P=0.04).

Clinical Status

Descriptive statistics and baseline data for enrolled subjects are summarized in Table 6.3. Intention-to-treat analysis, in which all subjects who withdrew from the trial were classified as nonresponders, showed a response rate of 16.7% (95% CI: 2%, 48%). The secondary as treated analysis, which included only subjects who competed the trial up to week 12, had a response rate of 25% (95% CI: 3%, 65%). Only two subjects who completed the trial achieved a response at week 12. The two subjects who were classified as responders achieved

Table 6.3. Psoriasis Trial: Baseline Demographic and Clinical Information

Subjects	Age (Median, IQR)	Sex (N, %) Male	Median (IQR)# of Prior Systemic Agents/Phototherapy Used	Race	Baseline PASI (Median, IQR)	Baseline Skindex (Median, IQR)
Completed trial						
N=8	50.5 (45, 55)	N=7 (87.5%) male	1.5 (1, 2.5)	N=7 White N=1 Asian	13.7 (9.7, 17.2)	34.6 (18.5, 50.9)
Did not complete trial						
N=4	50 (38.5, 62.5)	N=2 (50%) male	1.5 (0.5, 2.5)	N=2 White N=1 Black N=1 Other	14.6 (5.4, 8.3)	63.2 (52, 79.9)

Source: *J Am Acad Dermatol.* 2008 Apr;58(4):625–631.

a score of excellent on the PGA, were seen during the winter months, and were not exposed to sunlight during the trial based on patient report and physical examinations (Figure 6.6). No patients received a score of "cleared," "good," or "fair" at week 12, while two subjects received a PGA score of "slight," three of "unchanged," and one of "worse" at week 12. Both responders achieved a PASI 75 at week 12, while no other subjects achieved a PASI 75 or a PASI 50 (Table 6.4).

Four weeks after discontinuation of curcuminoid therapy, the responders maintained an excellent response based on PGA and PASI 75 at week 16. In those subjects who completed the trial, the median Skindex-29 score was reduced by 0.35 (IQR 5.5, 5.0) (a lower score signifies improvement in quality of life). In subgroup analysis, the two responders had a median reduction in Skindex-29 scores of 16 (IQR 5.1, 26.9) (n=2), whereas nonresponders had a median increase (worsening) in Skindex scores of 2.5 (IQR 0, 5.6) (n=6).

The efficacy of the study drug was low, with an intention-to-treat response rate of 16.7%. The confidence interval for the 16.7% response rate is wide because of the small sample size, and therefore the study cannot exclude the possibility that the response observed was caused by a placebo effect or the natural history of skin disease in these subjects rather than efficacy of the drug itself. The lack of any evidence of meaningful response (e.g., PASI 50) in all other subjects argues that the true response rate is very low, limited to a small subset of psoriasis patients, or not caused by curcuminoids but rather by other factors that cannot be accounted for in an uncontrolled study. Nevertheless, excellent responses were observed in two patients, and therefore, large, placebo-controlled trials will be necessary to definitively prove or disprove oral curcuminoids as a potential therapeutic agent for psoriasis.

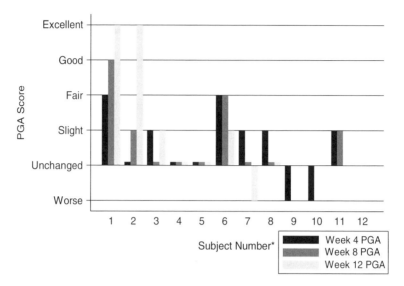

Figure 6.6. Psoriasis Trial: PGA Scores by Month

Week 12 PGA scores of "Good," "Excellent," and "Cleared" are classified as responders. Subjects 9–12 withdrew prior to week 12 and PGA scores, when available, are shown for these subjects for the weeks in which they were evaluated.

Source: *J Am Acad Dermatol.* 2008 Apr;58(4):625–631.

Table 6.4. Psoriasis Trial: Summary of Efficacy Endpoints at Week 12

Efficacy Outcome	Results of Subjects Who Completed Trial (n=8)	Results of Intention to Treat Analysis (n=12)*
Response rate based on achieving at least a PGA of "good"	25%, 95% CI (3%, 65%)	16.7%, 95% CI (2%, 48%)
PGA at week 12 (median, IQR)	Unchanged—slight improvement (unchanged, fair-good)	Unchanged (worse-unchanged, slight improvement)
PASI 75 at week 12	25%, 95% CI (3%, 65%)	16.7%, 95% CI (2%, 48%)
Change in PASI (baseline-week 12) (median, IQR)	5.4 (0.65, 7.6) p=0.04	0.65 (−1.25, 6.5) p=0.26
Change in Skindex** (median, IQR)	0.35 (IQR −5.5, 5.0) p=0.9	0.0 (−2.55, 4.95) p=0.63

*Change in PASI data of 2 of 4 subjects who withdrew are available (−11.1 and −4.1), whereas the other two subjects who withdrew had no follow-up PASI data and were given a score of zero to indicate no change.
   Change in Skindex data was only available for 1 of 4 subjects who withdrew and was 8.4. The other three subjects were given a score of zero to indicate no change.
**positive values indicate an increase in Skindex scores, suggesting a decrease in QOL.
Source: *J Am Acad Dermatol.* 2008 Apr;58(4):625–631.

CURCUMINOIDS IN PREVENTION AND TREATMENT OF NEURODEGENERATIVE CONDITIONS

Curcuminoids in Alzheimer's Disease: Ex Vivo Study

In 2004–2005, the Department of Medicine, Greater LA VA Medical Center and UCLA School of Medicine, Los Angeles, California, started testing a hypothesis that curcuminoids, which have epidemiologic and experimental rationale for use in Alzheimer's disease, may improve the innate immune system and increase amyloid clearance from the brain of patients with sporadic Alzheimer's disease (9, 10).

One of the most challenging fields in antiaging medicine is the management and treatment of chronic degenerative conditions as exemplified by Alzheimer's disease. This disease is increasingly seen as a defective response of the aging immune system to wear-and-tear damage and inflammation that occur with aging of the organism.

The aging immune system becomes progressively less efficient in dealing with inflammation. The innate and adaptive (acquired during lifetime) immune responses show age-related changes that could be decisive for healthy aging and survival. Natural or innate immunity is particularly important in the aging process and is based on macrophages, which are crucial for antimicrobial defense and removal of cellular and metabolic debris. Innate immunity functions result from a macrophage's ability to recognize a pattern of a pathogenic molecule through a code system called pathogen-associated molecular patterns (PAMPs). These potentially harmful molecules, for example, amyloid protein, when recognized by macrophages, trigger responses that also guide an appropriate adaptive immune response. The interaction between the innate and adaptive immune systems is critical for the clinical outcome of a pathogen molecule challenge to an organism—a difference between macrophages contributing to the body injury or to the healing process.

There is increasing evidence supporting a role for macrophages and the dependent innate immunity in Alzheimer's disease origins and progression. Brain amyloidosis is hypothesized to be a crucial pathogenic mechanism in the brain of a person with Alzheimer's disease, and many investigators of Alzheimer's disease pathogenesis believe that accumulation of amyloid-β (Aβ) is toxic to neurons. The immune system of patients with Alzheimer's disease is generally poorly responsive to Aβ and unable to remove amyloid from neurons. The amyloid hypothesis of Alzheimer's disease has increased interest in developing therapies that promote clearance of brain amyloidosis by macrophages leading to a novel strategy of immunotherapy with Aβ vaccine, or antibodies against the amyloid protein. It was established that the anti-Aβ antibodies were sufficient for reducing Aβ in the brain and that these reductions were accompanied by improvement in cognitive function in animal models of Alzheimer's disease.

The ex vivo study reported here was performed on peripheral blood mononuclear cells (PBMC) obtained from patients with Alzheimer's disease and healthy controls. All subjects gave informed consent approved by the UCLA Institutional Review Board for Human Studies. The diagnostic criteria for Alzheimer's disease satisfied the National Institute of Neurological and Communicative Disorders and the Alzheimer's Disease and Related Disorders Association (NINCDS/ADRDA) criteria for probable Alzheimer's disease as described. Normal age-matched control subjects were recruited from UCLA faculty and alumni. Peripheral blood mononuclear cells from six patients were separated from EDTA-anticoagulated blood by centrifugation on Ficoll-Hypaque gradient. Differentiated macrophages were treated with curcuminoids (0.1 mM) in the medium overnight and were then exposed to beta amyloid Aβ conjugated with fluorescein isothiocyanate (FITC) (FITC-Aβ) and examined by fluorescence or confocal microscopy.

Macrophages of a majority of patients with Alzheimer's disease did not phagocytose and did not efficiently clear amyloid from the brain, although they were able to phagocytose bacteria. In contrast, macrophages of normal subjects phagocytosed amyloid. Upon amyloid stimulation, macrophages of normal subjects accelerate synthesis of molecules and receptors that participate in the system of pathogen recognition, specifically, MGAT3 (beta-1,4-mannosyl-glycoprotein 4-N-acetylglucosaminyltransferase) and Toll-like receptors (TLRs), whereas mononuclear cells of patients with Alzheimer's disease generally down-regulate these genes. Defective phagocytosis of the amyloid may be related to suppression of these pathogen recognition molecules. In mononuclear, macrophage-like cells isolated from peripheral blood in patients with Alzheimer's disease, curcuminoids, especially bisdemethoxy-curcumin, may enhance defective phagocytosis of amyloid (see Figure 6.7) while restoring synthesis critical for phagocytic function molecules and receptors, MGAT3 and TLRs (9, 10). Therefore, curcuminoids may provide a novel approach to Alzheimer's disease immunotherapy that is safer than the recently suggested vaccine therapy.

The salient result of the current study is that macrophages of three patients, 50% of those tested, showed a significant increase in total Aβ uptake after curcuminoid treatment in vitro. The responding patients were younger and had a higher Mini Mental State Exam (MMSE) score, suggesting that patients in a less advanced stage of Alzheimer's disease may respond better. Further studies are needed to resolve the factors determining good response to curcuminoids. In vitro testing of curcuminoids in macrophage cultures may be useful in individualizing the treatment of patients with Alzheimer's disease. Testing Aβ phagocytosis in Alzheimer's disease macrophages might be helpful for assessing the ability of patients to respond to immunomodulatory therapy with curcuminoids.

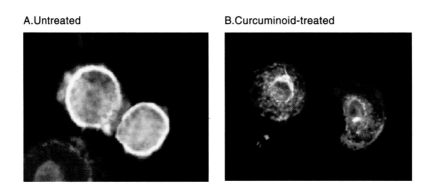

A.Untreated   B.Curcuminoid-treated

Figure 6.7. Alzheimer's Disease *ex Vivo*: Phagocytosis of Ab by AD Macrophages Is Increased by Curcuminoid Treatment

Confocal microscopy, FITC-Ab (green), phalloidin-FITC (red), colocalization (yellow). Note surface binding in (A) vs. intracellular uptake in (B).

Source: *J Alzheimers Dis.* 2006 Sep;10(1):1–7.

Curcuminoids in Alzheimer's Disease: Preliminary Clinical Study

In 2004–2008, a preliminary clinical trial of curcuminoids in Alzheimer's patients was conducted at the Mary S. Easton Center for Alzheimer's Disease Research in the UCLA Department of Neurology (22). The main objective of the study was to obtain tolerability and preliminary efficacy data of 2 g per day and 4 g per day of curcuminoids in mild to moderate Alzheimer's disease patients in a 24-week, randomized, double-blind study.

The group of 36 patients with Alzheimer's disease was evenly divided and randomized to receive placebo, 2 g, or 4 g per day of curcuminoids in two divided doses. The MMSE, ADAS-Cog (Alzheimer's Disease Assessment Scale-Cognitive subscale), NPI (Neuropsychiatric Inventory), and ADCS-ADL (Alzheimer's Disease Cooperative Study-Activities of Daily) scales were performed at baseline and at 24 weeks' time. Plasma samples and lumbar punctures were also performed at baseline and 24 weeks and Abeta40, Abeta42 measured in plasma and cerebrospinal fluid (CSF) and total tau and p-tau measured in CSF. Baseline and 24-week values were compared between groups using repeated measures ANOVA. Adverse events were recorded at each visit.

A total of 11 patients on placebo, 9 patients on 2 g of curcuminoids, and 10 patients on 4 g of curcuminoids completed the study. In an analysis of completers, there were no significant differences or favorable trends between placebo and treatment groups on clinical measures. No difference in plasma or CSF biomarkers were found between groups except for a tendency toward a lesser degree of increase in plasma Abeta40 in the combined group on 2 and 4 g per day of curcuminoids.

The curcuminoids were well tolerated except for some suggestions of gastrointestinal side effects in the form of diarrhea at both dose levels by the patients. However, this preliminary clinical trial does not support a large effect of orally administered curcuminoids on clinical and biomarker measures in patients with mild to moderate Alzheimer's disease at doses of 2 to 4 g per day. Limitations to the interpretation of this study include the small sample size, limited time of administration especially in view of interesting data on Abeta40 plasma levels, effective dose, and uncertain bioavailability of curcuminoids.

The interesting immunological mechanism of curcuminoids in Alzheimer's disease and safety of its clinical use calls for larger dose escalation clinical studies of longer duration in a population of patients who have mild to moderate Alzheimer's disease.

CURCUMINOIDS OVERVIEW OF CLINICAL USE, SAFETY, AND PHARMACOLOGY

The clinically effective and safe dose of curcuminoids and their form and route of administration to the body are the subject of ongoing controversy. In fact, mundane technical aspects of curcuminoid administration may separate success from failure in the therapy with these compounds.

In India and Ayurvedic traditions, turmeric is ingested with milk, especially when boiled with milk, and applied topically or ingested with oil preparations, for example, coconut oil, almond oil, mustard oil, or sesame oil. Curcuminoids are poorly absorbed from the gastrointestinal tract, with low nanogram levels of circulating curcuminoids detected in the plasma (43). Current clinical experience indicates that oral supplementation of curcuminoids is tolerated without toxicity at doses of up to 8 g daily for up to 18 months and that this dose may result in therapeutic activity in some patients with cancer (7, 16, 18, 19).

Dose Escalation Study

Dose escalation study was performed at the Division of Hematology-Oncology, Department of Internal Medicine, University of Michigan, to determine the maximum tolerated dose, safety profile, and resultant plasma concentration of a single dose of curcuminoids (43). The study protocol and the comprehensive written informed consent used in this study protocol were reviewed and approved by the University of Michigan Human Subject Review Board prior to the start of the study. Eligible participants were healthy male and female volunteers, 18 years of age or older, who had not consumed any curry- or curcumin-rich foods to their knowledge within the previous 14 days. Thirteen men and eleven women with mean age of 34 years (range: 19–74 years) were enrolled in the study. The racial distribution was 18 Caucasians and 6 African Americans.

After written informed consent was obtained, three subjects were entered consecutively at dose levels of 500, 1000, 2000, 4000, 6000, 8000, 10000, and 12000 mg. Subjects took the dose with 8 fl. oz. of water followed by a standard meal containing dietary fat (providing 34 g or 42 g fat, per 2200 kcal/day or 2500 kcal/day meal plan, respectively).

Safety was assessed for 72 hours following the curcuminoid dose. Toxicities were graded based on National Cancer Institute Common Toxicity Criteria version 2.0. The maximum tolerated dose was the highest dose that did not cause escalation to cease.

Blood specimens from all subjects on the escalation phase were obtained just prior to dosing and one, two, and four hours after completing dosing at each dose level tested.

Seven adverse events occurred, all were reported as grade 1, and none appeared to be dose related (Table 6.5). No curcumin was detected in serum of participants administered 500, 1000, 2000, 4000, 6000, or 8000 mg of curcuminoids. In two subjects taking 10000 mg and 12000 mg curcuminoids, respectively, plasma curcumin was detectable: 30.4 ng/ml after one hour (10000 mg), 39.5 after two hours (10000 mg), 50.5 after four hours (10000 mg), 29.7 after one hour (12000 mg), 57.6 after two hours (12000 mg), 51.2 after four hours (12000 mg) (Table 6.6). No plasma concentrations of curcumin were detected in the remaining subjects at the 10000 or 12000 mg dose levels.

Table 6.5.   Dose Escalation: All Adverse Events by Dose Levels

Dose Level[a]	Type	No. of Events	Toxicity Grade[b]
1000 mg	Diarrhea	1	1
4000 mg	Headache	1	1
8000 mg	Rash	1	1
	Yellow stool	1	1
10000 mg	Yellow stool	1	1
	Headache	1	1
12000 mg	Diarrhea	1	1

Source: *BMC Complement Altern Med.* 2006; Mar 17; 6–10.
[a]Total of 3 subjects at each level.
[b]National Cancer Institute. Common Toxicity Criteria v.2.0.

Table 6.6. Dose Escalation: Serum Curcumin Levels in Mg/Ml for Two Subjects

Dose	Baseline	One Hour	Two Hour	Four Hour
10000 mg	Approx .6.0	30.4	39.5	50.5
12000 mg	Approx trace	29.7	57.6	51.2

Source: *BMC Complement Altern Med.* 2006; Mar 17; 6–10.

Dose and Form of Curcuminoids in Relation to Efficacy

Reported low blood levels of curcumin may be caused in part by the extensive intestinal and hepatic metabolic biotransformation of curcuminoids. Preclinical and clinical work has demonstrated that avid sulfation, glucuronidation, and reduction of curcumin occur in the gastrointestinal tracts of rats and humans (45, 46, 47). Animal experiments suggest that 65% to 85% of orally administered curcuminoids are excreted unchanged in stool with negligible amounts excreted in the urine (48).

Interestingly, plasma concentrations of curcumin released from conjugated forms are surprisingly low, and there is little evidence for the biological activity of curcumin conjugates against malignant cell growth (45). Possibly there are other forms of conjugated curcumin or derivatives of curcuminoids that can better explain their biological activity and provide the future formulae for more effective clinical application. In an in vitro study, the anti-inflammatory and anticancer properties of curcumin (Cur) and its derivatives demethoxycurcumin (DMC) and bisdemethoxycurcumin (BDMC) were evaluated and compared. The results indicate that the relative potency for suppression of tumor necrosis factor was Cur > DMC > BDMC, thus suggesting the critical role of methoxy groups on the phenyl ring in a biological potential of curcuminoids (49).

It is also possible that curcuminoids may exert different biological properties at different doses in specific clinical conditions. In an experiment on prevention of Alzheimer-like pathology in mice, the effect of a low (160 ppm) and a high (5000 ppm) dose of dietary curcumin on inflammation, oxidative damage, and plaque pathology was evaluated. Low and high doses significantly lowered oxidized proteins and IL-1B, a proinflammatory cytokine usually elevated in the brains of these mice. With low-dose, but not high-dose, curcumin treatment, the astrocytic marker glial fibrillary acidic protein was reduced, and insoluble beta-amyloid (Aβ), soluble Aβ, and plaque burden were significantly decreased, by 43% to 50% (50).

Despite the discussed complexities of mechanism of action, the biological activity of curcuminoids is beyond question, with biomarkers of inflammation, for example, NF-κB and COX-2, suppressed by oral administration of curcuminoids with clinical improvement in the treated conditions (7, 16, 17, 18, 19, 20).

The above-presented clinical studies, for example, curcuminoids employed in pancreatic cancer patients, indicate that despite low levels of curcumin detectable in plasma (e.g., 22–41 ng/mL), some of the patients improved as evidenced by significantly lowered cytokine levels (NF-kappaB, COX-2, and pSTAT3) and shrinking of the tumor mass. Conceivably, the limited bioavailability of curcumin attenuated the response rate, because exposure to microgram amounts of curcumin is required to show antiproliferative effects in vitro. It should also be taken under consideration that circulating curcumin levels do not reflect tumor tissue curcumin levels. In another human trial, the glutathione *S*-transferase activity, a potential surrogate biomarker of curcumin activity, was significantly decreased in patients taking 440 mg curcuminoids per day despite the lack of measurable blood levels of curcumin (46). This finding suggests that the metabolites of curcumin and its derivatives, which may not have been detected, resulted in a systemic biological effect.

Route of Administration in Relation to Efficacy

The form and route of administration of curcuminoids are important aspects for future chemopreventive strategies with these compounds. Curcumin and its derivatives are hydrophobic and therefore cannot be given intravenously. However, because curcumin and its derivatives are lipophilic, they can be encapsulated in a liposome, and this preparation would allow IV administration, possibly leading to higher circulating levels of curcumin. It has been reported previously that liposomal curcumin has antitumor activity both in vitro and in vivo and has no overt toxicity in animal models when administered systemically (44). Therefore, development of liposomal curcuminoids for clinical trials in cancer patients is a worthwhile strategy. Another possibility under consideration involves a nanoemulsion of curcuminoids to bypass the gastrointestinal barrier to achieve higher plasma concentrations of the unaltered phenolic compounds (51).

Curcuminoids may have efficacy when applied topically as an anti-inflammatory, antioxidant, and anticancer preparation. One study evaluated topical gel delivery of curcuminoids for its anti-inflammatory effects (52). Carbopol 934P (CRB) and hydroxypropylcellulose (HPC) were used for the preparation of gels. The percutaneous flux and enhancement ratio of curcumin across rat epidermis was enhanced significantly by the addition of menthol to both types of gel formulations. Neither type of topical gel formulation, CRB or HPC, caused any skin irritation. CRB gel showed better anti-inflammatory effects in vivo as compared to HPC gel. Both formulations were comparable in their topical anti-inflammatory action to a standard diclofenac gel formulation.

Absorption- and Bioavailability-Enhancing Compounds

Administering curcuminoids combined with agents enhancing their absorption may result in better biological efficacy of these compounds. In a trial performed at the Department of Pharmacology, St. John's Medical College, Bangalore, India, the effect of piperine extracted from fruits of black pepper (standardized for a minimum 95% alkaloid piperine) on gastrointestinal absorption of curcuminoids was evaluated (53).

Ten healthy male volunteers, 20 to 26 years old and weighing 50 to 75 kg, participated in a randomized trial to determine the comparative bioavailability and pharmacokinetic profile of curcuminoids when given alone or with piperine. Complete physical examination and blood work were performed to confirm that the subjects were in good health when enrolled into the study. The study protocol was reviewed and approved by the Institutional Ethical Committee, and informed consent was obtained from all subjects.

Participants abstained from food from 10 PM of the previous evening and reported to the laboratory at 7 AM the following day. The blood samples were collected at times 0 (predrug time) and 25, 30, and 45 minutes and 1, 2, 3, 4, and 5 hours after intake of curcuminoids. Following the predrug time (time 0) blood sample collection, the dose of 2 g curcuminoids alone (four capsules each containing 500 mg of curcuminoids) or 2 g curcuminoids with 20 mg piperine (four capsules each containing 5 mg of piperine) were ingested by the participants of the study. The blood sampling and oral curcuminoids were repeated after two weeks of washout. The subjects were asked to refrain from smoking, drinking alcohol, and taking any drugs during the trial. Standard meals were given to all participants on the day of the test.

Curcuminoids alone or in combination with piperine were well tolerated by the volunteers with no subjective or objective side effects reported. Serum levels of curcumin when administered alone were very low at all time points in most of the subjects. However, when piperine was included in the formula, serum concentrations of curcumin were significantly increased at 25 minutes and 30 minutes ($p < 0.01$) and 45 minutes ($p < 0.001$) of blood testing time points. Subsequently, there was a rapid decline of serum levels of curcumin within the next one hour and gradual decline to undetectable levels by the three-hour time point. The pharmacokinetic parameters showed the mean Cmax of curcumin at 0.006 ug/ml when curcuminoids were administered alone, versus 0.18 ug/ml when curcuminoids were administered with piperine. The mean AUC (area under the curve) with curcuminoids administered alone was 0.004 ug/h/ml versus 0.08 ug/h/ml when curcuminoids were administered with piperine. Therefore, the relative bioavailability of curcuminoids when given with piperine was enhanced by 2000% as compared to values of curcuminoids alone.

The results of this study indicate that piperine may operate through any or all of the following mechanisms: (a) a nonspecific enhancement of gastrointestinal absorption, (b) a potent inhibition of drug metabolism via P450 enzymes, and (c) inhibition of glucuronidation altering the disposition of the drug. The postulated biological mechanisms suggest that piperine may be involved in inhibiting the metabolism of curcuminoids and enhancing their bioavailability. Piperine may enhance serum concentration of curcuminoids probably because of increased absorption, reduced metabolism, and decreased rate of elimination from the body. Therefore, piperine may be considered as a bioenhancer of curcuminoids administered orally. Because of its lipophylic nature, piperine may be considered in future parenteral formulations encased in liposomes with curcuminoids.

REFERENCES

[1]Ferri C, Croce G, Cofini V, De Berardinis G, Grassi D, Casale R, Properzi G, Desideri G. C-reactive protein: interaction with the vascular endothelium and possible role in human atherosclerosis. *Curr Pharm Des.* 2007;13(16):1631–1645.

[2]Ohshima H, Tazawa H, Sylla BS, Sawa T. Prevention of human cancer by modulation of chronic inflammatory processes. *Mutat Res.* 2005 Dec 11;591(1–2):110–122. Epub 2005 Aug 3.

[3]Fiala M, Cribbs DH, Rosenthal M, Bernard G. Phagocytosis of amyloid-beta and inflammation: two faces of innate immunity in Alzheimer's disease. *J Alzheimers Dis.* 2007 Jul;11(4):457–463.

[4]McKellar G, Madhok R, Singh G. The problem with NSAIDs: what data to believe? *Curr Pain Headache Rep.* 2007 Dec;11(6):423–427. Review.

[5]Santangelo C, Varì R, Scazzocchio B, Di Benedetto R, Filesi C, Masella R. Polyphenols, intracellular signalling and inflammation. *Ann Ist Super Sanita.* 2007;43(4):394–405.

[6]Shishodia S, Sethi G, Aggarwal BB. Curcumin: getting back to the roots. *Ann N Y Acad Sci.* 2005 Nov; 1056:206–217.

[6a]Majeed M, Badmaev V, Rajendran R. Bioprotectant composition, method of use and extraction process of curcuminoids. United States Patent 5,861,415 granted January 19, 1999.

[7]Sharma RA, Euden SA, Platton SL, Cooke DN, Shafayat A, Hewitt HR, Marczylo TH, Morgan B, Hemingway D, Plummer SM, Pirmohamed M, Gescher AJ, Steward WP. Oncology Department, University of Leicester, Leicester; Phase I clinical trial of oral curcumin: biomarkers of systemic activity and compliance. *Clin Cancer Res.* 2004 Oct;10:6847–6854.

[8]Aggarwal BB, Shishodia S, Takada Y, Banerjee S, Newman RA, Bueso-Ramos CE, Price JE. Curcumin suppresses the paclitaxel-induced nuclear factor-kappaB pathway in breast cancer cells and inhibits lung metastasis of human breast cancer in nude mice. *Clin Cancer Res.* 2005 Oct 15;11(20):7490–7498.

[9]Zhang L, Fiala M, Cashman J, Sayrec J, Espinosa A, Mahaniana M, Zaghia J, Badmaev V, Graves MC, Bernard G, Rosenthal M. Curcuminoids enhance amyloid-b uptake by macrophages of Alzheimer's disease patients. *J Alzheimers Dis.* 2006;10:1–7.

[10]Fiala M, Liu PT, Espinosa-Jeffrey A, Rosenthal MJ, Bernard G, Ringman JM, Sayre J, Zhang L, Zaghi J, Dejbakhsh S, Chiang B, Hui J, Mahanian M, Baghaee A, Hong P, Cashman J. Innate immunity and transcription of MGAT-III and Toll-like receptors in Alzheimer's disease patients are improved by bisdemethoxycurcumin. *Proc Natl Acad Sci USA.* 2007 Jul 31;104(31):12849–12854. Epub 2007 Jul 24.

[11]Kamat AM, Sethi G, Aggarwal BB. Curcumin potentiates the apoptotic effects of chemotherapeutic agents and cytokines through down-regulation of nuclear factor-kappaB and nuclear factor-kappaB-regulated gene products in IFN-alpha-sensitive and IFN-alpha-resistant human bladder cancer cells. *Mol Cancer Ther.* 2007 Mar;6(3):1022–1030.

[12]Sandur SK, Pandey MK, Sung B, Ahn KS, Murakami A, Sethi G, Limtrakul P, Badmaev V, Aggarwal BB. Curcumin, demethoxycurcumin, bisdemethoxycurcumin, tetrahydrocurcumin and turmerones differentially regulate anti-inflammatory and anti-proliferative responses through a ROS-independent mechanism. *Carcinogenesis.* 2007 Aug;28(8):1765–1773.

[13]Kunnumakkara AB, Guha S, Krishnan S, Diagaradjane P, Gelovani J, Aggarwal BB. Curcumin potentiates antitumor activity of gemcitabine in an orthotopic model of pancreatic cancer through suppression of proliferation, angiogenesis, and inhibition of nuclear factor-kappaB-regulated gene products. *Cancer Res.* 2007 Apr 15;67(8):3853–3861.

[14]Lin YG, Kunnumakkara AB, Nair A, Merritt WM, Han LY, Armaiz-Pena GN, Kamat AA, Spannuth WA, Gershenson DM, Lutgendorf SK, Aggarwal BB, Sood AK. Curcumin inhibits tumor growth and angiogenesis in ovarian carcinoma by targeting the nuclear factor-kappaB pathway. *Clin Cancer Res.* 2007 Jun 1;13(11):3423–3430.

[15]Aoki H, Takada Y, Kondo S, Sawaya R, Aggarwal BB, Kondo Y. Evidence that curcumin suppresses the growth of malignant gliomas in vitro and in vivo through induction of autophagy: role of Akt and extracellular signal-regulated kinase signaling pathways. *Mol Pharmacol.* 2007 Jul;72(1):29–39.

[16]Dhillon N, Aggarwal BB, Newman R, Wolff R, Kunnumakkara AB, Abbruzzese J, Ng C, Badmaev V, Kurzrock R. Phase II trial of curcumin, an NF-kappaB inhibitor, in patients with advanced pancreatic cancer (submitted to *Clin Cancer Res.* 2007).

[17]Vadhan Raj S, Weber D, Giralt S, Alexanian R, Thomas S, Zhou X, Patel P, Bueso-Ramos C, Newman R, Aggarwal BB. Curcumin downregulates NF-κB and related genes in patients with multiple myeloma: results of a phase1/2 study. Abstract presentation at American Society of Hematology meeting, 2007.

[18]Raza A, Lagmay P, Mehdi M, Mumtaz M, Upadhyay R, Butt A, Ali T, Galili N. Saint Vincent's Comprehensive Cancer Center, New York, NY, University of Massachusetts Medical Center, Worcester. Multi-lineage response to a combination of gingerol and curcumin in low risk myelodysplastic syndromes (MDS) (Abstract 2007; prepared for publication).

[19]Golombick T, Diamond T, Badmaev V. The potential role of curcumin in plasma cell dyscrasias/paraproteinemia. Dept. Endocrinology, St George Hospital, Sydney AU. Abstract P64 in 2nd International Symposium on Translational Research; December 9–12, 2007: Lonavala, Mumbai, India. Golombick T, Diamond T, Badmaev V, Manoharan A, Ramakrishna R. The potential role of curcumin in patients with MGUS: its effect on paraproteinemia and the uNTx bone turnover marker. Accepted for publication in *Clin Cancer Res.* October 2008.

[20]Kurd SK, Smith N, Vanvoorhees A, Troxel AB, Badmaev V, Seykora JT, Gelfand JM. Oral curcumin in the treatment of moderate to severe psoriasis vulgaris: a prospective clinical trial. *J Am Acad Dermatol.* 2008 Feb 2 [Eupub ahead of print].

[21]Kunnumakkara AB, Diagaradjane P, Guha S, Deorukhkar A, Shentu S, Aggarwal BB, Krishnan S. Curcumin sensitizes human colorectal cancer xenografts in nude mice to g-radiation by targeting NF-κB-regulated gene products. *Clin Cancer Res.* 2008 Apr 1;14(7):2128–2136.

[22]Ringman JM, Cole G, Teng E, Badmaev V, Bardens J, Frautschy S, Rosario E, Porter V, Vanek Z, Sugar C, Cummings JL. Oral curcuminoids for the treatment of mild-to-moderate Alzheimer's disease: tolerability and clinical and biomarker efficacy results of a 24-week study. UCLA Department of Neurology Kagan Alzheimer's Disease Treatment Development Program UCLA Alzheimer's Disease Center. Los Angeles, CA (Abstract 2008; prepared for publication).

[23]Kuttan G, Kumar KB, Guruvayoorappan C, Kuttan R. Antitumor, anti-invasion, and antimetastatic effects of curcumin. *Adv Exp Med Biol*. 2007;595:173–184. Review.

[24]Gautam SC, Gao X, Dulchavsky S. Immunomodulation by curcumin. *Adv Exp Med Biol*. 2007;595: 321–341. Review.

[25]Rao CV. Regulation of COX and LOX by curcumin. *Adv Exp Med Biol*. 2007;595:213–226. Review.

[26]Garg A, Aggarwal BB. Nuclear transcription factor-kappaB as a target for cancer drug development. *Leukemia*. 2002 Jun;16(6):1053–1068. Review.

[27]Garg AK, Hortobagyi GN, Aggarwal BB, Sahin AA, Buchholz TA. Nuclear factor-kappa B as a predictor of treatment response in breast cancer. *Curr Opin Oncol*. 2003 Nov;15(6):405–411. Review.

[28]Takada Y, Bhardwaj A, Potdar P, Aggarwal BB. Nonsteroidal anti inflammatory agents differ in their ability to suppress NF-kappaB activation, inhibition of expression of cyclooxygenase-2 and cyclin D1, and abrogation of tumor cell proliferation. *Oncogene*. 2004 Dec 9;23(57):9247–9258.

[29]Aggarwal BB, Sundaram C, Malani N, Ichikawa H. Curcumin: the Indian solid gold. *Adv Exp Med Biol*. 2007;595:1–75.

[30]Mehta K, Pantazis P, McQueen T, Aggarwal BB. Antiproliferative effect of curcumin (diferuloylmethane) against human breast tumor cell lines. *Anticancer Drugs*. 1997 Jun;8(5):470–481.

[31]Hong RL, Spohn WH, Hung MC. Curcumin inhibits tyrosine kinase activity of p185neu and also depletes p185neu. *Clin Cancer Res*. 1999 Jul;5(7):1884–1891.

[32]Poma P, Notarbartolo M, Labbozzetta M, Maurici A, Carina V, Alaimo A, Rizzi M, Simoni D, D'Alessandro N. The antitumor activities of curcumin and of its isoxazole analogue are not affected by multiple gene expression changes in an MDR model of the MCF-7 breast cancer cell line: analysis of the possible molecular basis. *Int J Mol Med*. 2007 Sep;20(3):329–335.

[33]Dorai T, Dutcher JP, Dempster DW, Wiernik PH.Therapeutic potential of curcumin in prostate cancer— V: interference with the osteomimetic properties of hormone refractory C4-2B prostate cancer cells. *Prostate*. 2004 Jun 15;60(1):1–17.

[34]Kiran MS, Kumar VB, Viji RI, Sherin GT, Rajasekharan KN, Sudhakaran PR. Opposing effects of curcuminoids on serum stimulated and unstimulated angiogenic response. *J Cell Physiol*. 2008 Apr;215(1):251–264.

[35]Bhandarkar SS, Arbiser JL. Curcumin as an inhibitor of angiogenesis. *Adv Exp Med Biol*. 2007;595:185–195. Review.

[36]Lao CD, Demierre MF, Sondak VK. Targeting events in melanoma carcinogenesis for the prevention of melanoma. *Expert Rev Anticancer Ther*. 2006 Nov;6(11):1559–1568. Review.

[37]Aggarwal BB, Kumar A, Bharti AC. Anticancer potential of curcumin: preclinical and clinical studies. *Anticancer Res*. 2003 Jan-Feb;2391:363–398.

[38]Johnson JJ, Mukhtar H. Curcumin for chemoprevention of colon cancer. Cancer Lett. 2007 Oct 8;255(2):170–181. Epub 2007 Apr 19.

[39]Cheng AL, Hsu CH, Lin JK, et al. Phase I clinical trial of curcumin, a chemopreventive agent, in patients with high-risk or pre-malignant lesions. *Anticancer Res*. 2001;21:2895–2900.

[40]Dhillon N, Aggarwal BB, Newman RA, Wolff RA, Kunnumakkara AB, Abbruzzese JL, Ng CS, Badmaev V, Kurzrock R. Phase II trial of curcumin in patients with advanced pancreatic cancer. *Clin Cancer Res*. 2008;14(14):4491–4499.

[41]Epelbaum R, Vizel B, Bar-Sela G. Phase II study of curcumin and gemcitabine in patients with advanced pancreatic cancer. *J Clin Oncol*. 2008;26(May 20 suppl; abstract 15619) (ASCO).

[42]Kurd SK, Smith N, VanVoorhees A, Troxel AB, Badmaev V, Seykora JT, Gelfand JM. Oral curcumin in the treatment of moderate to severe psoriasis vulgaris: a prospective clinical trial. *J Am Acad Dermatol*. 2008 Apr;58(4):625–631. Epub 2008 Feb 4.

[43]Lao CD, Ruffin MT 4th, Brenner DE. Dose escalation of curcuminoid formulation. *BMC Complement Altern Med*. 2006 Mar 17;6:10 (pp. 1–4).

[44]Li L, Braiteh FS, Kurzrock R. Liposome-encapsulated curcumin: in vitro and in vivo effects on proliferation, apoptosis, signaling, and angiogenesis. *Cancer*. 2005;104:1322–1331.

[45]Cheng AL, Hsu CH, Lin JK et al. Phase I clinical trial of curcumin, a chemopreventive agent, in patients with high-risk or pre-malignant lesions. *Anticancer Res*. 2001;21:2895–2900.

[46]Sharma RA, McLelland HR, Hill KA, Ireson CR, Euden SA, Manson MM, Pirmohamed M, Marnett LJ, Gescher AJ, Steward WP. Pharmacodynamic and pharmacokinetic study of oral Curcuma extract in patients with colorectal cancer. *Clin Cancer Res*. 2001;7(7):1894–1900.

[47]Ireson C, Orr S, Jones DJ, Verschoyle R, Lim CK, Luo JL, Howells L, Plummer S, Jukes R, Williams M, Steward WP, Gescher A. Characterization of metabolites of the chemopreventive agent curcumin in human and rat hepatocytes and in the rat in vivo, and evaluation of their ability to inhibit phorbol ester-induced prostaglandin E2 production. *Cancer Res*. 2001 Feb 1;61(3):1058–1064.

[48]Wahlstrom B, Blennow G. A study on the fate of curcumin in the rat. *Acta Pharmacol Toxicol (Copenh)*. 1978, 43(2):86–92.

[49]Sandur SK, Pandey MK, Sung B, Ahn KS, Murakami A, Sethi G, Limtrakul P, Badmaev V, Aggarwal BB. Curcumin, demethoxycurcumin, bisdemethoxycurcumin, tetrahydro curcumin and turmerones differentially regulate anti-inflammatory and anti-proliferative responses through a ROS-independent mechanism. *Carcinogenesis*. 2007 Aug; 28(8):1765–1773.

[50]Lim GP, Chu T, Yang F, Beech W, Frautschy SA, Cole GM. The curry spice curcumin reduces oxidative damage and amyloid pathology in an Alzheimer transgenic mouse. *J Neurosci*. 2001;21(21):8370–8377.

[51]Ganta S, Amiji M. Co-administration of paclitaxel and curcumin in nanoemulsion formulations to overcome multidrug resistance in tumor cells. *Mol Pharm*. 2009 Mar 11 [Epub ahead of print].

[52]Patel NA, Patel NJ, Patel RP. Formulation and evaluation of curcumin gel for topical application. *Pharm Dev Technol*. 2008 Sep 27;1–10.

[53]Shoba G, Joy D, Joseph T, Majeed M, Rajendran R, Srinivas PSSR. Influence of piperine on the pharmacokinetics of curcumin in animals and human volunteers. *Planta Med*. 1998;64:353–356.

Botanical Medicine: From Bench to Bedside
Edited by R. Cooper and F. Kronenberg
© Mary Ann Liebert, Inc.

Chapter 7

Use of Standardized Mixtures of Paw Paw Extract (*Asimina triloba*) in Cancer Patients: Case Studies

Jerry L. McLaughlin,[1], Gina B. Benson,[2]*
Tad A. Turgeon,[2] and James W. Forsythe[3]

The paw paw tree, *Asimina triloba* (L.) Dunal (Annonaceae), is native to the eastern United States (1). Its edible fruits (Indiana bananas) are popular in song and have nourished animals and mankind for thousands of years. Although a fluid extract of its seeds was sold by Eli Lilly and Company at the end of the 1800s as an emetic, paw paw has a history of safe human consumption, and paw paw festivals are held throughout the Midwest every September when the fruits are harvested. A small commerce has developed in the sale of the seedlings and grafted small trees for fruit tree growth and in the sale of the frozen fruit pulp as an ingredient for gourmet desserts and chutneys.

In 1976 at Purdue University, we prepared extracts of the leaves and twigs of paw paw and found them to be bioactive in antitumor screens for the U.S. National Cancer Institute (NCI). Over the past 30 years, our bioactivity-directed fractionations of paw paw extracts have resulted in the isolation and characterization of over 50 potent compounds in a new class of natural products called the annonaceous acetogenins.

CHEMICAL STRUCTURE FEATURES

These compounds have been found only in the Annonaceae, and they are derived biosynthetically from acetate units linked linearly. They are derivatives of C32 or C34, long-chain, fatty acids attached to a 2-propanol unit to form a terminal α,β-unsaturated γ-lactone or a ketolactone. They typically contain from zero to three adjacent or nonadjacent tetrahydrofuran (THF) or tetrahydropyran (THP) rings along the hydrocarbon chain; these

[1] Department of Medicinal Chemistry and Molecular Pharmacology, School of Pharmacy and Pharmaceutical Sciences, Purdue University, West Lafayette, Indiana 47904-2091
[2] Nature's Sunshine Products, Spanish Fork, Utah 84660
[3] Cancer Screening and Treatment Center of Nevada, Reno, Nevada 89511
* Corresponding author: jerrymcl1014@aol.com

rings and their flanking hydroxyls generate a number of chiral centers that result in a daunting and complex mixture of diastereomers. The different stereochemistries of the ring systems lead to subclasses within the major structural types. Various substituents (hydroxyls, carbonyls, acetoxyls, and double bonds) along the hydrocarbon chain create further chemical diversities. Several related tropical and subtropical species in the Annonaceae (e.g., species in the genera *Annona*, *Asimina*, *Disepalum*, *Goniothalamus*, *Rollinia*, *Uvaria*, *Xylopia*, etc.) have yielded over 350 additional compounds in this class. Our group at Purdue University has published five comprehensive reviews on the chemistry and biology of the annonaceous acetogenins (2–6). Four additional reviews focus progressively on our contributions to this area of study (7–10). The numerous acetogenins (50, so far) that we have found in paw paw are described in a series of research papers which are summarized in a recent review (11). Asimicin (12), bullatacin (13), bullatalicin (14), and trilobacin (15, 16) (Figures 7.1–7.4) are among the most potent and most abundant of the acetogenins of paw paw, and they represent the major parental structural types of the paw paw acetogenins.

MECHANISM OF ACTION

The annonaceous acetogenins are extremely potent biologically (with cytotoxic IC_{50} values sometimes as low as $< 10^{-13}$ mcg/ml), and, mechanistically, they are the most powerful inhibitors known of complex I (NADH:ubiquinone oxidoreductase) of the mitochondrial electron transport system (17–20), where they bind to specific protein subunits (21, 22). They also inhibit the NADH oxidase found in the plasma membranes of tumor cells (23). Thus, they inhibit both the substrate level and oxidative phosphorylations of adenosine diphosphate (ADP); their immediate effect is depletion of adenosine triphosphate (ATP) levels (17), and this quickly results in the depletion of all of the related nucleotides (11). The resulting paucity of ATP and related nucleotides (all of which are essential as precursors of DNA and RNA) upsets the timing of cell division and induces programmed cell death (apoptosis) (11, 24). The downstream consequences of apoptosis, such as caspase-3 activation and decreases in cyclic adenosine monophosphate (cAMP) and cyclic guanosine monophosphate (cGMP) levels, have been reported in human hepatic carcinoma cells treated with bullatacin (Figure 7.2) (25).

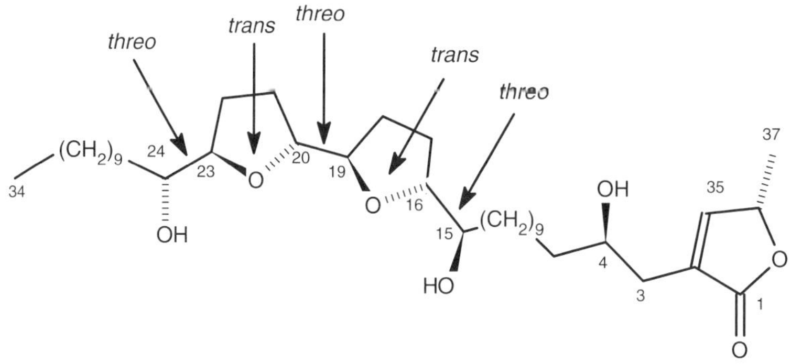

Figure 7.1. Asimicin

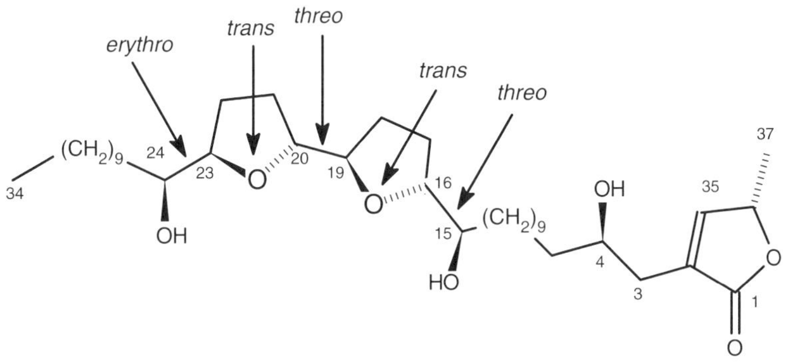

Figure 7.2. Bullatacin

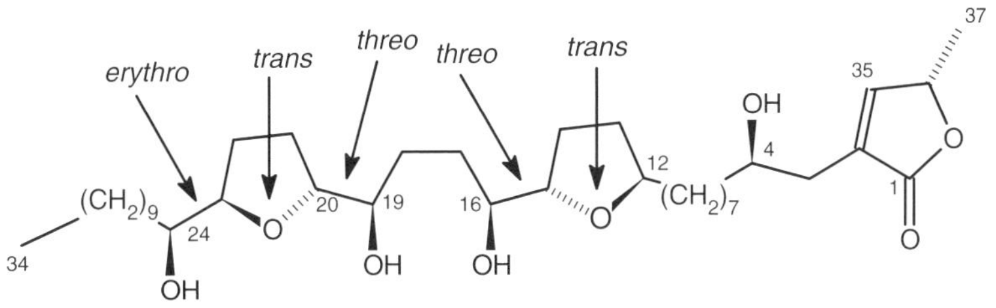

Figure 7.3. Bullatalicin

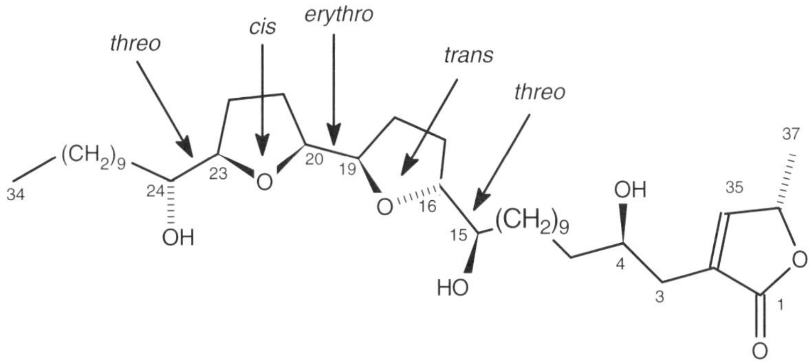

Figure 7.4. Trilobacin

Structure-activity relationships for the acetogenins have been evaluated in cultures of multiple drug resistant (MDR) and nonresistant cancer cells, brine shrimp, mosquito larvae, pesticide-resistant and nonresistant cockroaches, isolated mitochondria, and submitochondrial fragments (11), and the positioning of the acetogenins in biological membranes has been predicted using liposomes and intermolecular nuclear Overhauser effects with nuclear magnetic resonance spectrometry (26, 27). The acetogenins are especially effective against MDR cancer cells in which the drug resistance is due to ATP-dependent efflux pumps in the plasma membrane (28–31). The acetogenins circumvent MDR by decreasing the function of the efflux pump (P-170 glycoprotein) and increasing intracellular accumulation of anticancer agents (32, 33).

IN VIVO STUDIES

Our earlier studies, against murine leukemia in normal mice and human myeloma and ovarian cancer in athymic mice (4, 19), attested to the in vivo effectiveness of several of the acetogenins and demonstrated potencies in animals as high as 300 times that of Taxol; concurrent weight gain, rather than the drastic weight losses seen with Taxol and cisplatin (the positive controls), suggested that the acetogenins are well tolerated by the mice at the effective intraperitoneal dosages.

In spite of the success of the in vivo studies cited above, the inhibition of ATP production has been dogmatically deemed as too general a mechanism for systemic cancer chemotherapy. It has been argued that all cells require ATP, and thus ATP inhibitors would be simultaneously cytotoxic to essential normal tissues as well as cancer cells. However, the mice in the in vivo studies would have succumbed if this were true. Our studies with cell cultures of normal versus cancerous cells showed, early on, that the acetogenins are relatively less toxic to normal cells and more toxic to cancerous cells (34). Over 30 of our acetogenins have been repeatedly evaluated and show cytotoxic selectivities in the panel of 60 human tumor cell lines at the NCI and in the panel of 6 human tumor cell lines at the Cell Culture Laboratory of the Purdue Cancer Center. Thus, they are not generally cytotoxic agents. Furthermore, the endogenous biology of cancer cells is now understood to involve additional receptors for insulin and insulin-like growth factors (IGF-I and IGF-II) in the plasma membrane, which permit increased glucose uptake to fuel enhanced energy production and growth stimulation, respectively; this fact is the biochemical basis that supports insulin-potentiated chemotherapy (35). Breast cancer cells, for example, have an average of 7 times more insulin receptors (36) and 10 times more IGF receptors (37) than normal breast and other tissue cells within the host. Thus, these cancer cells can take up glucose 17 times faster than normal cells. To exploit this biochemical difference, mitochondrial inhibitors, such as the annonaceous acetogenins, should block the metabolism of the elevated glucose, deplete the ATP, induce apoptosis, and consequently show a selection for cancer cells, and they do. The depletion of ATP and the oxidized form of the pyrimidine, nicotinamide adenine dinucleotide (NAD), are finally being recognized as useful in the enhancement of cancer chemotherapy (38).

STANDARDIZATION

Several suppliers of botanical supplements are currently selling products that contain the powdered leaves and twigs of *Annona muricata* L. (guanabana, graviola, Brazilian paw paw); this species contains, predominantly, the less potent mono-THF acetogenins, and the producers have made no efforts to maximize acetogenin content or to standardize their products to assure consistent potency. Indeed, testing two of these products with the brine shrimp test alone reveals that as many as 20 to 50 capsules per serving would be necessary to achieve an effective dose level. Thus, standardized extracts, containing the natural complexes of the acetogenin mixtures as a botanical supplement, might be a solution to this problem and provide a beneficial adjuvant for the alleviation of clinical cancer.

To furnish the optimum in diversity of the most potent acetogenin structures, *Asimina triloba* (L.) Dunal, the paw paw tree, was first selected as the source of the biomass for preparation of the standardized extract. This species is native to the eastern United States and is abundant, and its edible fruit has a long history of safe human consumption (11). The potent acetogenins of paw paw have been isolated and individually characterized, using the brine shrimp lethality bioassay (7) to guide the isolation. The acetogenins have been found to be concentrated in the twigs, which thus serve as a convenient, renewable source of biomass (40). The brine shrimp assay and high-performance liquid chromatography/tandem mass spectrometry (LC/MS/MS) (41) have demonstrated that the concentrations of acetogenins in the twigs are maximal in the months of May through June; thus, collections of the biomass are best made at that time of year (42). The utility of biologically standardized extracts as botanical supplements containing mixtures of biologically active acetogenins rather than single chemical agents as drugs has not been previously reported.

EXTRACTION

Paw paw twigs (< 1/2 inch diameter) were collected in May through June from wild stands in the states of Indiana, Kentucky, and Missouri. The twigs were dried in a forced-air drier at < 50°C and reduced in a chipper/shredder through a 1/4 inch sieve. For testing purposes, small samples of the various lots were extracted with dichloromethane or methanol, and 20 mg portions were subjected to the brine shrimp assay. Only those lots that showed LC_{50} values of < 0.8 ppm were acceptable. In some cases, subpotent lots were combined with superpotent lots to furnish a blend that was acceptable.

Large-scale extractions of the plant material were initiated with hot water at one gallon per pound of twigs. After soaking the twigs for eight hours, the water was drained and discarded, and the water extraction was repeated three more times. The damp mass was then extracted with 95% ethanol, four times, in a similar manner. The ethanolic extracts were combined and concentrated, in vacuo, at < 40°C, to a syrup. The concentrate, upon sitting under refrigeration, formed a water layer that was removed and discarded, leaving a thick, black, syrupy, crude extract. The crude extract was standardized for 0% moisture, and the LC_{50} value was determined in the brine shrimp test. The standardized LC_{50} value was 0.5 ppm; generally, the crude extracts contained from 10% to 40% moisture, and the LC_{50} values ranged from 0.2 to 0.8 ppm. Adjustments were subsequently made in the amounts of extract per capsule to accommodate the standard value from lot to lot. The acetogenins in the crude extracts were monitored analytically by using LC/MS/MS on a Hewlett Packard (Palo Alto, California) model no. 1100 HPLC and a Finnegan Corporation (San Jose, California) model no. LCQ Duo MS/MS (40, 41) to be assured of the presence and amounts of the major bioactive acetogenins (asimicin, bullatacin, bullatalicin, and trilobacin) (Figures 7.1–7.4).

CAPSULE PREPARATION

The standardized crude extract was adsorbed onto microcrystalline cellulose, and vegetable magnesium stearate was added, as needed, to improve flow and to facilitate encapsulation. Analyses indicated that a two-year dating for shelf life would maintain potency.

SAFETY AND TOXICOLOGY

Previously we have shown that paw paw extracts and asimicin (Figure 7.1) are not significantly active as skin sensitizers in a modified guinea pig maximization test (43). For example, the Paw Paw Lice Remover Shampoo, which contains 0.5% of the standardized extract, passed the Draize test (44) for eye irritation in rabbits. The Ames test for mutagenicity was conducted with paw paw extracts, and the results were essentially negative; likewise, negative results have been reported for two purified acetogenins (squamocin and annonacin), although both were toxic to the bacteria in the absence of a metabolic activation system (45). In feeding experiments, mice tolerated 1% of the crude paw paw extract in their diets but succumbed when forced to eat the food containing 5% of the extract (11). Bullatacin (Figure 7.2) was emetic after injection at 185 mcg/kg to pigs; this was our first proof that the acetogenins are the emetic principles of paw paw, and this result might explain the use of the fluid extract of the seeds of paw paw as advertised and sold by Eli Lilly and Company a hundred years ago (46). Thus, emesis is a safety factor should someone ingest excessive amounts of the capsules or other paw paw products. Indeed, emesis is a common consequence of eating too many of the paw paw fruits.

Capsules containing the standardized paw paw crude extract were tested in male beagle dogs, in an ascending oral dosage schedule, ranging from 50 mg four times a day (QID) to 800 mg QID. Five to seven resting days were permitted between the days when doses were given. At the maximum dose (800 mg QID/dog), there were no severe effects other than emesis and loose stools. There was a gradual increase in signs of emesis and loose stools as the doses were increased, but it was impossible to reach a harmful or a fatal dose because of the emesis. There were no effects on alertness, appetite, or weight. Thus, any acutely toxic effects are conveniently avoided by emesis when oral dosing is used. The dogs were completely robust and normal after the study, and they were not sacrificed. Since the anti-tumor studies discussed above involved intraperitoneal injections and the mice (which could not possibly eliminate the acetogenins by vomiting) still survived, it was obvious that favorable therapeutic indexes must exist for the acetogenin products and that oral administration would be safe, provided no serious chronic toxicities would occur.

A type of atypical parkinsonism in which 75% of the patients do not respond to L-DOPA has been associated, epidemiologically, with the consumption of the fruits and teas (made from the leaves) of some tropical species of the Annonaceae. The species involved are *Annona muricata*, *A. squamosa*, and *A. reticulata* (47). The problem was first noticed on the island of Guadeloupe in the West Indies (48–50), but it has since been noted on the islands of Guam (51) and New Caledonia and in Afro-Caribbean and Indian populations now living in England (52). The condition appears to be caused by the chronic consumption of the fruits and teas, with the average age of the patients in the first Guadeloupe study of 74 years (a range from 42 to 84 years) (48). Especially in the younger patients, the symptoms show a regression after the patients stop consuming the annonaceous foods. At first the condition was blamed on the benzylisoquinoline alkaloids that are prevalent in the Annonaceae, but then the acetogenins were implicated as the causative agents. Annonacin, a mono-THF acetogenin, is the major acetogenin in *A. muricata* (53), and it causes damage (tau pathology) in cultured neurons (54–56) (involving ATP depletion) as well as in brain neurons in vivo after IV infusion in rats (57). The debate over this issue continues in the literature (11, 58).

Might the consumption of paw paw fruit or a supplement containing the paw paw extracts cause a similar problem? For several years, paw paws have been studied at Kentucky State University for their potential as a new fruit crop (59). The extracts of the ripe fruit pulp of paw paws were surprisingly potent in the brine shrimp assay, and LC/MS/MS analyses confirmed the presence of the major paw paw acetogenins (Figures 7.1–7.4) (60). In the consumption of paw paw fruit, the intake amount of the acetogenins is measurable; this is evident by the emesis caused when too many of the fruits are eaten. Yet, there has never been any association made between the consumption of paw paws and atypical parkinsonism or any other neurological affliction. The U.S. Food and Drug Administration has never received any such reports and suggests that paw paw consumption be continued. It should be noted that the major paw paw acetogenins are of the adjacent bis-THF type, while the mono-THF type predominate in *Annona muricata*; thus, the mono-THF acetogenins are chemically different and may have a peculiar affinity for brain neurons. Also, the alkaloids of the tropical Annonaceae are themselves known to be neurotoxic and may synergize with the mono-THF acetogenins to cause the neurotoxicity (61). Given the choice between dying of cancer and possibly experiencing the effects of atypical parkinsonism, after years of successful treatment of the cancer with the acetogenins, many cancer patients might choose the latter.

CLINICAL STUDIES

Previous clinical studies of the annonaceous acetogenins in cancer patients have been thwarted not so much by a lack of interest in these compounds and their novel mechanisms of action as by their unavailability in pure form. Several lengthy synthetic procedures have been reported (6, 11, 39), but these would be expensive to adapt to a commercial scale. The complexities of the mixtures of the acetogenins as found in nature would complicate an economical process for isolation and purification of individual acetogenins from their botanical sources, and the large number (over 400) of the individual acetogenins that could be developed as chemotherapeutic agents confuses the choice of which one is the best candidate to develop.

Selected Patient Case Studies

The state of Nevada permits terminal cancer patients and their physicians to use new approaches to cancer treatment. An initial group of 20 cancer patients, in the late stages of their illness, was recruited by one of us (JWF) from among the patient group. Additional volunteers were subsequently recruited by physicians and other health care practitioners. Only subjects diagnosed with clinical cancer were included, and many were those whose cancer at stage 4 was deemed to be terminal. Those who concurrently were undergoing chemotherapy and/or radiation were included along with those who had not had long-term success with their chemotherapy or radiation and those who had refused these options due to their known devastating effects on the immune system and general well-being. Patients suffering from a variety of tumor types were included in order to ascertain the tumor types that might be the most responsive.

Ninety-four cancer patients were enrolled as participants in the study. Each subject signed an informed consent and medical records release statement. Subjects were monitored by their health care provider for any adverse as well as positive effects. An Institutional Review Board, comprised of outside professionals, reviewed the protocols and found no concern for the safety of the subjects. The health care providers were instructed to discuss the possibility of adverse effects with the subjects and to report any adverse event within 24 hours. Precautions taken were more than necessary to conduct a study using a dietary supplement.

A preliminary study with three volunteers with terminal ovarian cancers revealed that a regimen of one capsule containing 12.5 mg of standardized paw paw extract, taken four times a day (QID) with food, was tolerable and avoided nausea and vomiting. Within one week the CA125 level of one of these volunteers was reduced by 66% from 3000 to 1000. Determinations of the usual blood parameters, for possible deleterious effects on liver and bone marrow, revealed no untoward effects. The study was continued over a period of approximately 18 months with new participants being added as the results with the earlier patients continued looking more and more promising.

Perusal of the records of the participants reveals some exciting observations. Over the 18-month period, of the 20 late-stage patients treated, 13 (65%) had survived and were in stable conditions taking the paw paw supplement every day. Longevities have increased. Levels of prostate specific antigen (PSA) have been held constant or lowered. Likewise, levels of breast tumor (CA 2729) and lung tumor (CEA) antigens have been significantly reduced. The rate of formation and sizes of primary and secondary tumors, for example, in bone, breast, lung, colon, pancreatic, and prostate cancers, melanoma, and cell counts in lymphomas, have decreased, and some have even disappeared. Stabilization was also achieved in a case of Waldenstrom's macroglobulinemia. Adverse effects are practically nonexistent when following the regimen of one 12.5 mg capsule taken four times a day (QID) with food over a period of 18 months or more. The participants showed no abnormalities in liver, kidney, electrolyte, blood sugar, or bone marrow functions. The only side effects reported were nausea and vomiting (three participants) and itching (one participant). Many patients reported having "increased energy." Some participants even chose to take as many as four capsules (50 mg) QID over several months without experiencing side effects. However, with one capsule, taken QID, most participants experienced positive responses within six to eight weeks. The results are, perhaps, best summarized by the presentation of ten case studies. Follow-up calls were made after five to six years to monitor the progress of these cases.

Ten Case Studies

Participant 1 had bone cancer. Prior treatment in 2002 involved radiation to the spine. She had not undergone any other conventional treatments. The levels of alkaline phosphatase were measured in the blood as a monitor of the progression of the disease. The normal range is from 0 to 136, and those with bone cancer have elevated levels. In September 2002, her test results showed 327. She started taking one paw paw capsule QID in November 2002. In December 2002, her alkaline phosphatase had decreased to 242, and by February 2003, it had decreased to 144. Her physician stated that as long as the levels remained stable, the cancer was being contained and not doing further damage. Over the next two years, her alkaline phosphatase levels varied between 144 and 150 as long as she took the paw paw, but if she stopped taking it the levels would increase. She reported that she had more energy and stamina when taking the paw paw. In September 2005, she was suffering severe emotional stress due to family problems, and she stopped taking paw paw. Her condition deteriorated and she passed away in March 2006, having survived a terminal condition for over three and one-half years by taking paw paw intermittently.

Participant 2 has a bone tumor on one of his neck bones. On July 30, 2002, the tumor, which was detected by X-ray, was measured as a 7 mm cavity with a 5 mm mass. He did not undergo any conventional treatments and elected only to take the paw paw capsules, which he began in September 2002. Another X-ray image, taken on March 13, 2003, showed a significant decrease in the tumor with a 4.5 mm cavity and a 3 mm mass. In the five-year follow up, he was reportedly doing well. He had continued with the paw paw capsules for a period of time and then stopped. The tumor grew in size, but it again regressed when he resumed taking paw paw. He remains in good health today taking the paw paw supplement.

Participant 3 has breast cancer. She has not undergone any conventional treatments since being diagnosed. She started taking the paw paw capsules in October 2002. She reported that the pain in her affected breast decreased, and her noncancerous fibrocystic lumps have reduced in size. Her physician reported that she has done "remarkedly well" considering that she has not had surgery. She reported that she feels good and has had some weight gain. In the five-year follow-up, she said that she had stopped taking the paw paw in lieu of some alternative treatments. Subsequently, cancer has formed in her other breast.

Participant 4 had breast cancer. She opted not to have any surgery, radiation, or chemotherapy. She started taking one paw paw capsule QID in November 2002. Her blood tests for the tumor antigen, CA2729, were consistent at 24 on September 12, 2002, and December 3, 2002. (In breast cancer patients, the CA2729 antigen is usually elevated above 15.) In March 2003, all of her blood tests were within the normal ranges. The tumor size had also reduced. She continued to take paw paw up to a week or two prior to her death on July 23, 2007. Although she passed away, her survival time for five years while taking paw paw is equivalent to the expected survival times of most breast cancer patients who opt for the expense and challenges to one's health of conventional treatments.

Participant 5 had breast cancer. She decided to undergo chemotherapy and take the paw paw capsules concurrently. The chemotherapy treatments lasted seven months. X-ray showed that the tumor had almost completely disappeared. She decided to undergo surgery as well to remove any traces of the tumor. Removal and examination of 14 subaxillary lymph nodes detected no metastatic cancer. This was followed by radiation treatments. Her subsequent screens have shown no detectable tumors in the breasts. She has retired from working and in the five-year follow-up is believed to be "cancer free."

Participant 6 has stage 4 breast cancer. After six weeks of taking paw paw, she saw a 50% reduction in her CA2729 tumor antigen levels, which went from 160 to 80 (< 15 is considered normal). The size of the tumor was also reduced. Since she had not changed any other treatment protocol, her physician was convinced that the paw paw supplement was responsible for her improvement. We were unable to locate this participant in the five-year follow-up.

Participant 7 has stage 4 lung cancer. He had previously undergone two years of chemotherapy, but the cancer had become resistant to the drugs. Within two months of taking the paw paw capsules (one capsule QID), his tumor marker (carcinoembryonic antigen, or CEA) had improved from 275 to 222. He also had a weight gain of five pounds and reported no side effects from the paw paw supplement. Prior to taking paw paw, he was bedridden or restricted to a wheelchair. His health improved to the point that he was able to walk and even play golf. We were unable to contact him in the five-year follow-up.

Participant 8 has stage 4 melanoma. The primary tumor had been surgically removed from his arm in 2001. By October 2002, the melanoma had metastasized to the lymph nodes and to the lungs. His physicians were not able to perform additional surgery and did not suggest chemotherapy or radiation as viable options. His breathing had become labored, and he could walk only with difficulty. In November 2002, he started taking one paw paw capsule QID and continued the paw paw supplement for one year. His breathing, mobility, and energy levels improved almost immediately, and he was able to return to work on his farm. In the spring of 2004, he had a follow-up X-ray of his lungs. His chest was completely clear, and there was no sign of the cancer. Interestingly, two fatty tumors on his arm have also decreased in size considerably, and the toenail fungus that had persisted for ten years has cleared up. At the time of the five-year follow-up, he was still doing well.

Participant 9 has prostate cancer, which was confirmed by a biopsy in July 2002. The tumor marker is prostate-specific antigen (PSA) with which normal values are <4. His PSA level was at 35 with two pea-sized tumors. In July 2002, he began a nutritional diet that consisted of lots of raw vegetables and fruits, no red meat, and low amounts of refined grains and sugars. He started taking four paw paw capsules per day in October 2002. His PSA level dropped to 2.08 by December 23, 2002, down from 3.85 when measured two months earlier. He continued to take the paw paw supplement, and his PSA levels through August 2004 remained stable. In the five-year follow-up, we learned that he has retired from work and continues to do well.

Participant 10 has stage 4 prostate cancer that has metastasized to several other parts of his body. Within six weeks of his starting QID consumption of paw paw, CT scans showed 25% reductions in the sizes of the tumors, while his PSA levels remained constant and did not increase. We were unable to contact him for the five-year follow-up.

OBSERVATIONS

Adjuvant Therapy

Due to the positive responses from the case studies above and from many other of the original 94 participants, it is apparent that the standardized paw paw extract is an effective supplement for the suppression of clinical cancers of various types. It appears that the extract may be an effective adjuvant to chemotherapeutic agents. When taken with chemotherapy, in some instances, an amount of tumor shrinkage beyond that expected with chemotherapy alone was noticed. The synergistic effect may be attributed to the novel action (ATP and nucleotide depletion) of the acetogenins working in conjunction with the cytotoxic actions of the chemotherapeutic agent. Also, the MDR cancer cells with their ATP-driven efflux pumps thwarted by the ATP-depleting action of the acetogenins would be expected to renew their cellular accumulation of the chemotherapeutic agent and become more susceptible to its cytotoxic effects. Thus, the combination of the paw paw extract with anticancer drugs should have not just additive but also synergistic effects.

Importance of Standardization

The standardized paw paw extract was effective, by both objective and subjective measurements, even when used alone and not combined with chemotherapy or radiation. Many participants who have exhausted the beneficial effects of these other modalities have enjoyed an extended longevity and improved their quality of life by taking this supplement. Many who were given only a couple of months to live have surpassed their physicians' predictions and have done so without the loss of hair, nausea and vomiting, bone marrow depression, or induction of new tumors by the carcinogenic actions of radiation and chemotherapeutic agents.

The standardized paw paw extract is unlike anticancer drugs because it is a complex mixture of compounds rather than a single entity. The compounds are natural and in the fruits of paw paw have been safely consumed by humankind for thousands of years. They even have a history of safe human use as an emetic.

Mode of Action

The mode of action (depletion of ATP with resulting apoptosis) gives these compounds selectivity for cancer cells because of the relatively more rapid rate of metabolism of cancer cells versus normal cells. They are especially effective against MDR cancer cells because of the increased demand that MDR cells have for ATP to run their efflux pumps. Thus, their actions focus on a fundamental biochemical difference between normal cells versus cancer cells and MDR cancer cells, that is, the voracious uptake of glucose and its accelerated metabolism to generate ATP and the related nucleotides.

Claims

The paw paw supplement is offered at reasonable cost in the United States as a dietary supplement. It costs less than $2.00 per day because the production from the paw paw twigs involves no elaborate separation steps but only simple extraction and analyses to assure potency and biological standardization. As the product is marketed as a dietary supplement, it avoids the tremendous costs in time, money, and labor that would be required in the United States for drug approval of one of its acetogenin components. However, it should be noted that as a dietary supplement, the paw paw product cannot be advertised as a treatment in the United States. The manufacturing company (Nature's Sunshine Products, Utah) only makes structure function claims that it is "selective for abnormal cells" and "slows the production of ATP in mitochondria of abnormal cells." Furthermore, a U.S. patent, assigned to Nature's Sunshine Products, is pending and protects the extract and its antitumor use in animals and humans (62).

SUMMARY

The selection of paw paw as an appropriate species and application of appropriate standardization led to a safe and effective supplement product. Specific chemical compounds (annonaceous acetogenins) in the paw paw were confirmed by in vitro and in vivo assays to have biological effects linked to the desired therapeutic outcome prior to entering clinical trial.

This dietary supplement, containing a standardized extract of paw paw, reduced tumor markers, reduced tumor sizes, and increased longevities among 94 subjects with clinical cancer while causing minimal side effects over a period of 18 months. Ten case studies are presented with five-year follow-ups. The product has been marketed for the past five years and has sold over 200,000 bottles, representing nearly 25,000,000 servings. Only 26 adverse events are reported. Inhibition of cellular energy (ATP), using the paw paw supplement, thus offers a novel, safe, inexpensive, and effective alternative for the control of clinical cancer.

ACKNOWLEDGMENTS

The authors thank the many health care workers who recruited the participants for this study, and the participants themselves deserve special acknowledgment for their courage. The earlier chemical and basic biological studies that made this study possible were largely funded by R01 grant no. CA30909 from the U.S. National Cancer Institute, National Institutes of Health. Additional support came from the Purdue Research Foundation and the Purdue Cancer Center. We thank John F. Kozlowski for his help in the preparation of this chapter.

REFERENCES

[1]Callaway MB. The paw paw (*Asimina triloba*). Frankfort, KY: Kentucky State University Publ.No. CRS-Hort 1–901, 1990.

[2]Rupprecht JK, Hui YH, McLaughlin JL. Annonaceous acetogenins: a review. *J Nat Prod*. 1990;62: 504–540.

[3]Fang XP, Rieser MJ, Gu ZM, Zhao GX, McLaughlin JL. Annonaceous acetogenins: an updated review. *Phytochem Anal*. 1993;4:27–48(part 1) and 49–67(part 2).

[4]Gu ZM, Zhao GX, Oberlies NH, Zeng L, McLaughlin JL. Annonaceous acetogenins: mitochondrial inhibitors with diverse applications. In: Arnason JT, Mata R, Romeo, JT, eds. *Recent Advances in Phytochemistry*. Vol 29. New York, NY: Plenum Press; 1995:249–310.

[5]Zeng L, Ye Q, Oberlies NH, Shi G, Gu ZM, He K, McLaughlin JL. Recent advances in annonaceous acetogenins. *Nat Prod Rep*. 1996;13:275–306.

[6]Alali FQ, Liu XX, McLaughlin JL. Annonaceous acetogenins: recent progress. *J Nat Prod*. 1999;62: 504–540.

[7]McLaughlin JL. Crown gall tumours in potato discs and brine shrimp lethality: two simple bioassays for higher plant screening and fractionation. In: Hostettmann K, ed. *Methods in Plant Biochemistry*. Vol 6. London: Academic Press; 1991:1–31.

[8]McLaughlin JL, Chang CJ, Smith DL. Simple bench-top bioassays (brine shrimp and potato discs) for the discovery of plant antitumor compounds: review of progress. In: Kinghorn AG, Balandrin MF, eds. *Human Medicinal Agents from Plants*. Washington, DC: American Chemical Society Symposium Series 534; 1993: 112–137.

[9]McLaughlin JL, Chang CJ, Smith DL. "Bench-top" bioassays for the discovery of bioactive natural products. In: Atta-ur-Rahman, ed. *Studies in Natural Products Chemistry*. Vol 9. Amsterdam: Elsevier; 1991: 383–409.

[10]McLaughlin JL, Chang CJ. Simple (bench-top) bioassays and the isolation of new chemically diverse antitumor and pesticidal agents from higher plants. In: Romeo JT, ed. *Recent Advances in Phytochemistry*. Vol 33. New York, NY: Kluwer/Plenum Publishers; 1999:89–132.

[11]McLaughlin JL. Paw paw and cancer: annonaceous acetogenins from discovery to commercial products. *J Nat Prod*. 2008;71:1311–1321.

[12]Rupprecht JK, Chang CJ, Cassady JM, McLaughlin JL, Mikolajczak KL, Weisleder D. Asimicin, a new cytotoxic and pesticidal acetogenin from the paw paw, *Asimina triloba* (Annonaceae). *Heterocycles*. 1986; 24:1197–1201.

[13]Hui YH, Rupprecht JK, Liu YM, Anderson JE, Smith DL, Chang CJ, McLaughlin JL. Bullatacin and bullatacinone: two highly potent bioactive acetogenins from *Annona bullata*. *J Nat Prod*. 1989;52:463–477.

[14]Hui YH, Rupprecht JK, Anderson JE, Liu YM, Smith DL, Chang CJ, McLaughlin JL. Bullatalicin, a novel bioactive acetogenin from *Annona bullata* (Annonaceae). *Tetrahedron*. 1989;45:6941–6948.

[15]Zhao GX, Hui YH, Rupprecht JK, McLaughlin JL, Wood KV. Additional bioactive compounds and trilobacin, a novel highly cytotoxic acetogenin, from the bark of *Asimina triloba*. *J Nat Prod*. 1992;55: 347–356.

[16]Zhao GX, Gu ZM, Zeng L, Chao JF, Wood KV, Kozlowski JF, McLaughlin JL. The absolute configuration of trilobacin and trilobin, a novel highly potent acetogenin from the stem bark of *Asimina triloba* (Annonaceae). *Tetrahedron*. 1996;51:7149–7160.

[17]Londerhausen M, Leicht W, Lieb F, Moeschler H, Weiss H. Molecular mode of action of annonins. *Pesticide Sci*. 1991;33:427–438.

[18]Lewis MA, Arnason JT, Philogene BJR, Rupprecht JK, McLaughlin JL. Inhibition of respiration at site I by asimicin, an insecticidal acetogenin of the paw paw, *Asimina triloba* (Annonaceae). *Pestic Biochem Physiol*. 1993;45:15–23.

[19]Ahammadsahib KI, Hollingworth RM, McGovren JP, Hui YH, McLaughlin JL. Mode of action of bullatacin: a potent antitumor and pesticidal agent. *Life Sci*. 1993;53:1113–1120.

[20]Hollingworth RM, Ahammadsahib KI, Gadelhak G, McLaughlin JL. New inhibitors of complex I of the mitochondrial electron transport chain with activity as pesticides. *Biochem Soc Trans*. 1994;22:230–233.

[21]Schuler F, Yano T, DiBernardo S, Yagi T, Yankovskaya V, Singer TP, Casida JE. NADH-quinone oxidoreductase: PSST subunit couples electron transfer from iron-sulfur cluster N2 to quinone. *Proc Nat Acad Sci USA*. 1999;96:4149–4153.

[22]Murai M, Ishihara A, Nishioka T, Yagi T, Miyoshi H. The ND1 subunit constructs the inhibitor binding domain in bovine heart mitochondrial complex I. *Biochemistry*. 2007;46:6409–6416.

[23]Morre DJ, de Cabo R, Farley C, Oberlies NH, McLaughlin JL. Mode of action of bullatacin, a potent antitumor acetogenin: inhibition of NADH oxidase activity of HELA and HL-60, but not liver, plasma membranes. *Life Sci*. 1995;56:343–348.

[24]Chih HW, Chiu HF, Tang KS, Chang FR, Wu YC. Bullatacin, a potent antitumor annonaceous acetogenin, inhibits proliferation of human hepatocarcinoma cell line 2.2.15 by apoptosis induction. *Life Sci*. 2001; 69:1321–1331.

[25]Chiu HF, Chiu TT, Hsian YM, Tseng CH, Wu MJ, Wu YC. Bullatacin, a potent antitumor annonaceous acetogenin, induces apoptosis through a reduction of intracellular cAMP and cGMP levels in human hepatoma 2.2.15 cells. *Biochem Pharmacol*. 2003;65:319–327.

[26]Shimada H, Grutzner JB, Kozlowski JF, McLaughlin JL. Membrane conformations and their relation to toxicity of asimicin and its analogues. *Biochemistry*. 1998;37:854–866.

[27]Shimada H, Kozlowski JF, McLaughlin JL. The localizations in liposomal membranes of the tetrahydrofuran ring moieties of the annonaceous acetogenins, annonacin and sylvaticin, as determined by ^{1}H NMR spectroscopy. *Pharmacol Res*. 1998;37:357–384.

[28]Oberlies NH, Croy VL, Harrison ML, McLaughlin JL The annonaceous acetogenin bullatacin is cytotoxic against multidrug-resistant human mammary adenocarcinoma cells. *Cancer Lett*. 1997;115:73–79.

[29]Oberlies NH, Chang CJ, McLaughlin JL Structure-activity relationships of diverse annonaceous acetogenins against multidrug resistant human mammary adenocarcinoma (MCF-7/adr) cells. *J Med Chem*. 1997; 40:2101–2106.

[30]Oberlies NH, Alali FQ, McLaughlin JL. Annonaceous acetogenins: thwarting ATP dependent resistance. In: Calis I, Ersoz T, Basaran AA, eds. *New Trends and Methods in Natural Products Research, Proceedings of the 12th International Symposium on Plant Originated Crude Drugs, May 20–22, 1998*. Ankara: The Scientific and Technical Research Council of Turkey; 1999:192–223.

[31]Johnson HA, Oberlies NH, Alali FQ, McLaughlin JL. Thwarting resistance: annonaceous acetogenins as new pesticidal and antitumor agents. In: Cutler H, Cutler S, eds. *Biologically Active Natural Products: Pharmaceuticals, ACS Symposium Book*. Boca Raton, FL: CRC Press; 1999:173–183.

[32]Fu LW, He LR, Liang YJ, Chen LM, Xiong HY, Yang XP, Pan QC. Experimental chemotherapy against xenografts derived from multidrug resistant KBv200 cells and parental drug-sensitive KB cells in nude mice by acetogenin 89-2. *Yao Xue Xue Bao*. 2003;38:565–570.

[33]Fu LW, Tan BY, Liang YJ, Huang H. The circumvention of tumor multidrug resistance by bullatacin. *Acta Pharm Sin*. 1999;34:268–271.

[34]Oberlies NH, Jones JL, Corbett TH, Fotopoulos SS, McLaughlin JL. Tumor cell growth inhibition of annonaceous acetogenins in an *in vitro* disk diffusion assay. *Cancer Lett*. 1995;96:55–62.

[35]Ayre SG, Garcia y Bellon DP, Garcia Jr DP. Insulin, chemotherapy, and the mechanisms of malignancy: the design and the demise of cancer. *Medical Hypothesis.* 2000;55:330–334.

[36]Papa V, Pezzino V, Constantino A, Belfiore A, Giuffrida D, Frittitta L, Vannelli GB, Brand R, Goldfine ID, Vigneri R. Elevated insulin receptor content in human breast cancer. *J Clin Investig.* 1990;86:1503–1510.

[37]Cullen KJ, Yee D, Sly WS, Perdue J, Hampton B, Lippman MF, Rosen N. Insulin-like growth factor expression and function in human breast cancer. *Cancer Res.* 1990;50:48–53.

[38]Martin DS, Bertino JR, Koutcher JA. ATP depletionn+pyrimidine depletion can markedly enhance cancer therapy: fresh insight for a new approach. *Cancer Res.* 2000;60:6776–6783.

[39]Das S, Li LS, Abraham S, Chen Z, Sinha SC. A bidirectional approach to the synthesis of a complete library of adjacent bis-THF annonaceous acetogenins. *J Org Chem.* 2005;70:5922–5931.

[40]Ratnayake S, Rupprecht JK, Potter WM, McLaughlin JL. Evaluation of various parts of the paw paw tree, *Asimina triloba* (Annonaceae), as commercial sources of the pesticidal annonaceous acetogenins. *J Econ Entomol.* 1992;85:2353–2356.

[41]Gu ZM, Zhou D, Wu J, Shi G, Zeng L, McLaughlin JL. Screening for annonaceous acetogenins in bioactive plant extracts by liquid chromatography/mass spectrometry. *J Nat Prod.* 1997;60:243–248.

[42]Gu ZM, Johnson HA, Zhou D, Wu J, Gordon J, McLaughlin JL. Quantitative evaluation of annonaceous acetogenins in monthly samples of paw paw (*Asimina triloba*) twigs by liquid chromatography/electrospray ionization/tandem mass spectrometry. *Phytochem Anal.* 1999;10:32–38.

[43]Avalos J, Rupprecht JK, McLaughlin JL, Rodriguez E. Guinea pig maximization test of the bark extract of paw paw. *Contact Dermatitis.* 1993;29:33–35.

[44]Draize JH, Woodard G, Calvery H. Methods for the study of irritation and toxicity of substances applied topically to the skin and mucous membranes. *J Pharmacol Exp Ther.* 1944;82:377–390.

[45]Guadano A, Gutierrez C, de la Pena E, Cortes D, Gonzales-Coloma A. Insecticidal and mutagenic evaluation of two annonaceous acetogenins. *J Nat Prod.* 2000;63:773–776.

[46]Anonymous. *Lilly's Handbook of Pharmacy and Therapeutics.* 13th ed. Indianapolis, IN: Eli Lilly and Company; 1898:89.

[47]Morton J. *Fruits of Warm Climates.* Greensboro, NC: Media, Inc.; 1987:65–90.

[48]Caparros-Lefebvre D, Elbaz A. Possible relation of atypical parkinsonism in the French West Indies with consumption of tropical plants: a case-control study. *Lancet.* 1999;354:281–286.

[49]Caparros-Lefebvre D, Sergeant N, Lees A, Camuzat A, Daniel S, Lannuzel A, Brice A, Tolosa E, Delacourte A, Duyckaerts C. Guadeloupean parkinsonism: a cluster of progressive supranuclear palsey-like tauopathy. *Brain.* 2002;125:801–811.

[50]Caparros-Lefebvre D, Lees AJ. Atypical unclassifiable parkinsonism on Guadeloupe: an environmental toxic hypothesis. *Movement Disord.* 2005;20(Suppl 12):S114-S118.

[51]Caparros-Lefebvre D, Steele J. Atypical parkinsonism on Guadeloupe, a comparison with the parkinsonism-dementia complex of Guam, an environmental toxic hypothesis. *Environ Tox Pharmacol.* 2005;19:407–413.

[52]Chaudhuri KR, Hu MT, Brooks DJ. Atypical parkinsonism in Afro-Caribbean and Indian origin immigrants to the UK. *Mov Disord.* 2000;15:18–23.

[53]Champy P, Melot A, Guerineau V, Gleye C, Fall D, Hoglinger GU, Ruberg M, Lannuzel A, Laprevote O, Laurens A, Hocquemiller R. Quantification of acetogenins in *Annona muricata* linked to atypical parkinsonism in Guadeloupe. *Mov Disord.* 2005;20:1629–1633.

[54]Lannuzel A, Michel PP, Caparros-Lefebvre D, Abaul J, Hocquemiller R, Ruberg M. Toxicity of Annonaceae for dopaminergic neurons: potential role in atypical parkinsonism in Guadeloupe. *Mov Disord.* 2002; 17:84–90.

[55]Lannuzel A, Michel PP, Hoglinger GU, Champy P, Jousset A, Medja F, Lombes A, Darios F, Gleye C, Laurens A, Hocquemiller R, Hirsch EC, Oertel WH, Ruberg M. The mitochondrial complex I inhibitor annonacin is toxic to mesencephalic dopaminergic neurons by impairment of energy metabolism. *Neuroscience.* 2003;121:287–296.

[56]Escobar-Khondiker M, Hollerhage M, Muriel MP, Champy P, Bach A, Depienne C, Respondek G, Yamada ES, Lannuzel A, Yagi T, Hirsch EC, Ortel WH, Jacob R, Michel PP, Ruberg M, Hoglinger GU. Annonacin, a natural mitochondrial complex I inhibitor, causes tau pathology in cultured neurons. *J Neurosci.* 2007; 27:7827–7837.

[57]Champy P, Hoglinger GU, Feger J, Gleye C, Hocquemiller R, Laurens A, Guerineau V, Laprevote O, Medja F, Lombes A, Michel PP, Lannuzel A, Hirsch EC, Ruberg M. Annonacin, a lipophilic inhibitor of mitochondrial complex I, induces nigral and striatal neurodegeneration in rats: possible relevance for atypical parkinsonism in Guadeloupe. *J Neurochem.* 2004;88:63–69.

[58]Lannuzel A, Hoglinger GU, Champy P, Michel PP, Hirsch EC, Ruberg M. Is atypical parkinsonism in the Caribbean caused by the consumption of Annonaceae? *J Neural Trans Suppl.* 2006;70:153–157.

[59]Pomper KW, Layne DR. The North American paw paw: botany and horticulture. *Hort Rev.* 2005;31: 351–364.

[60]Pomper KW, Lowe JD, Crabtree SB, Keller WJ. Assessment of annonaceous acetogenin activity in paw paw fruit. *Hort Sci*. 2007;42:939.

[61]Caparros-Lefebvre D, Steele J, Kotake Y, Ohta S. Geographic isolates of atypical parkinsonism and tauopathy in the tropics: possible synergy of neurotoxins. *Mov Disord*. 2005;21:1769–1771.

[62]McLaughlin JL, Benson GB. Control of cancer with annonaceous extracts. U.S. Patent (pending), serial no. 10\717,746, November 20, 2003.

Botanical Medicine: From Bench to Bedside
Edited by R. Cooper and F. Kronenberg
© Mary Ann Liebert, Inc.

Chapter 8

Valerian and Hops: Synergy, Mode of Action, and Clinical Evidence

Uwe Koetter

Valerian and hops are among the most widely used herbal medicines to induce sleep and treat insomnia. Advances in research on valerian and hops in regard to sleep depend first of all on the current knowledge of sleep and the underlying physiological processes. Short-comings in understanding how these herbal substances work may be a result of the ongoing scientific debate on sleep mechanisms and patterns rather than on the absence of a good night's sleep. Recent advances in understanding physiological processes involved in regulating sleep offer new explanations on the mode of action of valerian and hops. Both appear to work as naturally occurring sleep-regulating substances.

Sleep can be well described, but little is known about its function. Freemon wrote in his book on sleep research in 1972 that "an unequivocal definition of sleep evades us. There are about as many theories of sleep as there are sleep researchers. For every research worker who has restrained himself from publishing his theoretical ideas on sleep, another investigator has advanced two or more different, often competing theories. Some sciences and medieval medicine is an example, have been affected by premature and extensive theorization. The development of sleep research, however, has reached the point where some type of general theory is desperately needed to hold together such disparate findings" (1).

Thirty years on and the situation has changed little. In 2000, Benington wrote in his introduction in an article about sleep homeostasis and the function of sleep: "We still do not know the function of sleep. . . . Sleep represents a global alteration of brain functioning that occupies about one-third of each day and appears to be indispensable. As long as we do not understand the function of sleep, we also do not understand some very important and as yet undiscovered physiological requirements of neural tissue" (2).

Sleep is an essential part of everyday life maintained by physiological processes. The brain appears to use the time of sleep to reorganize itself. Both mood and learning benefit from sleep, and it is also important for physical health. Poor sleep is associated with greater psychological distress and higher levels of biomarkers associated with elevated risk of heart disease and type 2 diabetes (3).

Two separate types of sleep can be observed: sleep with rapid eye movement (REM) and sleep without—so-called non-REM sleep (NREM). Sleep proceeds in cycles, with each

---

Dr. Koetter Consulting, 8592 Uttwil, Switzerland; koettu@mac.com

cycle lasting about 100 minutes. Deeper sleep during these cycles occurs earlier during the night, while REM sleep occurs more toward the end of night. Each type has its own physiological and psychological features and may benefit overall health in a different way.

To make matters more complex, sleep changes during life. Older people spend more time in unwanted wakefulness during the night than do younger adults (4). Therefore, physiological changes need to be taken into account when insomnia is investigated. Finding appropriate volunteers for mild to moderate insomnia is a particular challenge, as sleep perception may differ from the actual sleep problem.

According to Borbély, sleep architecture and sleep propensity are determined by a history-dependent homeostatic process and a circadian process. The homeostatic process rises during wakefulness and declines during sleep (Process S). Process S interacts with a circadian process (Process C) that is independent of sleep and waking. The conceptual framework of the two-process model was first published by Borbély in 1982 and appears to explain the processes of sleep initiation and continuation (5).

The time course of Process S is derived from electroencephalogram (EEG) slow-wave activity (6), while Process C seems closely related to melatonin secretion (7). Prolonged wakefulness decreases the degree of arousal in the frontal cortex. Both the propensity to sleep and the intensity of delta EEG waves upon falling asleep have been shown to be proportional to the duration of prior wakefulness. Evidence has been provided that the basal forebrain and mesopontine cholinergic neurons, whose discharge activities play an important role in EEG arousal, are under the tonic control of endogenous adenosine. The local concentration of adenosine at the basal frontal cortex neurons increases with prolonged wakefulness. Therefore, local adenosine concentration is related to sleep mechanisms and is consequently attributed as somnogen (8).

Important for research on valerian and hops is that for Process S and Process C to occur, chemical compounds in these plants may play a role. These compounds are found in either or both of these herbal preparations, which together may mimic their action. Advances in understanding how valerian and hops contribute to a good night's sleep through their potential mode of action are described in the following sections.

MODE OF ACTION OF VALERIAN

More than 200 plant species belong to the genus *Valeriana*, but the one most commonly used as an herb is *Valeriana officinalis*. The root is used for medicinal purposes. Preparations of valerian (*Valeriana officinalis* L.) are today well established for the relief of mild nervous tension and sleep disorders. They have been used traditionally for the relief of mild symptoms of stress as well (9).

Extract from valerian root has been widely used in Europe for decades. In the United States, it is estimated that approximately 1% of the population use valerian as a self-prescribed treatment for insomnia (10). The typical preparation of valerian employed as a sleep aid is a tea, a tincture, or an extract produced with an alcohol-water mixture. The preparation as such is considered the "active ingredient" for which the extract ratio should be provided. For identification and quality control, valerenic acid is used as the marker compound. The content of these sesquiterpenic acids ranges (for just valerenic acid) from 0.04% to 0.9%, or for the combination of valerenic acid, acetoxyvalerenic acid, and hydroxyvalerenic acid, from 0.17% to 0.9% (11).

However, the general acceptance that valerian provides an effective treatment option has remained open for discussion. For a long time, it was believed that the intense and heavy odor plays an important role in the sleep-promoting properties. Evidence from animal studies supported this thesis, as inhalation of valerian produced a distinct sedative effect in rats (12). The lack of correlation between the volatile oil and a sedative effect prompted research for other constituents contributing to this activity. In the 1960s, much attention was directed to the valepotriates. A standardized mixture was developed and marketed with preclinical research supporting it (13). It is now known, however, that valepotriates are not stable in tinctures and extracts. For that reason, their contributions to the sleep-promoting effects of traditionally used formulas were disputed (14).

According to another theory, valerenic acid is responsible for sedative activity (15). Valerian extract and valerenic acid were shown to have an effect on neuronal activity mediated by the GABAergic system (16). Gamma-aminobutyric acid (GABA), as a neurotransmitter, participates in the thalamus in sleep induction and maintenance. It exerts its action through three different types of receptors, namely, $GABA_A$, $GABA_B$, and $GABA_C$. $GABA_A$ receptors are ligand-activated ion channels with different subunits, which mediate fast synaptic transmission.

Very recently it was confirmed that valerenic acid positively modulates the $GABA_A$-induced chloride currents. Its content in extracts is proportionally related to their $GABA_A$ receptor modulation (17). $GABA_A$ receptors containing the β_3 subunit were identified as a target mediating the anxiolytic action of valerenic acid (18). In this context it was demonstrated that anxiolytic and antidepressant properties of valerian may contribute to the sleep-inducing effect of valerian (19).

Recently, compounds structurally similar to adenosine have been isolated from valerian. Adenosine is involved in sleep induction mediated via G protein–coupled receptors. Specifically the adenosine A_1 receptor was found to play a part in homeostatic sleep regulation (20).

From a methanolic valerian extract, lignans were isolated and investigated for their pharmacological activity on various receptors of the central nervous system. Olivil was identified as a lignan derivative with partial agonistic affinity to human adenosine A_1 receptors in meaningful concentrations (21).

This effect on adenosine A_1 receptors was confirmed in commercially available extracts, which are typically employed in sleep aids. Valerian was extracted by maceration with methanol/water 45% at ambient temperature for two hours with stirring followed by evaporation and spray drying. The ratio of dried herbal material employed to spray-dried extract with 25% maltodextrin as a carrier was about 4–6:1. The valerian roots employed were of European Pharmacopeia quality. The resulting extract contained 0.37% to 0.39% valerenic acids (sum of valerenic acid and acetoxyvalerenic acid). It was free of valepotriates.

Affinity for adenosine A_1 receptors was determined in radioligand binding assay at rat brain cortical membranes versus [^{3}H] 2-chloro-N^6-cyclopentyladenosine [^{3}H]CCPA. Individual extracts and a combination with hops exhibited affinity in a low concentration range (K_i values 0.15–0.37 mg/mL). In order to investigate whether valerian extract acts as an agonist, its effect on [^{35}S]GTPgS binding to human recombinant adenosine A_1 receptors was measured. Valerian extract exhibited a concentration-dependent stimulation of [^{35}S] GTPgS. The maximal effect was about 30% over baseline with EC_{50} values of 0.85 mg/mL. Adenosine A_1 receptors are negatively coupled to adenylate cyclase as a second messenger system. The agonist N^6-cyclopentyladenosine (CPA) and valerian extract inhibit dose dependently cAMP accumulation, confirming the agonistic activity of valerian extract (22). Thus, adenosine activity reported earlier (23) is confirmed by this detailed work and the function on the receptor explained.

Lignans were isolated prior to the work of Schumacher et al. 2002. They were investigated at various central nervous system (CNS) receptors (24) and presented as potentially active substances (25). However, several years later, Müller made the link between lignans and adenosine receptor activity of valerian (22). This finding triggered further preclinical and clinical work described in the following paragraphs.

The agonistic activity of the valerian extract was confirmed in ex vivo experiments with brain slices. The extract employed was of similar quality as that used by Müller et al. 2002, produced with methanol/water 45% and the content of valerenic acids was determined by HPLC (22).

Postsynaptic potentials were dose-dependently inhibited by valerian extract with a minimum concentration of 0.1 mg/ml and saturation at 10 mg/ml. The inhibition reached around 50%, and its extent was comparable to the inhibition by the selective agonist CPA. The effect could be blocked by a specific adenosine A_1 receptor antagonist (26).

The results were confirmed in a second study with a similar design. It appears, however, that the extraction solvent—in this case, methanol—is essential for adenosine agonistic effects in this model, as ethanol extracts from valerian did not show affinity (27). It is notable that this is in accordance with independent findings of a second group, in that pharmacological profiles of valerian preparations are linked to the polarity of their extraction solvents (28).

With the evidence from the analytical work, together with the in vitro and ex vivo results, a potential adenosine-like action of valerian can be concluded. Establishing a link to in vivo results provides further proof and is discussed in a later section.

MODE OF ACTION OF HOPS

Hop is a member of the Cannabaceae family. It is a dioecious perennial plant native to the Northern Hemisphere. The flower cones of the plant, known as hops, are used in the production of beer to impart bitterness and flavor and for their preservative qualities. The aromatic odor of the hop strobiles is caused by a volatile oil, present in a yield of about 0.3% to 1.0%. Among the actives that are thought to be responsible for its medicinal effects are 15% to 30% resins (such as humulon and lupulon and its derivatives 2-methyl-3-butenol), tannins, flavonoids, and essential oils (with its main constituents myrcene, alpha- and beta-caryophyllene, and farnesene) (29).

Preparations of hops (*Humulus lupulus* L.) or of hop strobiles are today traditionally used for the relief of mild symptoms of stress and to aid sleep (30). Preparations are made of infusions, tinctures, and extracts. Despite the long-standing use of hop preparations as sedatives in traditional medicine, data on the effects of hops are rare (31). Therefore, the sedative activity is still under investigation to elucidate the active principles responsible for the neuropharmacological effects.

In an analogous manner to valerian, it was believed earlier that hops acted through their strong and heavy odor. Pillows filled with hops have been successfully employed for many years, according to the literature. There is anecdotal evidence that goes back to the reign of George III (32). The aroma of hops causes somnolence, which led to the use of "sleep pillows" filled with hops and placed in the bed (and thus close to the head). Reference to such successful use can be found in the literature (33, 34).

Reports on the systematic investigation of hops and their ingredients can be found as early as 1820. Ives coined the name *lupulin* for the fine, yellow, resinous substance of the female flowers from hops and investigated it chemically. As a physician, he was most convinced of its effects and reported that it frequently induced sleep and "quiets great nervous" irritation (35). Despite this early praise, little work was published on sleep in subsequent years. Nevertheless, hops have been consistently employed in combination products with other sleep-promoting herbal preparations.

Some recent in vitro work with hops was conducted with lipophilic extracts. The $GABA_A$ response was measured using a Xenopus oocyte expression system. Two hop oils, alpha-humulene and mycrene, caused a small potentiation of the $GABA_A$ receptor response. However, these compounds did not work as agonists. Beta-acid fractions from hops were found to modulate GABA response inversely (36).

It appears the effects of hop fragrance were more pronounced in causing potentiation of the $GABA_A$ receptor response. This result links to the traditional use of hops in sleep pillows (37) but has little relevance for hydrophilic hop extracts typically used in sleep aids.

Perhaps more relevant is a study on hops as a sleep aid using a recently conducted systematic screening for activity on receptors of the CNS. The screening included 5-hydroxytryptamine (5-HT) and melatonin (ML) receptors. The 5-HT receptors on the cell membrane of nerve cells are receptors for the signal mediator serotonin in the CNS and on the periphery. They affect the release and activity of other neurotransmitters such as dopamine and are known for their role in cognitive performance, depression, and sleep disorders (38).

The effects of melatonin are mediated by specific, high-affinity melatonin receptors (ML1/ML2). Melatonin is an endogenous hormone released from the pineal gland in response to light and dark signals. It stimulates melatonin receptors, which appear to contribute to the sleep-wake cycle modulating the circadian rhythm (39).

Hop extract used for the following experiments was produced by maceration of hops (European Pharmacopeia quality) with methanol/water 45% at ambient temperature followed by evaporation under vacuum and spray drying. The ratio of dried herbal material employed to spray-dried extract with 30% maltodextrin as a carrier was about 5–7:1. The extract contained about 0.48% of flavonoids calculated as rutin determined spectrophotometrically. Because of the hydrophilic solvent, hop bitter acids were not detectable.

The screening assays were performed using published procedures with human cloned receptors where available. The receptors selected for screening are involved in various mental functions related to relaxation, stress, cognition, maintenance of circadian rhythm, and sleep. Pharmacological details regarding the receptors are listed in Table 8.1.

Of all the selected receptors, the tested extracts showed considerable affinities toward the $5\text{-}HT_{4e}$, $5\text{-}HT_6$, $5\text{-}HT_7$, ML_1, and ML_2. For these receptors, a determination of IC_{50} was conducted. The results are as follows: 21mg/ml for the $5\text{-}HT_6$ and 71mg/ml for the ML_1 receptor. This is the first report of hops' interaction with these receptors. $5\text{-}HT_6$ antagonists are thought to improve cognition, while melatonin, through binding to its receptor, is responsible for maintaining the diurnal circadian rhythm in vertebrates (40).

Table 8.1. Affinity of Hops to Selected CNS Receptors and Their Function in the Body; Gs = G Stimulatory

Receptor Type	Nonspecific Binding	Affinity for Hops $IC_{50}(m/ml)$	Molecular Function	Pharmacodynamic / Pharmacological Activity
5-HT$_{4e}$	serotonin		Gs protein, coupled to the stimulation of adenylyl cyclase, increasing cellular levels of cAMP	CNS: neuronal excitation, learning, memory
5-HT$_6$	serotonin	21	Gs protein, coupled to the stimulation of adenylyl cyclase increasing cellular levels of cAMP	May be involved in neuropsychiatric disorders; high affinity for various antipsychotic and antidepressant drugs
5-HT$_7$	serotonin		Gs protein, coupled to the stimulation of adenylyl cyclase increasing cellular levels of cAMP	Mood and learning, neuroendocrine and vegetative behavior; 5-HT7-selective agents might be effective in the treatment of jet lag or sleep disorders of a circadian nature
ML$_1$	melatonin	71	G protein–coupled receptor	Regulation of circadian and seasonal responses, some retinal, cardiovascular, and immunological functions; antidepressant/anxiolytic activity
ML$_2$	melatonin		G protein–coupled receptor	Regulation of circadian and seasonal responses, some retinal, cardiovascular, and immunological functions; antidepressant/anxiolytic activity

PRECLINICAL EVIDENCE FOR VALERIAN

With the evidence from in vitro and ex vivo studies, adenosine-like action was demonstrated, which is most likely mediated by lignans. Because of the many lignans that are present as aglycones or as the glycosides—and they are present in low concentrations—measurement of pharmacodynamic properties is a necessary substitute for testing of bioavailability. Adenosine-like action of lignans from valerian extract might reduce alertness that should be reflected in an increase of the slow-wave activity in the frontal cortex. To test this hypothesis, changes in field potentials were measured from the depth of the brain in conscious adult Fisher rats. The animals carried bipolar concentric steel electrodes. Signals were transmitted, amplified, and processed to give power spectra of 0.25 Hz resolution. During the recordings, the rats could move freely. Experiments were started after adaptation and control experiments with saline. The trials were authorized according to German Health Guidelines, and the principles of laboratory animal care were followed in all trials.

The rats received a fixed combination of valerian and hop extracts, both manufactured with methanol/water 45%. The valerenic acid content and flavonoid content were determined respectively. The extracts were suspended in 20% Solutol (BASF, Mannheim, Germany). Research presented earlier had already confirmed that hops do not contribute to the adenosine agonistic affinity. Hence the results of this study can be attributed to valerian only. Slow-wave activity of field potentials was recorded in the frontal cortex. Application of 200 and 250 mg/kg resulted in an increase of delta and alpha2 power in the cortex and hippocampus starting after 60 minutes. The results became statistically significant in the last hour of recording (4 h). This action is similar to the increased slow-wave activity related to sleep deprivation. Therefore, such an increase in slow-wave activity in the frontal cortex might indicate an elevation of sleep propensity induced by the valerian fraction of the fixed combination. Additionally, the bioavailability of the extract is related to the reaction of the target organ, that is, the central nervous system with a short latency after oral administration (41).

PRECLINICAL EVIDENCE FOR HOPS

Animal studies were conducted in the past using frogs, pigeons, mice, goldfish, and golden carp to better understand the sedative effects of hops. However, an understanding of the biochemical mechanism and a conclusive identification of the compounds responsible for such activity have not yet been achieved (42). In mice, hypothermic, analgesic, anticonvulsant, and hypnotic properties were recorded after intraperitoneal injection of a hop extract (43). Hop extracts, prepared either with ethanol (40%, 90%) or with CO_2, were investigated for their sedating activities. The preparations reduced spontaneous locomotor activity, increased the ketamin-induced sleeping time, and reduced body temperature. The lipophilic extract from hops was superior to the ethanolic extract (44). Another hop extract using CO_2 prolonged the pentobarbital-induced sleeping time without influencing the motor behavior of rats and exerted antidepressant activity. The same effects were elicited by the administration of the hop fraction containing alpha-acids (45). In contrast, administration of the beta-acid-enriched fraction increased exploratory activity in the open field, reduced the pentobarbital hypnotic activity, and worsened the picrotoxin-induced seizures. In the anxiety elevated plus maize test, a reduction in anxiety was clearly demonstrated (36). Therefore, the relationship between the different, bitter acids may influence the overall action. Whether the results obtained with the lipophilic CO_2 extract can be transferred to the extracts employed in medicines is debatable. These extracts are produced with water or mixtures of alcohol and water.

To understand the mode of action of hops, the in vitro finding on melatonin receptor activity provides an excellent starting point. Building on the in vitro results published by Abourashed et al. in 2004, an animal study was designed to investigate the melatonin-like activity further and to confirm the relevance of the findings in a living organism.

The spray-dried hop extract was prepared from dried cones of *Humulus lupulus* L. of European Pharmacopeia quality by maceration with methanol/water 45%. Qualitative and quantitative phytochemical analysis of the extract was performed by HPLC. The hops extract was standardized to an amount of 0.48% flavonoids calculated as rutin. Bitter acids were not detectable.

First, mice received either a hop extract or control, orally, one hour before the measurements, by means of a feeding needle. Melatonin and control were given intraperitoneally. The rectal temperatures were measured at hourly intervals for three hours. Melatonin (50 mg/kg) and hop extract (250 mg/kg) both had significant hypothermic effects in male mice. The decrease of body temperature was $0.75 \pm 0.07°C$ for hop extract versus $0.66 \pm 0.06°C$ with melatonin. Less (125 mg) or more (500 mg) hop extract induced a smaller effect. The response curve was U-shaped.

In a second set of experiments, the hypothermic effect was antagonized with the competitive melatonin receptor antagonist, luzindole. The data suggest that potential sleep-inducing effects of hop extract are mediated through activation of melatonin receptors (46). This is the first study on hops providing evidence that the affinity on melatonin receptors is an effect that is relevant for a living organism.

CLINICAL EVIDENCE

Postulating adenosine-like action for valerian is an exciting topic. It would mean that valerian could act instead of or alongside adenosine, increasing the adenosine effects on sleep propensity. Sleep would initiate naturally; hence, evidence for such an effect in humans would be helpful.

Because of the immense screening work to find subjects with comparable sleep problems for such a trial and the exploratory nature of such a trial, a study design with healthy volunteers appears advisable. It should be noted, however, that earlier research has shown that effects of sleep aids are difficult to detect in non-sleep-deprived normal volunteers (47).

Hence, a well-known adenosine antagonist was employed to create a standardized artificial state of arousal, restlessness, and agitation. Healthy volunteers received orally 200 mg caffeine and were divided into three groups. One group received valerian extract, again in a fixed combination with a hop extract; a second group received three times the dose; and a third group received a placebo. A quantitative pharmacological EEG was employed for measurement of the effects.

The extracts of valerian and hops were produced similarly to the previously described experiments with methanol/water 45% by maceration followed by evaporation, addition of a carrier, and spray drying to drug-to-extract ratios of 4–6:1 and 5–7:1, respectively. Content of valerenic acid was determined by HPLC-DAD, and flavonoids were measured photometrically.

In the placebo group, the caffeine action was reflected in a typical change of EEG parameters. Because of the faster disintegration time of the caffeine tablets, the caffeine effect was seen in all groups after 30 minutes. The active medication was capable of reducing (one dose) or inhibiting (three doses) the caffeine-induced arousal. The pharmacodynamic interaction was observed from 60 minutes on. The offset of these effects was dose dependent after the coated valerian tablets had disintegrated and were absorbed. These results provide evidence that the mode of action is mediated via the adenosine receptor by competitive behavior. Second, the results confirm a rather fast bioavailability in humans supporting the posology "to be taken half to one hour before bedtime" (48).

The results on valerian and hops indicate that preparations of both herbal substances support sleep but by different modes of action. This should result in an additive effect when taken in combination. To test this hypothesis, a clinical trial with a fixed combination of both herbals versus a monopreparation and placebo as control was designed.

For a three-arm, parallel-group, double-blind, randomized, and placebo-controlled trial, 43 patients were screened. Thirty patients (16 female, 14 male) were eligible to participate in the trial. The volunteers had nonorganic insomnia (ICD 10, F51.0–F51.2) with sleep latency longer than 30 minutes. They received a combination of 120 mg of dry extract from hop strobile and 500 mg of dry extract from valerian root, placebo, or just 500 mg dry extract from valerian root. Both of the extracts are manufactured with methanol/water 45% with drug-to-extract ratios of 5.3:1 for valerian and 6.6:1 for hops, respectively. The fixed valerian combination is similar to the combinations described in earlier trials referred to as Ze 91019.

Study duration was four weeks, and all measurements were taken in the familiar environment at home. Objective sleep parameters were registered with a portable recording device. Polysomnographic recordings were obtained twice at baseline and a third time after four weeks at the end of the trial period. The study protocol was approved by the German authorities, Federal Institute for Drugs and Medical Devices (BfArM) No. 4022772, and received the EudraCT number 2005-005296-15 PILOT ZE 91019.

At the end of the treatment period, 27 patients were available for statistical analysis. No serious adverse events were reported, and no difference in safety parameters between groups could be detected. As the main efficacy outcome, the trial showed a significant reduction of sleep latency when hops were added to the valerian formulation. Sleep latency with valerian alone was reduced by 22.1 minutes ($p = 0.19$), while the addition of hops increased the reduction to 44.5 minutes ($p = 0.05$). Additionally, it could be shown that the sum of sleep stages S3 and S4 increased in the valerian-hops group and the clinical global impression was superior.

Under real-life conditions in a home setting, sleep aids with hops and valerian are safe and effective. The additive effects of hops were demonstrated using objective measurements (49).

CONCLUSION

Insomnia is a widespread health complaint in the general population. An estimated one-third of the adult population present insomnia symptoms at least occasionally, and about 15% are dissatisfied with their sleep, thus qualifying for use of complementary and alternative medicines such as herbal and dietary supplements. Herbal products such as valerian, hops, chamomile, and passionflower are widely marketed as natural sleep aids. Most evi-

Table 8.2. Link between Findings in in Vitro Studies, Results of Animal Trials and Clinical Studies

Herbal Substance	In Vitro Results	Animal Studies	Clinical Research
Valerian	Adenosine A_1 receptor agonist	Increase of slow-wave activity in the cortex and hippocampus as an indicator of adenosine-like action	Has an opposite effect to caffeine, which is an adenosine A_1 receptor antagonist
Hops	Affinity to ML_1 receptor	Reduction of body temperature–like melatonin, which could be blocked by a melatonin receptor antagonist	Addition of hops to valerian reduces sleep latency, supporting theory of separate mode of action for hops

dence from randomized trials suggests that with repeated administration, valerian produces a mild sleep-initiating effect without causing alteration of sleep architecture or significant residual effects (50–53). Sleep improvements with a valerian-hops combination are associated with improved quality of life. In a recent randomized, placebo-controlled trial, the treatment appears safe and did not produce rebound insomnia upon discontinuation during the study (54).

With the results presented for valerian and hops, a scientific rationale is provided that confirms the long-established use of both as sleep aids. Owing to the increasing understanding of sleep and the physiological processes, the mode of action of valerian and hops can be explained better. The established use of combination products is justified. Their synergistic action seems obvious. Valerian appears to the homeostatic process of sleep initiation by supporting adenosine in its activity. Hops play a role in the circadian process via their melatonin-like action (Table 8.2).

Treatment of insomnia should improve the physiological basic mechanism instead of simply turning off wakefulness, as is the case with some prescription and over-the-counter drugs. Even if prescription medication is effective in shortening sleep latency and reducing waking after sleep onset, improvement of the physiological sleep regulation is not documented (55). Additionally, drug therapy is frequently burdened with adverse effects (56).

Working with the natural processes of sleep, valerian and hops come close to imitating biological sleep rhythm and are therefore the ideal drugs at least for mild and transient insomnia. They work in synergy via different mechanisms within the body, not against it.

ACKNOWLEDGMENTS

For all the colleagues and collaborators in ten years of research on increasing evidence for and proof of efficacy of valerian and hops.

REFERENCES

[1]Freemon FR. *Sleep Research: A Critical Review*. Springfield, IL: Charles C Thomas; 1972.

[2]Benington JH. Sleep homeostasis and the function of sleep. *Sleep*. 2000;23(7):959–966.

[3]Duke University Medical Center (2008, March 11). Poor Sleep More Dangerous for Women. ScienceDaily. Retrieved April 22, 2008, from http://www.sciencedaily.com /releases/2008/03/080310131529.htm.

[4]Cajochen C, Munch M, Knoblauch V, Blatter K, Wirz-Justice A. Age-related changes in the circadian and homeostatic regulation of human sleep. *Chronobiol Int*. 2006;23(1–2):461–474.

[5]Borbély AA. From slow waves to sleep homeostasis: new perspectives. *Archives Italiennes de Biologie*. 2001;139(1–2):53–61.

[6]Finelli LA, Baumann H, Borbély AA, Achermann P. Dual electroencephalogram markers of human sleep homeostasis: correlation between theta activity in waking and slow-wave activity in sleep. *Neuroscience*. 2000;101(3):523–529.

[7]Cajochen C, Krauchi K, Wirz-Justice A. Role of melatonin in the regulation of human circadian rhythms and sleep. *J Neuroendocrinol*. 2003;15(4):432–437.

[8]Porkka-Heiskanen T, Alanko L, Kalinchuk A, Stenberg D. Adenosine and sleep. *Sleep Med Rev*. 2002; 6(4):321–332.

[9]HMPC. *Community herbal monograph on* Valeriana officinalis *L., Radix*. In: EMEA, ed. European Medicines Agency; 2006.

[10]Bent S, Padula A, Moore D, Patterson M, Mehling W. Valerian for sleep: a systematic review and meta-analysis. *Am J Med*. 2006;119(12):1005–1012.

[11]Health Canada. Drug and Health Products. Product licensing. Compendium of Monographs. Retrieved March 11, 2009 from http://www.hc-sc.gc.ca/dhp-mps/alt_formats/hpfb-dgpsa/pdf/prodnatur/mono_valerian -eng.pdf.

[12]Macht DI, Ting GC. Experimental inquiry into the sedative properties of some aromatic drugs and fumes. *J Pharmacol Exp Ther*. 1921;18:361–372.

[13]Houghton PJ. The biological activity of valerian and related plants. *J Ethnopharmacol*. 1988;22(2): 121–142.

[14]Hänsel R, Schulz H. Beitrag zur Qualitätssicherung von Baldrianextrakten. *Die Pharmazeutische Industrie*. 1985;47(5):531–533.

[15]Hendriks H, Bos R, Woerdenbag HJ, Koster AS. Central nervous depressant activity of valerenic acid in the mouse. *Planta Med*. 1985(1):28–31.

[16]Yuan CS, Mehendale S, Xiao Y, Aung HH, Xie JT, Ang-Lee MK. The gamma-aminobutyric acidergic effects of valerian and valerenic acid on rat brainstem neuronal activity. *Anesth Analg*. 2004;98(2): 353–358.

[17]Trauner G, Khom S, Baburin I, Benedek B, Hering S, Kopp B. Modulation of GABAA receptors by valerian extracts is related to the content of valerenic acid. *Planta Med*. 2008;74(1):19–24.

[18]Benke D, Barberis A, Kopp S, Altmann KH, Schubiger M, Vogt KE, et al. GABA(A) receptors as in vivo substrate for the anxiolytic action of valerenic acid, a major constituent of valerian root extracts. *Neuropharmacology*. 2009 Jan;56(1):174–181.

[19]Hattesohl M, Feistel B, Sievers H, Lehnfeld R, Hegger M, Winterhoff H. Extracts of *Valeriana officinalis* L. s.l. show anxiolytic and antidepressant effects but neither sedative nor myorelaxant properties. *Phytomedicine*. 2008;15(1–2):2–15.

[20]Elmenhorst D, Meyer PT, Winz OH, Matusch A, Ermert J, Coenen HH, et al. Sleep deprivation increases A1 adenosine receptor binding in the human brain: a positron emission tomography study. *J Neurosci*. 2007; 27(9):2410–2415.

[21]Schumacher B, Scholle S, Holzl J, Khudeir N, Hess S, Muller CE. Lignans isolated from valerian: identification and characterization of a new olivil derivative with partial agonistic activity at A(1) adenosine receptors. *J Nat Prod*. 2002;65(10):1479–1485.

[22]Müller CE, Schumacher B, Brattström A, Abourashed EA, Koetter U. Interactions of valerian extracts and a fixed valerian-hop extract combination with adenosine receptors. *Life Sci*. 2002;71(16):1939–1949.

[23]Balduini W, Cattabeni F. Displacement of [3H]-N6-cyclohexylahdenosine binding to rat cortical membranes by an hydroalcoholic extract of *Valeriana officinalis*. *Med Sci Res*. 1989;17:639–640.

[24]Bodesheim U, Holzl J. Isolation and receptor binding properties of alkaloids and lignans from Valeriana officialis L. *Die Pharmazie*. 1997;52(5):386–391.

[25]Scholle S, Holzl J. Lignan: active substances in valerian roots? *Zeitschrift für Phytotherapie*. 1997;18(4): 221–222.

[26]Vissiennon Z, Sichardt K, Koetter U, Brattstrom A, Nieber K. Valerian extract Ze 911 inhibits postsynaptic potentials by activation of adenosine A1 receptors in rat cortical neurons. *Planta Med.* 2006;72(7): 579–583.

[27]Sichardt K, Vissiennon Z, Koetter U, Brattstrom A, Nieber K. Modulation of postsynaptic potentials in rat cortical neurons by valerian extracts macerated with different alcohols: involvement of adenosine A(1)- and GABA(A)-receptors. *Phytother Res.* 2007. 2007 Oct;21(10):932–937.

[28]Lacher SK, Mayer R, Sichardt K, Nieber K, Muller CE. Interaction of valerian extracts of different polarity with adenosine receptors: identification of isovaltrate as an inverse agonist at A1 receptors. *Biochem Pharmacol.* 2007;73(2):248–258.

[29]Schilcher H, Kammerer S, Wegener T. *Leitfaden Phytotherapie.* 3rd ed. Munich: Urban & Fischer; 2007.

[30]HMPC. *Community Herbal Monograph on Humulus lupulus L., Flos.* In: EMEA, ed. European Medicines Agency; 2007.

[31]ESCOP. *Lupuli Flos: Hop strobile.* In: ESCOP Monographs. 2nd ed.; 2003: 306–311.

[32]Braungart R. *Der Hopfen als Braumaterial.* Munich: Verlag von R. Oldenbourg; 1901.

[33]Schulz H. *Vorlesungen über Wirkung und Anwendung der deutscher Arzneipflanzen.* 2nd ed. Leipzig: Georg Thieme Verlag; 1929.

[34]Schilcher H, Dorsch W. *Phytotherapie in der Kinderheilkunde: Ein Handbuch fur Arzte und Apotheker.* 4. Auflage ed. Stuttgart: Wissenschaftliche Verlagsgesellschaft mbH. 2006.

[35]Ives AW. An experimental inquiry into the chemical properties and economical and medicinal virtues of the Humulus Lupulus, or the common hop. *Am J Sci.* 1820:302–312.

[36]Zanoli P, Zavatti M, Rivasi M, Brusiani F, Losi G, Puia G, et al. Evidence that the beta-acids fraction of hops reduces central GABAergic neurotransmission. *J Ethnopharmacol.* 2007;109(1):87–92.

[37]Aoshima H, Takeda K, Okita Y, Hossain SJ, Koda H, Kiso Y. Effects of beer and hop on ionotropic gamma-aminobutyric acid receptors. *J Agric Food Chem.* 2006;54(7):2514–2419.

[38]Wesolowska A. In the search for selective ligands of 5-HT5, 5-HT6 and 5-HT7 serotonin receptors. *Polish J Pharmacol.* 2002;54(4):327–341.

[39]Morin AK, Jarvis CI, Lynch AM. Therapeutic options for sleep-maintenance and sleep-onset insomnia. *Pharmacotherapy.* 2007;27(1):89–110.

[40]Abourashed E, Koetter U, Brattstrom A. In vitro binding experiments with a valerian, hops and their fixed combination extract (Ze 91019) to selected central nervous system receptors. *Phytomedicine.* 2004;11: 633–638.

[41]Dimpfel W, Brattström A, Koetter U. Central action of a fixed valerian-hops extract combination (Ze 91019) in freely moving rats. *Eur J Med Res.* 2006;11(11):496–500.

[42]Chadwick LR, Pauli GF, Farnsworth NR. The pharmacognosy of *Humulus lupulus* L. (hops) with an emphasis on estrogenic properties. *Phytomedicine.* 2006;13(1–2):119–131.

[43]Lee KM, Jung JS, Song DK, Krauter M, Kim YH. Effects of *Humulus lupulus* extract on the central nervous system in mice. *Planta Med.* 1993;59:691.

[44]Schiller H, Forster A, Vonhoff C, Hegger M, Biller A, Winterhoff H. Sedating effects of *Humulus lupulus* L. extracts. *Phytomedicine.* 2006;13(8):535–541.

[45]Zanoli P, Rivasi M, Zavatti M, Brusiani F, Baraldi M. New insight in the neuropharmacological activity of *Humulus lupulus* L. *J Ethnopharmacol.* 2005;102(1):102–106.

[46]Butterweck V, Brattström A, Grundmann O, Koetter U. Hypothermic effects of hops are antagonized with the competitive melatonin receptor antagonist luzindole in mice. *J Pharm and Pharmacol.* 2007;59(4): 549–552.

[47]Balderer G, Borbély AA. Effect of valerian on human sleep. *Psychopharmacology.* 1985;87(4):406–409.

[48]Schellenberg R, Sauer S, Abourashed EA, Koetter U, Brattström A. The fixed combination of valerian and hops (Ze 91019) acts via a central adenosine mechanism. *Planta Med.* 2004;70(7):594–597.

[49]Koetter U, Schrader E, Käufeler R, Brattström A. A randomized, double blind, placebo-controlled, prospective clinical study to demonstrate clinical efficacy of a fixed valerian hops extract combination (Ze 91019) in patients suffering from non-organic sleep disorder. *Phytother Res.* 2007;21(9):847–851.

[50]Gyllenhaal C, Merritt SL, Peterson SD, Block KI, Gochenour T. Efficacy and safety of herbal stimulants and sedatives in sleep disorders. *Sleep Med Rev.* 2000;4(3):229–251.

[51]Stevinson C, Ernst E. Valerian for insomnia: a systematic review of randomized clinical trials. *Sleep Med.* 2000;1(2):91–99.

[52]Hallam KT, Olver JS, McGrath C, Norman TR. Comparative cognitive and psychomotor effects of single doses of Valeriana officianalis and triazolam in healthy volunteers. *Hum Psychopharmacol.* 2003;18(8): 619–625.

[53]Mcoli AL, Rosen C, Kristo D, Kohrman M, Gooneratne N, Aguillard RN, et al. Oral nonprescription treatment for insomnia: an evaluation of products with limited evidence. *J Clin Sleep Med.* 2005;1(2): 173–187.

[54]Morin CM, Koetter U, Bastien CH, Ware JC, Wooten V. Valerian-hops combination and diphenhydramine for treating insomnia: a randomized placebo-controlled clinical trial. *Sleep.* 2005;28(11):1307–1313.

[55]Vignola A, Lamoureux C, Bastien CH, Morin CM. Effects of chronic insomnia and use of benzodiazepines on daytime performance in older adults. *J Gerontol.* 2000;55B(1):P54–P62.

[56]Mitler MM. Nonselective and selective benzodiazepine receptor agonists: where are we today? *Sleep.* 2000; 23(Suppl 1):S39–S47.

Botanical Medicine: From Bench to Bedside
Edited by R. Cooper and F. Kronenberg
© Mary Ann Liebert, Inc.

Chapter 9

Development of Iberogast: Clinical Evidence for Multicomponent Herbal Mixtures

Bettina Vinson

Functional gastrointestinal (GI) diseases like functional dyspepsia (FD) and irritable bowel syndrome (IBS) are characterized by a broad spectrum of variable symptoms of the upper (FD) or lower (IBS) GI tract which are caused by several functional disorders in the GI system (1, 2). Therefore, therapeutic management of these diseases is still difficult, and at this time no curative treatment is available. Complete treatment would require targeting every distinct underlying disorder, and therefore, success of a monodrug approach targeting only one specific disorder as a therapeutic intervention is limited (3). An optimal treatment would be a combination of monodrug preparations that are each effective in the essential GI functions and offer the chance to target the multiple causes of the diseases (4). Simultaneously, a good benefit-to-risk ratio for these preparations is necessary. Compared to synthetically derived monodrugs, herbal extracts contain multiple substances that are assessed as one active agent. The substances in each extract and especially within a combination of these extracts can perform synergistic and additive effects that multiply and expand efficacy. Herbal medicinal combination products therefore offer the chance to treat the multifactorial pathophysiology of multicausal diseases like IBS and FD while reducing the concentration of any one single component. The result may lead to a reduction of potential side effects and to a positive benefit-to-risk ratio of the herbal combination preparation (5). Because herbal drugs are from natural sources, the development, quality assurance, and pharmacological and clinical characterization of an herbal medicinal product are major challenges for ensuring consistently high-quality and scientific evidence.

STW 5 (Iberogast, Steigerwald Arzneimittelwerk GmbH, Darmstadt, Germany) is an herbal combination product consisting of nine plant extracts. STW 5 contains an alcoholic fresh plant extract of *Iberis amara totalis* (bitter candytuft) and alcoholic extracts of *Angelica archangelica* (angelica) root, *Matricaria recutita* (chamomile) flowers, *Carum carvi* (caraway) fruits, *Silybum marianum* (milk thistle) fruit, *Melissa officinalis* (lemon balm)

Department of Clinical Research, Steigerwald Arzneimittelwerk GmbH, 64925 Darmstadt, Germany; vinson@steigerwald.de

Table 9.1. Components of STW 5, Drug Extract Ratio, and Amount in 100 ml of the Finished Product

Extract	Drug Extract Ratio (DER)	In 100 ml Iberogast
Iberis amara (alcoholic fresh plant extract)	1:1.5–2.5	15.0 ml
Angelica root (alcoholic drug extract)	1:2.5–3.5	10.0 ml
Chamomile flowers (alcoholic drug extract)	1:2.5–4	20.0 ml
Caraway fruits (alcoholic drug extract)	1:2.5–3.5	10.0 ml
Milk thistle fruits (alcoholic drug extract)	1:2.5–3.5	10.0 ml
Lemon balm leaves (alcoholic drug extract)	1:2.5–3.5	10.0 ml
Peppermint leaves (alcoholic drug extract)	1:2.5–3.5	5.0 ml
Greater celandine (alcoholic drug extract)	1:2.5–3.5	10.0 ml
Licorice root (alcoholic drug extract)	1:2.5–3.5	10.0 ml

leaves, *Mentha X piperita* (peppermint) leaves, *Chelidonium majus* (greater celandine), and *Glycyrrhiza glabra* (licorice) root (see Table 9.1 and Figures 9.1a–9.1i).

Iberogast is approved in Germany and several other European and non-European countries for the treatment of functional GI disorders like FD and IBS and has been available on the German market since 1961. The development of STW 5 included the development and validation of harvesting, processing, and manufacturing techniques; the proof that each plant is efficacious in the GI tract regarding functional GI disorders; and an extensive toxicology, pharmacology, and clinical study program to show efficacy and safety of STW 5. During 47 years of development and use, STW 5 has become the most extensively investigated herbal medicinal product and is verified at the highest level of scientific evidence for the treatment of functional GI diseases.

HARVESTING, MANUFACTURING, AND QUALITY ASSURANCE OF STW 5

The required consistent quality, efficacy, and safety of STW 5 as an herbal medicinal combination product can be derived only by the strict control of the growing, harvesting, and manufacturing processes.

Good Agricultural Practice (GAP)

A major challenge for the manufacturing process of herbal extracts compared to synthetically derived drugs is that the origin of the drug is a living subject which responds to environmental influences (temperature, light, soil, humidity, etc.). These environmental influences change during the year and influence continuously the content and composition of ingredients of a plant. To ensure consistently good quality, agricultural conditions such as soil quality, light intensity, suitable cultivation, and harvesting time and methods and the exact plant parts that should be harvested have to be specified and standardized. International regulations like Good Agricultural Practice (GAP), the German Drug Book (DAB), and Pharmacopoe Europe (Ph. Eur.), as well as in-house specifications based on detailed experience about the extract constituents and their chemical behavior, determine these specific factors for each plant extract of STW 5. After the plant material is harvested, milled, and stored as dried or frozen drug, the quality of that drug has to be analyzed and identified according to its individual specification. Only original material in perfect condition is used for further processing (6).

Good Manufacturing Practice (GMP)

The extraction of drug material is carried out under standardized manufacturing conditions and using "in-process" controls. Relevant quality parameters are the drug-to-extract ratio (DER), the quality of the herbal drug (grade of comminution, water content, content of extractable substances), the extraction solvent (type, concentration, amount, flow speed), the procedure (type of extraction, time, temperature, pressure, batch size, filtration), and the equipment (type, level of filling, static pressure) (6, 7). All parameters are defined for each drug by standard operating procedures (SOPs) and all steps of the manufacturing process are validated. The quality of each extract is tested according to the individual specifications.

Specifications

Extraction of the dried herbal drugs is carried out under controlled conditions whereby temperature, the extracting agent, and the extraction time are exactly determined for each plant extract. Therefore, specific methods have been developed and validated by Steigerwald Arzneimittelwerk GmbH. The specific properties of the individual plant species and the properties of the plant extract constituents regarding quality (purity, identity) are determined with individual in-house specifications. The quality of each extract is tested according to the individual specification. Characteristic parameters of the extract include the general properties of the extract (color, odor), the content of ethanol and residual solvents, the density, the identity of the used drug (thin layer chromatography [TLC]—the fingerprint of the chromatographic profile), and the content of the analytical marker substances within a defined range. For analyzing the characteristic marker substances, Steigerwald has developed high-performance liquid chromatography (HPLC) and gas liquid chromatography (GLC). These methods comply with the relevant guidelines with

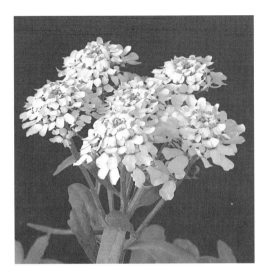

Figure 9.1a. Bitter candytuft (*Iberis amara*). Glucosinolates, flavonoids. Specific effects on tone of gastrointestinal tract, influencing gastrointestinal peristalsis.

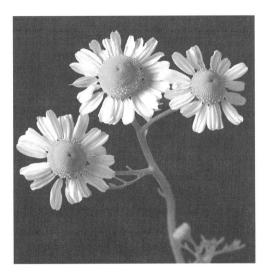

Figure 9.1b. Chamomile flowers (*Matricariae flos*) volatile oils (0.3–3%), organic acids, flavonoids. Anti-inflammatory, spasmolytic, carminative, ulcer protection.

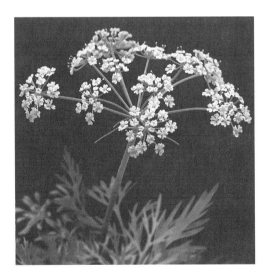

Figure 9.1c. Caraway fruits (*Carvi fructus*) volatile oils (2–7%), coumarins, flavonoids. Carminative, spasmolytic, bacteriostatic.

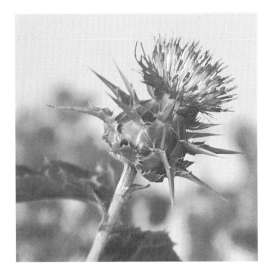

Figure 9.1d. Milk thistle fruits (*Cardui mariae fructus*) Flavonolignans (silymarin, silybin) neolignans, flavonoids. Antidyspeptic, carminative, cytoprotective in stomach and liver.

Figure 9.1a–i. Plants Used in STW 5 and Their Known Pharmacological Properties [9–23].

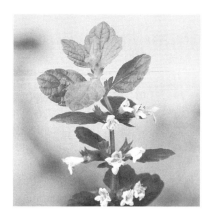

Figure 9.1e. Lemon balm leaves (*Melissae folium*). Volatile oil, Lamiaceae tannins, Triterpenic acids, amaroids, flavonoids. Sedative, carminative, spasmolytic, anti-inflammatory.

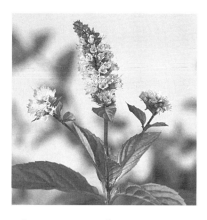

Figure 9.1f. Peppermint leaves (*Menthae pip. folium*). Volatile oil (0.7%), Lamiaceae tannins, amaroids, flavonoids. Slightly anesthetic, antiemetic, spasmolytic, carminative, disinfectant.

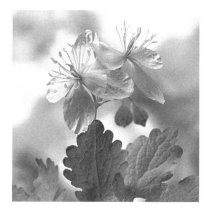

Figure 9.1g. Greater Celandine (*Chelidonii herba*). Alkaloids, organic acids, flavonoids. Spasmolytic, tonicizing in the stomach, cholekinetic, anti-inflammatory, bacteriostatic.

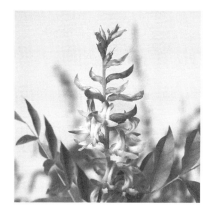

Figure 9.1h. Licorice root (*Liquiritiae radix*). Glyzyrrhicinic acid (5–15%), flavonoids, phytosterols, coumarins. Antiulcerative, anti-inflammatory, spasmolytic.

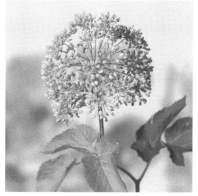

Figure 9.1i. Angelica root (*Angelicae radix*). Volatile oils (0.35–1%), amaroids, flavonoids, coumarins. Spasmolytic, especially in the stomach; inhibiting acid-secretion, stimulating gastric secretion.

respect to precision and robustness for the individual extracts and the complex herbal matrix of the final combination product. Therefore, it is essential that an active substance responsible for the pharmacological action is identified or a marker substance is chosen that can be analyzed well and is quantitatively dominant. These compounds may be used for the quantification of the single extracts and the finished product. For example, carvone in caraway fruit is a characteristic marker substance. The specification of the drug and the standardized manufacturing process ensure high batch-to-batch reproducibility and conformity of the extracts. Also, the content and quality of the active ingredient(s) for each of the nine extracts of STW 5 are continuously characterized via chromatographic fingerprints during the manufacturing process, according to GMP and validated "in-process" controls, determined by national and international guidelines (e.g., Ph. Eur. and DAB; see Figure 9.2).

Only after exact definition and strict analysis of each plant extract can the extracts be defined as suitable for manufacturing of the finished-product STW 5. The manufacturing process is fixed and determines the sequence as well as the ratios of the mixing process (6).

"In-Process" Controls

The quality and reproducibility of an herbal multicomponent product are achieved by defined processing and in-process-controls, in concordance with (a) the GMP standards (8) and (b) the analytical control of all intermediate products and the finished product. For excellent quality of the finished product, the right sequence of mixture, mixing time, interim storage, and filtration process are essential to avoid side reactions and interactions between the different extracts (major precipitations) and to ensure stability. Test parameters of the extracts include TLC fingerprint chromatograms within the complete polarity range, the appearance (color, clearness), the density, the content of ethanol, the microbiological purity, and the content of all nine components by the assay of the characteristic marker substances. These measurements are carried out by validated HPLC or GLC methods. This has to be fulfilled for every processed plant (Figure 9.3).

The Finished Product

The manufactured product STW 5 has finally to be analyzed for quality and quantity. For the quality of the whole combination product, it is essential that the amount of the marker substances for each extract is in the range of the calculated amount. The proportion of each component in the final product has to be in a range of 95% to 105% of the specified content. The efficiency of separation of the methods has to be in view of the great number of different substances of very high quality. To meet these requirements, most of the analytical methods were especially developed for manufacturing and quality assurance of Iberogast. To achieve approval from the official authorities, the herbal medicinal product had to fulfill the same guidelines and regularities recommended for quality, safety, and efficacy recommended for synthetically derived drugs. In 2005, Iberogast received approval from the competent authorities in Germany.

Specification

Iberis amara

Geographical origin	Germany
Fresh-plant procedures	GAP
Harvesting	June–August
Postharvesting processing	Directly deep-freeze after harvesting

Criteria	Methods	Nominal Size
Properties	validated STW method	validated STW monograph
Identity	validated STW method	validated STW monograph
Purity	validated STW method	validated STW monograph
Loss at drying	Ph. Eur. 2.2.32	max 87.5% (m/m)
Ash	Ph. Eur. 2.4.16	max 10% (m/m)
Microbial contamination	Ph. Eur. 2.2.6.12/13	according Ph.Eur.5.1.4. Kat. 4A
Aflatoxines	Ph. Eur. 2.2.29	according aflatoxines regul.
Heavy metals	Ph. Eur. 2.2.23	according AM. Cont. regul.

Figure 9.2. Parts of an In-House Specification of *Iberis amara* for Assurance of Consistent Quality

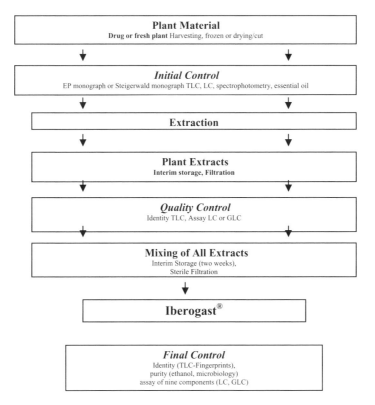

Figure 9.3. Overview of the "In-Process" Controls during Manufacturing of STW 5

Source: Adopted from Kroll and Cordes 2006 [6].

RATIONALE FOR DEVELOPMENT OF STW 5 FOR FUNCTIONAL GI DISEASES

Investigational Data

In monographs of Commission E and German Bundesanzeiger, as well as from the documentation in *Hagers Handbook*, all plants are known traditionally to have effects in the GI tract (see Figure 9.1) (9–23).

During the first years on the German market, STW 5 was officially registered and traditionally used for various GI disorders. Furthermore, during this time, it was successfully investigated for treatment of diseases such as nonulcer dyspepsia, gastroentheropathia, and various GI disorders that were, in the late 1980s for the first time, exactly defined as functional GI diseases (e.g., IBS and FD). FD and IBS were then characterized by a broad spectrum of GI symptoms for which no evidence for an underlying organic disease or lesion can be detected with common diagnostic measurements (24, 25). Although these diseases are not life threatening, the well-being and quality of life as well as the ability to work are persistently and significantly impaired for the patients. The incidence in Western countries is almost 30%, and both diseases stand for the most frequent diagnoses in gastroenterological practice (26). Impaired ability to work and early retirement cause significant socioeconomic impact (27, 28). Various functional disorders may be responsible for the symptoms of FD and IBS: dysfunctions of acid secretion or disturbed motoric reaction of the GI tract to acid secretion, as well as dysfunctions in the sensoric or neuromotoric signal-transduction resulting in hypersensitivity to stimuli-like distension of the fundus or corpus of the stomach (29). Also, dysmotility of specific areas of the GI tract like hypomotility of the antrum resulting in delayed gastric emptying or spasms of the fundus area causing impaired

Table 9.2. Various Symptoms of Functional GI Diseases in Relationship to Underlying Functional Disorder of the GI Tract

Symptoms	Acid	Hypersensitivity	Hypermotility	Hypomotility	Inflammation
Epigastric pain / upper abdominal pain	X	X		X	X
Abdominal cramps		X	X		
Retrosternal discomfort	X	X	X	X	X
Early satiety		X		X	
Fullness / meteorism obstipation		X		X	
Nausea		X	X	X	
Retching		X	X	X	
Vomiting		X	X	X	
Acid regurgitation / heartburn	X			X	

Table 9.3. Effects of the Single Extracts of STW 5 on Several Multiple Functional Disorders of FD or IBS and Their Contribution to the Whole Efficacy of STW 5 in FD and IBS

Multiple functional disorders of IBS or FD	Hypomotility	Hypermotility	Acid secretion	Inflammation	Oxydative processes
Bitter candytuft	moderate effect	weak effect	moderate effect	strong effect	weak effect
Angelica	no effect	strong effect	no effect	moderate effect	moderate effect
Caraway	no effect	moderate effect	no effect	strong effect	moderate effect
Milk thistle	no effect	moderate effect	no effect	moderate effect	moderate effect
Celandine	moderate effect	no effect	moderate effect	moderate effect	moderate effect
Licorice	moderate effect	no effect	no effect	strong effect	weak effect
Chamomile	moderate effect	strong effect	moderate effect	moderate effect	moderate effect
Lemon balm	no effect	moderate effect	moderate effect	moderate effect	strong effect
Peppermint	no effect	moderate effect	moderate effect	strong effect	strong effect

Legend: no effect / weak effect / moderate effect / strong effect

Source: Modified from Wagner 2006 (5).

accommodation to ingested food (30) and various postinflammatory conditions (induced by oxygen radicals, for example, gastritis or *Helicobacter pylori* infections) are noted to cause symptoms of FD or IBS (31) (Table 9.2). Pharmacological investigations on underlying functional disorders of the functional GI diseases have been conducted on STW 5. With these investigations, the mechanistic activity of STW 5 and its components in all dysfunctions were verified, whereas the contribution of each plant extract was of individual magnitude (Table 9.3). Each of these investigations has been published elsewhere. Below, a brief overview is presented.

PHARMACOLOGICAL DATA AND SAFETY/TOXICOLOGY

Motility

Motility disorders in the stomach can impair accommodation of fundus and corpus to ingested food, which can result in FD symptoms like early satiety, nausea, cramps, and epigastric pain. An impaired tone of the lower esophagus-sphincter during this situation increases the possibility of acidic ingested food to reflux into the esophagus, potentially increasing the development of symptoms like dyspeptic heartburn (32). On the other hand, a low muscle tone of the antrum can lead to an impaired gastric emptying process and symptoms like bloating and feeling of fullness. Spastic colon or high muscle tone can lead to either constipation or diarrhea symptoms of IBS.

STW 5 and GI Motility

Stomach

In a pharmacological model with muscle strips of different stomach areas from guinea pig and with human stomach tissue, Schemann et al. 2006 (33) demonstrated an area-specific effect of STW 5. In the fundus and corpus area of the stomach where ingested food is received from the esophagus, stomach volume has to accommodate to food volume via relaxing of the muscle tissue. STW 5 acts in a spasmolytic way, mainly because of the presence of angelica extract. In the antrum region, where food has to be transported via the pylorus to the duodenum and the muscle tissue should be tonicized, STW 5 showed tonicizing effects, which were mainly stimulated by the *Iberis amara* extract and greater celandine (Figure 9.4).

This effect could be clinically verified by Pilichiewicz et al. 2007 (34). In a double-blind, placebo-controlled investigation with 19 probands, the persons received either STW 5 or placebo via an oral gastric tube. During ingestion of a standardized meal, the proximal stomach volume and the antropyloroduodenal motility were continuously measured. With STW 5 treatment, the volume of the proximal stomach was increased and the antropyloroduodenal motility was significantly enhanced, compared to probands receiving placebo (Figure 9.5).

Intestine

Investigations with unstimulated ileum muscle strips of guinea pig showed an increasing effect of STW 5 on the basic tonus. The effect was spasmolytic when muscle strips already were tonicized by acetylcholine, histamine, or prostaglandin F2. The investigations could be confirmed with isolated tissue of duodenum, jejunum, ileum, and colon of rats and mice as well as with human colon tissue in vitro. The most tonicizing effects were caused by the *Iberis amara* extract (35, 36).

Esophagus

In experimental investigations with esophagus-sphincter of guinea pigs, STW 5 was tonicizing significantly the tone of the lower esophagus-sphincter (37).

In conclusion, STW 5 in vitro showed the potential to influence motility of the whole GI tract.

Hypersensitivity

Neuromotoric sensitivity disorders in the GI tract can manifest as disorders in the neuromuscular signal transduction level or can be disorders in signal transduction from enteric nervous system of the gut-brain axis. Also, differences in neuroreceptor quality and quantity were discussed for IBS or FD patients (38). The patients suffering from FD as well as IBS perceive stimuli from ingested food as well as from digestion processes much stronger than adequate.

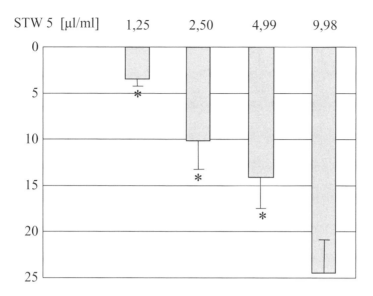

1) Decrease of Tone [Δm N] in the Fundus

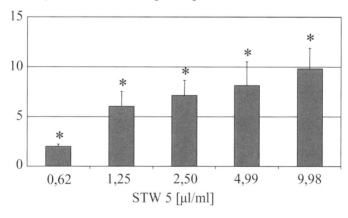

2) Contractile Force [Δm N] in the Antrum

STW 5 [μl/ml]

Figure 9.4. Muscular Tone in Muscle Strips of Corpus and Fundus (1) and in the Gastric Antrum of Guinea Pigs (2) after Dose-Dependent Application of STW 5 (*p ≤ 0.05) [23]

STW 5 Was Investigated for Effects in Hypersensitivity

In a pharmacologic hypersensitivity model, Liu et al. 2004 (39) measured the effect of STW 5 on the sensitivity of afferent nerves of narcoticized rats after mechanic distension and application of serotonin and the agent bradykinin, which all have stimulating effects on afferent signal transduction. STW 5 led in all models to a significant reduction of the impulse rate of the neuro-gramme signal of the stimulated nerve (Figure 9.6). STW 5 in these investigations reduced sensitivity for stimuli from the upper GI tract.

Motoric as well as sensoric reactions in the GI tract are transferred via mediator substances binding at specific receptors. Conversely, substances similar to serotonin and opiate

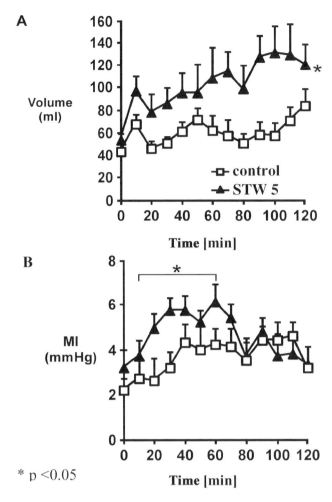

Figure 9.5. Course of the Proximal Stomach Volume (A) and Phasic Activity of the Antrum (B) over Time after Application of STW 5 or Placebo in Healthy Subjects [34]

play a predominant role. For STW 5, it could be evaluated that components of the single extracts show binding properties of different strength and concentration on serotonergic and muscarinic receptors. These properties could explain the way the effects of STW 5 on motility and sensitivity could be mediated (40).

Acid Secretion

Increased acid secretion as well as an increased sensitivity to acid in the GI tract can lead to symptoms like cramping, pain, and heartburn. In a pharmacological model of indomethacin-induced ulcer in rats, STW 5 showed a protective effect in acid-related dysfunctions. Acid secretion was reduced: different extracts showed different contributions to the whole effect. Also, secretion of the mucosa protective mucine was increased with application of STW 5 in different intensities by each extract (Figure 9.7) (41, 21). Furthermore, the concentration of the anti-inflammatory prostaglandin E2 was stimulated, indicating an increased potential for mucosa protection as well as a protective function in inflammation processes.

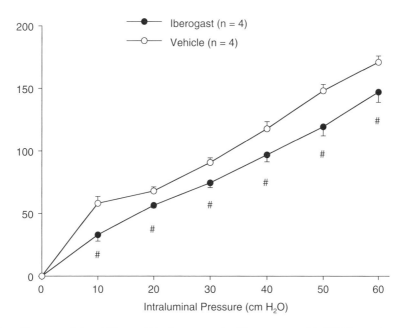

Figure 9.6. Change of the Afferent Discharge under Treatment with STW 5 or 30.8% Ethanol (Vehicle) after Mechanic Distension of the Rat Ileum (*p < 0.05) [39]

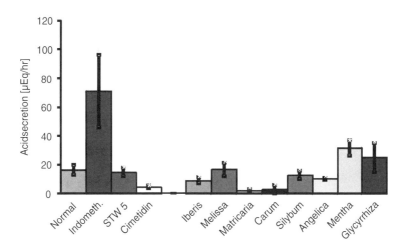

Figure 9.7. Indomethacin Induced Acid Secretion per Hour in Stomach Tissue of Pyloric Ligated Rats after Application of STW 5, Cimetidine, and the Single Extracts of STW 5 [41]

Inflammation

During the development of functional GI diseases, especially IBS, several postinflammatory conditions are discussed with possible manifestations in altered intestinal flora or altered mucosa properties. This can possibly lead to an increased sensitivity to GI stimuli

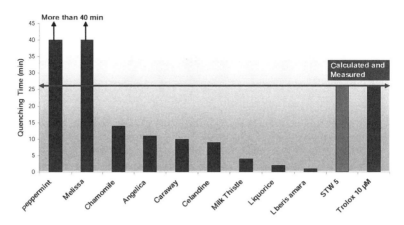

Figure 9.8. Initiated Quenching Time of the Single Extracts of STW 5 (1:5000) in the in Vitro AAPH-Model (2-2' amidinoazopropane dihydro-chloride) Indicating the Individual Free Radical–Scavenging Properties [45]

in healthy persons (42). In several inflammation models measuring the antioxidative potential of single extracts, effects in reducing inflammation and oxidative potential could be verified for the single extracts (Figure 9.8) (43). In a model of trinitrobenzene sulphonate (TNBS)-induced colitis (a standardized model for inflammatory bowel diseases), STW 5 showed similar effects to the standard therapeutic sulfasalazine (44). In specific in vitro models, free radical–scavenging properties of the single extracts could be verified, which might explain partially the anti-inflammatory properties (45).

The pharmacological data so far evaluated for STW 5 show a broad spectrum of effects regarding the underlying functional disorders of FD and IBS, offering a multitarget approach for the treatment of these diseases (see Table 9.3).

CLINICAL DATA

Pharmacological evaluations confirmed mechanistic activity of the single extracts as well as the combination product in every functional disorder considered as causes of FD and IBS. Clinical studies and analyses at the highest scientific evidence level (46) confirmed the clinical efficacy in FD and IBS. These studies have been conducted since the 1980s and now include randomized, double-blind clinical trials, open trials, postmarketing surveillances, experience reports, and a cohort study, as well as meta-analyses. Scientific evidence (46) is given as follows and is summarized in Table 9.4:

- Evidence from meta-analyses of randomized, controlled clinical trials
- Evidence from at least one suitably planned, randomized, controlled trial
- Evidence from suitably planned, nonrandomized, controlled trials
- Evidence from suitably planned cohort studies or case reports
- Evidence from comparisons of therapy time ranges or centers with or without intervention (e.g., postmarketing surveillances)
- Evidence from opinion leaders, based on clinical experience, case reports, or reports from expert panels

Table 9.4.   Clinical Studies on STW 5

Clinical Study/Surveillance (Indication)	Number of Patients	Scientific Evidence
2 meta-analyses (FD)	661	I-1
5 controlled, randomized studies (FD) 1 controlled, randomized study (IBS)	1,095	I-2
12 partially open, nonrandomized studies, 2 postmarketing surveillances (various GI diseases, FD, IBS)	5,163	II-1
Retrospective cohort study (FD)	961	II-2 / II-3
2 retrospective surveillances with children up to 12 years (GI complaints, FD, IBS)	43.311	II-3

Randomized, Double-Blind, Controlled Trials of STW 5 in Patients with FD and IBS

There were five randomized, double-blind, controlled trials conducted with STW 5 in FD and one trial conducted in patients with IBS (Table 9.5). All clinical phase III studies have been published as well as briefly summarized in reviews (47–57). Some pivotal studies are presented.

Functional Dyspepsia

In four clinical trials, STW 5 was tested versus placebo. One trial tested noninferiority of STW 5 to the prokinetic drug Cisapride. A gastroenterologic expert panel of leading German gastroenterologists gave recommendations during the study planning and for the primary target criteria. They also developed the GI symptom score (GIS), a summary score consisting of ten dyspepsia-specific symptoms that were evaluated with a 5-point Likert scale, as well as the abdominal symptom score with eight IBS-specific symptoms. The GIS was validated during a research project regarding sensitivity, responsibility, and specificity for functional dyspepsia (58), and the change of the GIS during treatment was used as the primary target parameter in all functional dyspepsia studies. Below, the comparison of STW versus Cisapride (55) and the placebo-controlled study with eight weeks' treatment duration (57) is presented.

Equivalent Efficacy to Prokinetics

The trial of Rösch et al. (2002) was a comparative trial testing noninferiority of Iberogast versus Cisapride. Because of the different application form, it was designed as a double dummy comparison. One hundred eighty-six patients with functional dyspepsia of the dysmotility type were enrolled to be treated after a seven-day washout phase with Cisapride, an herbal research preparation, or Iberogast for four weeks. After the treatment period, patients were followed up for six months. The primary target parameter was the change of the GIS during treatment period, and the secondary end point included efficacy

Table 9.5. Controlled, Randomized, Double-Blind Studies with STW 5 since the 1990s (52–57)

Author / Year	Study Title	Design	Patients (n)	Efficacy
Buchert 1994	Efficacy and tolerability of Iberogast in patients with non-ulcus dyspepsia	Double-blind, placebo-controlled, 4 weeks of treatment	243	Significant superior efficacy vs. placebo
Madisch et al. 2001	Efficacy and therapeutic safety of Iberogast in patients with functional dyspepsia	Double-blind, placebo-controlled, 4 weeks of treatment	60	Significant superior efficacy vs. placebo
Rösch et al. 2002	Efficacy of Iberogast (STW 5) or Iberogast N (STW 5 II) compared to Cisapride in the treatment of patients with functional dyspepsia of the dysmotility type	Double-blind, double-dummy verum-controlled, 4 weeks of treatment, follow-up at 6 months	183	Comparable efficacy to Cisapride
Von Arnim et al. 2007	Efficacy and tolerability of the herbal medicinal product STW 5 vs. placebo in patients with functional dyspepsia	Double-blind, placebo-controlled, 8 weeks of treatment, follow-up at 6 months	308	Significant superior efficacy vs. placebo after 8 weeks of treatment
Schneider et al. 2007	A double-blind, randomised, multicenter study to compare efficacy and safety of STW 5 versus placebo in patients with functional dyspepsia with respect to gastric emptying	Double-blind, placebo-controlled, 4 weeks of treatment	93	Significant superior efficacy vs. placebo after 4 weeks of treatment
Madisch et al. 2004	Efficacy and tolerability of Iberogast (STW 5) or Iberogast N (STW 5 II) in patients with irritable bowel syndrome	Double-blind, placebo-controlled, 4 weeks of treatment	208	Significant superior efficacy vs. placebo after 4 weeks of treatment

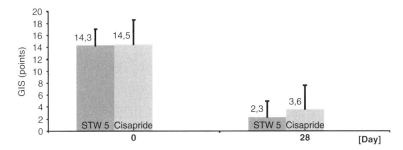

Figure 9.9. Change of the Gastrointestinal Summary Score during 4 Weeks of Therapy with STW 5 or Cisapride in Patients with Functional Dyspepsia of the Dysmotility Type [55]

and tolerability assessments by the physician and patient as well as the documentation of adverse events and laboratory parameters. The patient groups were not significantly different regarding demographic and anamnestic parameters. During treatment in both groups, the GIS decreased significantly. The mean summary score in the Iberogast group decreased during four weeks of treatment from 14.3 ± 4.7 to 2.3 ± 2.1 points and in the Cisapride group from 14.4 ± 4.1 to 3.6 ± 4.0 score points. These differences between the groups were not significant, confirming equivalent efficacy of Iberogast to the prokinetic Cisapride in patients with functional dyspepsia of the dysmotility type (Figure 9.9). The patients who were symptom free after treatment remained recurrence free during the six-month follow-up period without any significant difference between the groups. There were no clinically relevant changes in laboratory parameters documented. Two adverse events with Iberogast during treatment were seen in a probable or possible causal relationship to study medication but were classified as nonserious. The tolerability of Iberogast was assessed by 96.7% of the physicians and 93.5% of the patients as being very good or good. A previous open trial in 1984 comparing metoclopramide and Iberogast in patients with GI complaints (59) as well as a modern retrospective cohort study comparing Iberogast with metoclopramide regarding efficacy and times to be off from work (60) further confirmed the equivalent efficacy of Iberogast to prokinetics of this randomized, double-blind study.

Significant Superior Efficacy versus Placebo during Eight-Week Treatment

In a randomized, double-blind, placebo-controlled study, von Arnim et al. (2007) treated, after a washout period of seven days, 315 patients with functional dyspepsia according to ROME II criteria for eight weeks with either STW 5 or placebo. The patients were afterward followed up for six months. The main target parameter was the change of the GIS over the treatment period. After eight weeks of treatment, a significantly better improvement of the GIS was observed in the patient group that had been treated with STW 5. The mean values of the GIS changed in the STW 5 group from 11.0 ± 3.4 to 4.1 ± 4.5 points and in the placebo group from 11.2 ± 4.0 to 5.3 ± 5.2 points, revealing a significant difference in favor of STW 5 (p = 0.041) (Figure 9.10). In five patients, the following adverse events were assessed to be in causal relationship to STW 5 (abdominal pain,

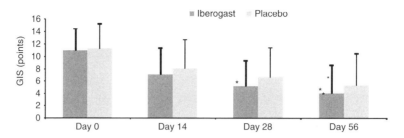

Figure 9.10. Change of the Gastrointestinal Summary Score During Eight Weeks of Therapy with STW 5 or Placebo in Patients with Functional Dyspepsia [57]

pruritus, sore throat, alopecia, hypersensivity, hypotension, and GI pain). None of these events were classified as serious. Tolerability was assessed by the patients and physicians as comparable to placebo. No clinically relevant changes of laboratory or vital parameter were detected.

Evaluation of the number of recurrence-free patients during the follow-up period indicates that after treatment with STW 5, patients stay recurrence free longer than patients who were treated with placebo (61). This effect is interesting for future evaluation regarding the clinical mechanism of efficacy of STW 5.

The studies of STW 5 with patients suffering from functional dyspepsia were sufficient comparable to start meta-analyses. Two meta-analyses were conducted with different approaches. Gundermann et al. (2004) (48) analyzed from the pooled data of four dyspepsia trials the overall efficacy of STW 5 versus placebo. They found significant superior efficacy of Iberogast. Melzer et al. (2004) (47) analyzed the efficacy of STW 5 regarding the prevailing, most bothersome symptom. In this analysis, they also showed significant superior efficacy of Iberogast versus placebo.

In a meta-analysis regarding all herbal medicinal products for which randomized, double-blind, placebo-controlled clinical trials were published, Holtmann et al. 2007 (51) defined for STW 5 significant efficacy in functional dyspepsia versus placebo verified with the highest number of published clinical studies of the analyzed medicinal preparations.

Iberogast for Patients with IBS

In a randomized, double-blind, placebo-controlled clinical trial, 208 patients with IBS were treated after a washout phase of seven days with either STW 5 or placebo for four weeks (53). The main target parameter was the change of an abdominal symptom score consisting of eight IBS-specific symptoms that were evaluated with a five-point Likert scale as a summary score. In the patient group treated with STW 5, the abdominal symptom score changed from 5.5 to 2.1 points, whereas in the placebo group it ranged from 5.1 to 3.2 points. The difference to STW 5 was statistically significant ($p < 0.0004$) in favor of STW 5 (Figure 9.11). Tolerability was evaluated by patients and physicians to be excellent. No clinically relevant changes of laboratory and vital parameter were detected.

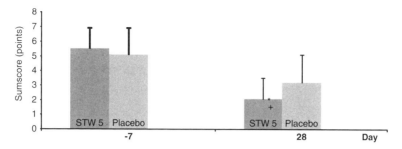

Figure 9.11. Change of the Abdominal Summary Score during Four Weeks of Therapy with STW 5 or Placebo in Patients with Irritable Bowel Syndrome [53]

Postmarketing Surveillances

In one postmarketing surveillance, 2,267 patients with FD were treated, and in another study, 2,548 patients with IBS were treated with STW 5 for an optional treatment duration of four weeks if the symptoms had not improved significantly earlier. In both surveillances, all symptoms of the patients improved in a range from 65% to 80%. The patients assessed efficacy and tolerability as being very good. There were no adverse drug effects or interactions documented in these surveillances (62, 63).

Using the retrospective surveillances with more than 40,000 children up to 12 years old, the frequent application of STW 5 in common practice in that age group was documented and an excellent safety profile was further confirmed (64, 65).

Safety of STW 5

The safety of STW 5 was extensively evaluated. Toxicity evaluations regarding acute, subchronic, and chronic toxicity are documented (66–68). Reproductive toxicity, mutagenic testing, and cytotoxicological measurements all showed no or very low toxicity of STW 5 (69–75). The clinical safety profile of STW 5 during 47 years of marketing and clinical evaluations is excellent. Table 9.6 summarizes the adverse events that were assessed to be in probable or possible causal relation to STW 5 during clinical trials and of spontaneous reports. The data gave no indication of any systemic side effects. There are few reports indicating a minimal allergic potential probably caused by a known effect of a substance class being common ingredients of asteraceae.

CONCLUSION

During its 47 years of development and continuous improvement and optimization, STW 5 has been evaluated with investigations that make this herbal medicinal product one of the most extensively investigated herbal medicines. From its start as an empirically used herbal at market launch in 1961, it has developed into an evidence-based medicinal product, verified on the highest level of scientific evidence. The data support the product approval from the leading authorities in Germany and several European countries for therapy

Table 9.6. Adverse Events during Clinical Studies and Spontaneous Reports since Market Launch (Assessed in a Possible or Probable Causal Relationship to STW 5)

Clinical Trial / Surveillance (Indication)	Number of Patients Treated with STW 5	Number of Adverse Events Assessed in a Possible or Probable Causal Relationship to STW 5
6 controlled, randomized studies (FD, IBS)	413	15
12 partially open, nonrandomized studies, 2 postmarketing surveillances (various GI diseases, FD, IBS)	5.092	14
1 retrospective cohort study (FD)	490	-
2 retrospective surveillances with children up to 12 years (GI complaints, FD, IBS)	43.311	-
Calculated treated patients in Germany—spontaneous reports since market launch	>20.000.000	19

of functional and motility-related GI diseases like FD and IBS. The combination of nine plants contributes to extensive efficacy in the sense of a multitarget approach, possibly for treating the various functional disorders underlying the diseases. This approach also makes it suitable to sufficiently treat FD and IBS. Furthermore, the combination of nine herbal drugs for achieving a high-quality medicinal product was possible only through extensive development of manufacturing methods, in-process controls, and validation of methods necessary to guarantee quality continuously on the highest level. Growing, harvesting, and manufacturing processes have to be controlled continuously to produce a medicinal product of confirmed safety and efficacy. STW 5 is therefore in Germany the only medicinal product that is approved as a combination phytopharmacon, consisting of nine components, and because of its multitarget properties, it is additionally in Germany the only medicinal product that is approved for both functional diseases—FD and IBS. It is therefore mentioned in the German Gastroenterology Guidelines as a treatment opportunity for FD and IBS. Iberogast has made its way successfully.

REFERENCES

[1]Camilleri M, Talley NJ. Pathophysiology as a basis for understanding symptom complexes and therapeutic targets. *Neurogastroenterol Motil.* 2004;16:135–142.

[2]Thompson WG, Longstreth GF, Drossman DA, Heaton KW, Irvine EJ, Müller-Lissner SA. Functional bowel disorders and functional abdominal pain. *Gut.* 1999;(Suppl II):43–47.

[3]Talley NJ, Lauritsen K. The potential role of acid suppression in functional dyspepsia: the BOND, OPERA, PILOT, and ENCORE studies. *Gut.* 2002;50 (Suppl IV):iv36–iv41.

[4]Allescher HD. Functional dyspepsia: a multi-causal disease and its therapy. *Phytomedicine.* 2006;13, S V:2–11.

[5]Wagner H. Multitarget therapy: the future of treatment for more than just functional dyspepsia. *Phytomedicine*. 2006;13, S V:122–129.

[6]Kroll U, Cordes C. Pharmaceutical prerequisites for a multi-target therapy. *Phytomedicine*. 2006;13, S V:12–19.

[7]Gaedcke F. Production, quality, analysis and use of extracts of St. John's wort. *Z Arzn Gew Pfl*. 1997;2:63–72.

[8]Good Manufacturing Practice (GMP). 2003. Medicinal Products for Human and Veterinary Use, Eudralex, Vol 4 (2003/94/EC).

[9]Monography of Commission E of the BGA. Angelicae radix (Angelica root), Bundesanzeiger 1.6.1990.

[10]Monography of Commission E of the BGA. Chelidonii herba (Greater Celandine), Bundesanzeiger 6.5.1985.

[11]Monography of Commission E of the BGA. Matricariae flos (Chamomile flowers), Bundesanzeiger 13.03.1990.

[12]Monography of Commission E of the BGA. Melissae folium (Lemon balm leaves), Monography of Commission E of the BGA. Menthae piperitae folium (Peppermint leaves), Bundesanzeiger 1.9.1990.

[13]Monography of Commission E of the BGA. Cardui mariae fructus (Milk thistle fruits), Bundesanzeiger 18.2.1986.

[14]Monography of Commission E of the BGA. Carvi fructus (Caraway fruits), Bundesanzeiger 1.2.1990.

[15]Monography of Commission E of the BGA. Liquiritiae radix (Licorice root), Bundesanzeiger 21.9.1991.

[16]Okpanyi SN, Mark M, Wahl MA. Gastrointestinal motility modulation with Iberogast. *Acta Horticulturae*. 1993;332:227–235.

[17]Reichling J, Saller R. Iberis amara L. (bitter candy tuft): profile of an herbal medicine. *Forsch Komplementärmed Klass Naturheilkd*. 2002;9(Suppl 1):21–33.

[18]Reichling J, Saller R. Iberis. In: Blaschek W, Ebel S, Fricke U, Hackenthal E, Holzgrabe U, Keller K, Reichling J, Schulz V (Hrsg): Hager ROM 2006. *Hagers Handbook of Drugs and Medicinal Products*. Berlin: Springer; 2006.

[19]Hohenester B, Rühl A, Kelber O, Schemann M. The herbal preparation STW5 (Iberogast) has potent and region specific effects on gastric motility. *Neurogastroenterol Motil*. 2004;16:765–773.

[20]Heinle H, Hagelauer D, Pascht U, Kelber O, Weiser D. Intestinal spasmolytic effects of STW 5 (Iberogast) and its components. *Phytomedicine*. 2006;13, S V:75–79.

[21]Khayyal MT, El-Ghazaly MA, Kenawy SA, Seif-El-Nasr M, Mahran LG, Kafafi YAH, Okpanyi, SN. Antiulcerogenic effect of some gastrointestinally acting plant extracts and their combination. *Arzneimittel Forsch/Drug Res*. 2001;51:545–553.

[22]Storr M, Sibaev D, Weiser D, Kelber O, Schirra J, Allescher HD. Herbal extracts modulate amplitude and frequency of small intestinal slow waves in circular smooth muscle of mouse small intestine. *Digestion*. 2004;70:257–264.

[23]Hohenester B, Rühl A, Kelber O, Schemann M. Effect mechanism of STW 5 (Iberogast) and the region specific effects of the single components on stomach motility of the guinea pig. *Z Gastroenterol*. 2004;42:814.

[24]Talley NJ, Zinsmeister AR, Schleck CD, Melton LJ 3rd. Dyspepsia and dyspepsia subgroups: a population-based study. *Gastroenterology*. 1992 Apr;102(4 Pt 1):1259–1268.

[25]Talley NJ, Stanghellini V, Heading RC, Koch KL, Malagelada JR, Tytgat GNJ. Functional gastroduodenal disorders. *Gut*. 1999;45(Suppl II):37–42.

[26]Talley NJ, Weaver AL, Zinsmeister AR. Impact of Functional Dyspepsia on Quality of Life. *Dig Dis Sci*. 1995;40(3)584–589.

[27]Nyren O, Lindberg G, Lindström E, Marke LA, Seensalu R. Economic costs of functional dyspepsia. *Pharmaco Economics*. 1992;1(5):312–324.

[28]Talley NJ, Meineche-Schmidt V, Pare P, et al. Efficacy of omeprazole in functional dyspepsia: double-blind, randomized, placebo-controlled trials (the Bond and Opera studies). *Aliment Pharmacol Ther*. 1998;12:1055–1065.

[29]Schwartz MP, Samsom M, Smout AJPM. Duodenal motor activity in response to acid and different nutrients. *Gastroenterology*. 1999;116:A1079.

[30]Talley NJ, Verlinden M, Jones M. Can symptoms discriminate among those with delayed or normal gastric emptying in dysmotility-like dyspepsia. *Am J Gastroenterol*. 2001;96(5):1422–1428.

[31]Cremonini F, Talley NJ. Irritable bowel syndrome: epidemiology, natural history, health care seeking and emerging risk factors. *Gastroenterol Clin N Am*. 2005;34:189–204.

[32]Quigley EMM. Motility, heartburn and dyspepsia. *Aliment Pharmacol Ther*. 1997;11(2):41–50.

[33]Schemann M, Michel K, Hohenester B, Rühl A. Region-specific effects of STW 5 and its components in gastric fundus, corpus and antrum. *Phytomedicine*. 2006;13, S V:90–99.

[34]Pilichiewicz AN, Horowitz M, Russo A, Maddox AF, Jones KL, Schemann M, Holtmann G, Feinle-Bisset C. Effects of Iberogast on proximal gastric volume, antropyloroduodenal (APD) motility and gastric emptying in healthy men. *Am J Gastroenterol*. 2007;102:1–8.

[35]Okpanyi SN. Evaluation of the effect of Iberogast (STW 5) or Iberogast N-II (STW 5-II) on the histamine-induced contraction of the guinea pig ileum. Research Report 11/91, Steigerwald Arzneimittelwerk GmbH, Darmstadt, 1991.

[36]Ammon HTP. Evaluation of the effect of STW5 (Iberogast), STW6 (Iberis amara fresh plant extract) und STW 7 (Iberogast-drug extracts without Iberis amara) on the acetylcholine-induced contraction of the isolated guinea pig ileum. Research report 01/86, Steigerwald Arzneimittelwerk GmbH, Darmstadt, 1986.

[37]Krüger D, Gruber L, Angay O, Zeller F, Kelber O, Schemann M. Efficacy profile of STW 5 (Iberogast) offers new options for treatment of gastrointestinal diseases. Z Phytother. 2008;29:S29.

[38]Camilleri M. Enteric nervous system disorders: genetic and molecular insights for the neurogastroenterologist. Neurogastroenterol Mot. 2001;13:277–295.

[39]Liu CY, Müller MH, Glatzle J, Weiser D, Kelber O, Enck P, Grundy D, Kreis ME. The herbal preparation STW 5 (Iberogast) desensitizes intestinal afferents in the rat small intestine. Neurogastroenterol Motil. 2004;16:759–764.

[40]Simmen U, Kelber O, Okpanyi SN, Jaeggi R, Bueter B,Weiser D. Binding of STW 5 and its components to intestinal 5-HT, muscarinic M3, and opioid receptors. Phytomedicine. 2006:13, S V:51–55.

[41]Khayyal MT, Seif-El-Nasr M, El-Ghazaly MA, Okpanyi SN, Kelber O, Weiser D. Mechanisms involved in the gastro-protective effect of STW 5 (Iberogast) and its components against ulcers and rebound activity. Phytomedicine. 2006:13, S V: 56–66.

[42]Kassinen A, Krokius-Kurikka L, Mäkivuokko H, Rinttilä T, Paulin L, Corander J, Malinen E, Apajalahti J, Palva A. The fecal microbiota of irritable bowel syndrome patients differs significantly from that of healthy subjects. Gastroenterology. 2007;133:24–33.

[43]Michael S, Kelber O, Vinson B, Nieber K. Herbal preparations STW 5 and STW 6 inhibit inflammation-mediated motility disorders in the ileum. Gut. 2006;55, S V:A206.

[44]Abdel-Aziz H, WadieW, Kelber O, Vinson B, Weiser D, Khayyal MT. Antiinflammatory effect of STW5 in colonic inflammation in vivo. Gut. 2007b, 56:A154.

[45]Schempp H, Weiser D, Kelber O, Elstner EF. Radical scavenging and anti-inflammatory properties of STW 5 and its components. Phytomedicine. 2006;13, S V:36–44.

[46]Woolf SH. Practice Guidelines, a new reality in medicine. II. methods of developing guidelines. Arch Int Med. 1992;152:946–952.

[47]Melzer J, Rösch W, Reichling J, Brignoli R, Saller R. Meta-analysis: phytotherapy of functional dyspepsia with STW 5 (Iberogast). Aliment Pharmacol Ther. 2004;20:1–9.

[48]Gundermann K-J, Godehardt E, Ulbrich M. Efficacy of a herbal combination preparation for treatment of functional dyspepsia: metaanalysis of the randomised double blind studies based on a validated gastrointestinal symptom score. MMW-Fortschr Med. 2004;146,Nr.33/34.

[49]Holtmann G, Adam B, Vinson B. Evidence based medicine and phytotherapy for functional dyspepsia: an analysis of the evidence for the herbal medicinal preparation Iberogast. Wiener Medizinische Wochenschrift. 2004;Nr.154:21–22.

[50]Rösch W, Vinson B, Gundermann K-J, Holtmann G. Phytotherapy for functional dyspepsia: a review of the clinical evidence for the herbal preparation STW5. Phytomedicine. 2006;13 S V:114–121.

[51]Holtmann G, Nandurkar S, Talley N, Moayyedi P. Herbal medicine for the treatment of functional dyspepsia: a systematic review of the literature and meta-analysis. Gastroenterology. 2007;132(4):W1204.

[52]Buchert D. Efficacy of a fixed herbal combination for treatment of non-ulcer dyspepsia. Z Phytother. 1994;15:24–25.

[53]Madisch A, Holtmann G, Plein K, Hotz J. Treatment of irritable bowel syndrome with herbal preparations, results of a double-blind, randomized, placebo-controlled, multi-centre trial. Aliment Pharmacol Ther. 2004;19:271–279.

[54]Madisch A, Melderis H, Mayr G, Sassin I, Hotz J. A phytotherapeutics and his modified research preparation for treatment of functional dyspepsia. Z Gastroenterol. 2001;39:511–517.

[55]Rösch W, Vinson B, Sassin I. A randomised clinical trial comparing the efficacy of a herbal preparation STW 5 with the prokinetic drug cisapride in patients with dysmotility type of functional dyspepsia. Z Gastroenterol. 2002;40:401–408.

[56]Schneider A, Caspary W, Börner N, Vinson B, Braden B. Application of the Octanoat-breath-test for measurement of the gastral motility in patients with functional dyspepsia and delayed gastric emptying: results of a multicenter double blind randomised placebo-controlled study with STW 5 (Iberogast). Z Gastroenterol. 2007;45:P069.

[57]von Arnim U, Peitz U, Vinson B, Gundermann KJ, Malfertheiner P. STW 5, a phytopharmacon for patients with functional dyspepsia: results of a multicenter, placebo-controlled doubleblind study. Am J Gastroenterol. 2007;102:1268–1275.

[58]Adam B, Liebregts T, Saadat-Gilani K, Vinson B, Holtmann G. Validation of the gastrointestinal symptom score for the assessment of symptoms in patients with functional dyspepsia. Aliment Pharmacol Ther. 2005;22:357–363.

[59]Nicolay K. Treatment of functional gastroenteropathia with Metoclopramide compared to the phytotherapeutics Iberogast: a single blind study. *Gastro-Entero-Hepatol.* 1984;2:24–28.

[60]Raedsch R, Hanisch J, Bock P, Sibaev A, Vinson B, Gundermann KJ. Wirksamkeit und Unbedenklichkeit eines des Phytopharmakons STW 5 versus Metoclopramid oral bei funktioneller Dyspepsie unter Praxisbedingungen. *Z Gastroenterol.* 2007;45:1041–1048.

[61]von Arnim U, Vinson BR, Malfertheiner P, Saller R. Functional dyspepsia: are relapse rates influenced by active treatment. *Gastroenterology.* 2008;134:W1085.

[62]Sassin I, Buchert D. Efficacy and tolerability of the herbal preparation Iberogast in the therapy of functional dyspepsia. *Phytomedicine.* 2000;7(Suppl II):91–92 (69P).

[63]Klein-Galczinsky C, Sassin I. Post marketing surveillance of efficacy and tolerability of Iberogast in patients with irritable bowel syndrome. *Phytotherapie an der Schwelle zum neuen Jahrtausend* (Abstracts). 1999;125:(P25).

[64]Leichtle K. Experience reports of the application of Iberogast in children. Research report, Steigerwald Arzneimittelwerk GmbH, 1999.

[65]Gundermann K-J, Vinson B, Hänicke S. Functional dyspepsia in children: a retrospective study with a phytotherapeutics. *Päd.* 2004;(10):1–6.

[66]Okpanyi SN. Acute oral toxicity of Iberogast in the rat. Research report 17/86, Steigerwald Arzneimittelwerk GmbH, Darmstadt, 1986a.

[67]Okpanyi SN. Acute oral toxicity of Iberogast in mice. Research report 18/86, Steigerwald Arzneimittelwerk GmbH, Darmstadt, 1986b.

[68]van Rozendaal AWM. 3-month oral gavage toxicity study in male and female beagle dogs followed by a one-month recovery period. Study report Nr. 330222, Notox B.V.,'s-Hertogenbosch, NL, 2003.

[69]Burns L. Oral (gavage) fertility and early embryonic development study in the rat. Study report Nr. VEB0007, Sequani, Ledbury, UK, 2003.

[70]Burns L. Oral (gavage) developmental toxicity study in the rat. Study report Nr. VEB0008, Sequani, Ledbury, UK, 2003.

[71]Burns L. Oral (gavage) pre- and postnatal developmental toxicity study in the rat. Study report Nr. VEB0009, Sequani, Ledbury, UK, 2003.

[72]Miltenburger HG. Report of the study LMPZyt 10 (STW 6). Research report, Laboratory for Mutagenicity Investigation, Technische Hochschule Darmstadt, 1986.

[73]Völkner W, Arenz M, Hermann F, Miltenburger HG. Micronucleus assay in bone marrow cells of the mouse with STW 5. Test report, Proj. No. 538 204, Cytotest Cell Research GmbH & Co. KG, Roßdorf, 1996.

[74]Völkner W, Arenz M, Hermann F, Miltenburger HG. In vivo / in vitro unscheduled DNA synthesis in rat hepatocytes with STW 5. Test report, Proj. No. 538 203, Cytotest Cell Research GmbH & Co. KG, Roßdorf, 1996.

[75]Völkner W, Arenz M, Hermann F, Miltenburger HG. Micronucleus assay in bone marrow cells of the mouse with STW 6. Test report, Proj. No. 538 104, Cytotest Cell Research GmbH & Co. KG, Roßdorf, 1996.

Botanical Medicine: From Bench to Bedside
Edited by R. Cooper and F. Kronenberg
© Mary Ann Liebert, Inc.

Chapter 10

Biological Activity of Cranberry Proanthocyanidins: Effects on Oxidation, Microbial Adhesion, Inflammation, and Health

Jess D. Reed and Amy B. Howell

The link between food and health is firmly established, and consumers are keenly interested in utilizing "functional foods" to help manage their health. One such food is the American cranberry (*Vaccinium macrocarpon* Ait), which has demonstrated a wide array of health benefits in research studies. Cranberries are native to North America and were utilized for hundreds of years as food and medicine and for trading in New England by the Native Americans and Colonial settlers (1). Native Americans used cranberries to treat urinary disorders and blood poisoning and in poultices for wounds. Since citrus fruits were not grown in New England, American sailors brought cranberries along on ships to prevent scurvy on the sailing trips to Europe and England (1). Interestingly, recent research is demonstrating that cranberries may have multiple health benefits, ranging from prevention of urinary tract infections (UTIs) and bacterial adhesion to reducing risk factors associated with heart disease.

Cranberries possess a tart taste because of the level of the natural organic acids. Early work on cranberry juice and cranberry fruit extracts related to percentage of organic acids' content. More recently, there is evidence to show that cranberries contain many polyphenolic compounds that have anti-inflammatory, bacterial antiadhesion, and antioxidant activity in cell culture, animal models, and clinical research (2). Bacterial antiadhesion properties of cranberries are further discussed in Chapter 11, "Cranberry Products Prevent Urinary Tract Infections in Women: Clinical Evidence," by Tempesta and Barrett. These properties suggest that cranberry consumption may reduce the risk of cancer, cardiovascular disease, and infections of the mouth, stomach, and urinary tract and are discussed herein (3).

Cranberries contain at least 10 hydroxycinnamic acids, including the recently identified 3-O-p-hydroxycinnamoyl ursolic acid, which is cytotoxic to cervical and prostate tumor cell

[1] Department of Animal Sciences, University of Wisconsin, Madison, Wisconsin 53706-1481; jdreed@wisc.edu

[2] Marucci Center for Blueberry Cranberry Research, Rutgers University, New Jersey 07102; ahowell@aesop.rutgers.edu

lines (4); more than 20 flavonols, glycosides of quercetin, myricetin, and kaempferol and their aglycones; 6 anthocyanins, cyanidin-3-galactoside, cyanidin-3-glucoside, cyanidin-3-arabinoside, peonidin-3-galactoside, peonidin-3-glucoside, and peonidin-3-arabinoside; and a complex mixture of oligomeric flavonoids known as proanthocyanidins (PACs) that may exceed one thousand individual compounds (5). In this chapter, we discuss the chemistry of PACs and their relationship to cranberry health benefits. In Chapter 11, effects of cranberry extracts, which were standardized to PACs, against UTIs are presented.

TANNIN AND PROANTHOCYANIDIN NOMENCLATURE AND STRUCTURE

Tannins are defined as water-soluble oligomeric polyphenols that precipitate proteins (6). There are two groups of tannins: hydrolyzable tannins (HTs) and PACs. HTs include gallic acid and ellagic acid esters of core molecules that consist of polyols such as sugars. However, cranberries do not contain HTs. PACs are polymers of flavan-3-ols and flavans linked through an interflavan carbon bond between carbon 4 of the C-ring and carbon 8 of the A- ring (Figure 10.1). This bond is not susceptible to hydrolysis. PACs are also referred to as condensed tannins. The nomenclature for PACs is derived from the acid-catalyzed oxidation reaction, which produces anthocyanidins upon heating PACs in acidic alcohol solutions (6). The most common anthocyanidins produced are cyanidin and delphinidin from the corresponding PACs, procyanidin and prodelphinidin. However, most food PACs are heteropolymers with monomers that vary in the number and pattern of hydroxylation (5). PACs may also have substitution with sugars, such as the glycosylated 3-deoxyproanthocyanidins in sorghum, and gallic acid, such as in grape seed PACs (7, 8). PACs may have an additional interflavan ether bond through carbon 2 of the C-ring and carbon 7 of the A-ring (Figure 10.1). This type of interflavan bond is referred to as an "A-type" bond, which does not yield an anthocyanidin in the acid-catalyzed autoxidation reaction (9). Cranberry PACs have one or more A-type linkages.

Foo et al. elucidated the trimeric structures of cranberry A-type PACs that are associated with the inhibition of adhesion of P-fimbriated *Escherichia coli* to uroepithelial cells (10, 11). In our studies, we isolated cranberry PACs over Sephadex LH-20 to determine any association with low-density lipoprotein in serum and subsequent inhibition of Cu^{2+}-induced oxidation (12). The fraction that eluted with methanol contained trimers through heptamers with at least one A-type interflavan bond. This series of molecular weights closely resembled the epicatechin structures reported by Foo et al. (11). Our mass spectrometric (MS) results also showed the presence of more complex heteropolymers for PACs with a degree of polymerization greater than four (5, 12). The pentamer and hexamer also had masses corresponding to PACs with two A-type linkages. The fraction that eluted in aqueous acetone contained pentamers through nonamers with either two or three A-type interflavan bonds in each oligomer.

Pigmentation in fruits such as cranberries and grapes is attributed to anthocyanins. However, in grapes, Kennedy et al. reported that anthocyanins are incorporated into PACs during fruit ripening (13). While there are few reports of anthocyanin-PAC oligomers occurring in fruits and unfermented beverages, there are accounts of complex pigments in alcoholic beverages such as red wine and rose cider (14–17). Our MS studies indicate that cranberries and cranberry juice contain pigments that are anthocyanins linked to PACs (18). The large

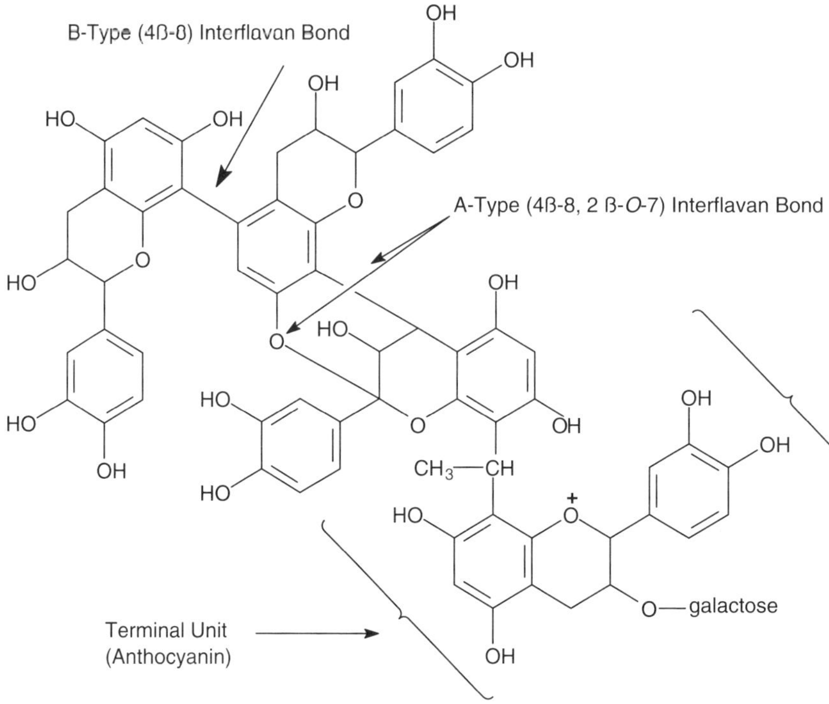

Figure 10.1. Representative Cranberry Proanthocyanidin Oligomer Showing the Main Features That Lead to Variation in Structure

A proanthocyanidin trimer, with one "A-type" and one "B-type" interflavan bond, is shown linked to cyanidin galactoside through an ethyl bridge.[50]

number of individual PAC compounds and anthocyanin-PAC pigments creates difficulty in obtaining high MS resolution of any individual compounds. The combination of liquid chromatographic separation and mass spectrometry indicates that the structural heterogeneity of cranberry pigments is much greater than previously described (5). Structural heterogeneity exists in the degree of polymerization, nature of the interflavan bonds (A and B type), pattern of hydroxylation of flavan units, and substitution with anthocyanins. In addition, there is isomerization within each degree of polymerization that is not detected by mass spectrometry. Therefore, cranberries probably contain several hundred individual PAC oligomers. This structural heterogeneity creates difficulty in relating structure to bioactivity. Biomedical research on the health benefits and risks of increased consumption of cranberry PACs is limited by lack of information on structure or bioactivity relationships that can be used in standardization of cranberry products.

CRANBERRY PACS AND OXIDATION OF LOW-DENSITY LIPOPROTEINS

Tannins are active in redox reactions and scavenge free radicals in biologically induced or metal catalyzed oxidation of lipids (19, 20). Diluted cranberry extracts inhibited in vitro oxidation of low-density lipoprotein (LDL) (21). Research in our laboratory indicated that cinnamic acids, anthocyanins, and flavonol glycosides in cranberries do not bind to LDL and do not inhibit Cu^{2+}-induced LDL oxidation when mixed with serum prior to LDL isolation (12). However, cranberry PACs, specifically associated with LDL in serum, inhibited oxidation of the isolated LDL (12). PACs of five to nine catechin units appeared to have greater affinity for LDL and greater antioxidant capacity than oligomers of a lower degree of polymerization (12).

CRANBERRY PACS AND MICROBIAL ADHESION

Potential for Promotion of Urinary Tract Health

Adhesion of bacteria to mucosal surfaces in the body is an important step in the pathogenesis of infection (22). An infection is initiated by bacterial adhesion to cells followed by bacterial multiplication and colonization. For example, UTIs are predominantly caused by adhesion of uropathogenic strains of *Escherichia coli* (*E. coli*) bacteria to uroepithelial cells (23). Adhesins (P fimbriae and type 1 fimbriae) adhere to carbohydrate receptors on the surface of uroepithelial cells and are important virulence factors in the pathogenesis of UTIs (22). Most uropathogenic strains of *E. coli* express type 1 fimbriae that bind to mannose-like receptors (24). P-fimbriated *E. coli* adhere to oligosaccharide receptor sequences (α-Gal[1→4]b-Gal) (25) and are important in both cystitis and pyelonephritis (26).

Methods for inhibiting bacterial adhesion are being explored for prevention of UTIs and other bacterial infections rather than prescribing low-dose antibiotic regimes, as the antiadhesion mechanism does not kill bacteria and therefore does not lead to significant selection pressure favoring survival of antibiotic-resistant bacterial strains (27).

A study on cranberry, a dietary inhibitor of bacterial adhesion, found that susceptible and antibiotic-resistant P-fimbriated *E. coli* were no longer able to adhere to bladder cell receptors following incubation in urine of human participants after 240 mL of cranberry juice cocktail had been consumed (28). Thus cranberry, used to prevent UTIs, could potentially slow the pace of antibiotic resistance development, as the ultimate use of antibiotics to treat infections would be lower. This type of preventative strategy could become more important as antibiotic resistance rates continue to increase because of excessive use of antibiotics (29).

Cranberries also contain the monosaccharide fructose together with PACs, which have both been associated with prevention of bacterial adhesion. Fructose inhibits type 1 (mannose-sensitive) fimbrial adhesion to uroepithelial cells in vitro, but this effect has yet to be demonstrated in vivo (30). Cranberry PACs inhibit mannose-sensitive adhesion of P-fimbriated *E. coli* to uroepithelial cells (11, 31, 32) both in vitro and in vivo (33). The cranberry PAC structures contain a number of unusual A-type double interflavan bonds (11). A-linked dimers from cranberry have higher in vitro bacterial antiadhesion activity than the B-linked dimers, suggesting that the conformational rigidity of the A linkage may be important in imparting the activity (11). The antiadhesion activity is not associated with PACs from other food sources that do not have A-type interflavan bonds, such as chocolate, grape, apple, and green tea (34).

The bacterial antiadhesion mechanism of cranberry is currently under investigation. PACs bind readily to proteins (35), which suggests that the cranberry PACs and/or their metabolites may be binding to the proteinaceous fimbrial tips on *E. coli* and act as receptor analogs. Cranberry PACs may inhibit the specific receptor-ligand adhesion to uroepithelial cells favored by hydrophobic interactions (36, 37). In culture, cranberry juice reduced P-fimbriated *E. coli* fimbrial length and density and changed bacterial shape from rods to spheres (38). More research is needed to determine if and how these induced conformational changes influence the adhesion activity of the bacteria.

The daily dose of cranberry PACs is currently based on the amount of PAC in a glass of cranberry juice cocktail (200–300 mL). More effective methods for quantification of PACs are needed, as the heterogeneous nature of the cranberry PACs (molecular weight and linkage type) makes analysis among cranberry products unreliable (39). The most reliable way to estimate daily dosage of cranberry is to examine clinical trial data on whole-cranberry products. Clinical trials on cranberry indicate reduction in recurrent UTIs when cranberry juice or powder is consumed on a daily basis (40–42). The Cochrane Database Systematic Review (43) states that there is positive evidence from clinical trials indicating that consumption of cranberry juice can decrease the number of symptomatic UTIs over a 12-month period in women; however, cranberry cannot treat a UTI once an infection progresses. Daily intake of 240 to 300 mL of cranberry juice cocktail can prevent about 50% of recurrence of UTI and reduce bacteriuria and pyruria (40). Twice-daily dosing (two 240 mL/day) may offer more protection over a 24-hour period according to an ex vivo study on human urine following cranberry juice cocktail consumption (28). Dried cranberry powder (41, 44, 45), sweetened dried cranberries (46), and cranberry sauce (47) may also provide some benefits, although further clinical research is needed. Additional studies sponsored by the National Center for Complementary and Alternative Medicine at the U.S. National Institutes of Health (NIH) are underway on the role of cranberry and urinary tract health.

Further details are presented in Chapter 11.

Potential for Promotion of Gastrointestinal Health

Adhesion of *Helicobacter pylori* (*H. pylori*) to stomach epithelial cells leads to chronic infection associated with peptic ulcers (48). Bacteria colonize the gastric mucus in asymptomatic subjects, making them potential sources of infection. Clearance of the *H. pylori* from the gastric mucosa may be an effective way of preventing infection. Cranberry extract containing PACs prevented *Helicobacter pylori*, the bacterium that causes stomach ulcers, from attaching to isolated stomach cells (48). In a study of 83 *H. pylori* isolates, there was no relationship between resistance to the antiadhesion effect of this cranberry extract and antibiotic resistance, suggesting that the combination of treatment with this PAC cranberry extract and antibiotic may improve eradication (49). In a clinical study with patients receiving triple therapy for *H. pylori* infection (omeprazole, amoxicillin, and clarithromycin), addition of cranberry juice drink (250 ml/day) to the treatment improved rate of eradication in females (50). In a randomized, placebo-controlled clinical study in China, consumption of two 250 ml servings of cranberry juice cocktail (27% cranberry) per day accounted for a 15% eradication of *H. pylori* (51). A recent double-blind, placebo-controlled clinical trial in Chile found a 200 ml serving of cranberry juice or *Lactobacillus* probiotic for three weeks inhibited *H. pylori* in 15% of asymptomatic children (52). Given that the standard therapy for acute ulcers is quite intense, involving multiple antibiotic regimes and proton pump inhibitors over several months, the use of cranberry could be an attractive alternative. However, additional research is necessary to determine long-term prophylaxis and preventative effectiveness of cranberry.

Potential for Promotion of Oral Cavity Health

Adhesion and coaggregation of over 30 species of bacteria to biofilms in the oral cavity are associated with the development of periodontal disease (53). Cranberry PAC extract (nondialyzable material, or NDM) has demonstrated activity in the oral cavity preventing biofilms associated with coaggregation and adhesion of bacteria to teeth and gums (53, 54), as well as prevention of adhesion of *Streptoccocus sobrinus* to hydroxyapatite (55). This extract inhibited the glycosyltransferases involved in biofilm formation and promoted desorption of the bacterium from biofilms (55, 56). In addition, it reduced the capacity of *Porphyromonas gingivalis* (*P. gingivalis*) to colonize periodontal sites by inhibiting biofilm formation (57). More research is needed to study the effect of contact time of cranberry PACs on adhesion prevention of oral bacteria. Cranberry juice may not be a viable product for adhesion prevention in the oral cavity, as the acidity could potentially harm teeth. PAC-based products would need to be developed for consumer use such as gums, mouthwashes, or lozenges with sufficient contact time between the PACs and the oral bacteria.

CRANBERRY PACS

Inflammation

Inflammation is associated with atherosclerosis and cardiovascular disease, several cancers (including colorectal, prostate, and skin), arthritis, and Alzheimer's disease. The role of cyclooxygenase-2 (COX-2) in the production of proinflammatory prostaglandins and their association with pain and fever suggest that COX-2 has a role in the etiology of these diseases. Our preliminary results presented herein show that cranberry PACs attenuate the increased expression of COX-2 and inducible nitric oxide synthase (iNOS) in macrophage cells after stimulation with bacterial lipopolysaccharide (LPS). Periodontitis is an inflammatory disease caused by macrophage response to periodontopathogens (58). Cranberry NDM (65% proanthocyanidin) inhibited proinflammatory cytokine response of macrophages to LPS from periodontalpathogens (58). Cranberry NDM also dose dependently inhibited the proteinases and other enzymes involved in periodontopathogen proliferation in periodontal pockets (59).

Cardiovascular Disease

The relationship between cranberry consumption and reduced risk of cardiovascular disease was recently reviewed (2, 60). Clinical and epidemiological research indicates that consumption of tannins in foods and beverages may decrease the risk of developing atherosclerosis. Research in our laboratory determined the effect of feeding cranberry spray-dried juice powder (CJP) on blood cholesterol in normal (N) and familial hypercholesterolemic (FH) swine (61). Feeding CJP for four weeks lowered LDL-C in FH sows by 94 mg/dl, a 22% decrease from baseline (reference). Feeding CJP to FH pigs also returned the endothelium-dependent relaxation dose-response to bradykinin toward values observed in vessels from normal pigs. These results indicate that feeding CJP may improve vascular relaxation responses in FH pigs with atherosclerosis. Consumption of cranberry juice improved flow-mediated dilation in human subjects (62, 63). Studies with proanthocyanidin supplements (hawthorn and grape seed extracts) and red wine polyphenols indicate that PACs improve endothelial-dependent vaso-relaxation (64, 65).

Cancer

A review of literature on anticancer properties of cranberries concluded that the fruit has a potential role as a dietary chemopreventive (66). Cranberry PAC fractions inhibited the growth of eight tumor cell lines at GI(50) concentrations from 20 to 80 µg ml^{-1} and inhibited the expression of metalloproteinases in a prostate carcinoma cell line (3). A cranberry fraction containing anthocyanins, flavonols, and PACs prepared from a water extract of the press cake inhibited the proliferation of eight human tumor cell lines of multiple origins at GI(50) of 10 to 250 mg L^{-1} (67). The same flavonoid extract and a more purified extract containing PACs were tested in an in vivo mouse model for inhibition of explant tumors (68). The PAC fraction (100 mg kg^{-1}) and the flavonoid fraction (250 mg kg^{-1}) were administered by intraperitoneal (i.p.) injection. The flavonoid and PAC fractions slowed the growth of glioblastoma multiforme (U87). The PAC fraction inhibited growth of colon carcinoma (HT-29) and prostate carcinoma (DU145) and induced complete regression of two of the DU145 explants.

BIOAVAILABILITY OF PACS

Research suggests that PACs are poorly absorbed and are therefore not bioactive at the cellular and tissue levels. Beecher reviewed the literature on bioactivity of PACs in relation to human health and concluded that research is needed "to identify further biologically active components of PAC so that mechanism of action at the tissue, cellular and subcellular levels can be elucidated" (69). The author emphasized the need to determine compounds that are absorbed and their tissue distribution. The research showing that PACs reach only low peripheral blood concentrations (<50 nM) does not preclude them from affecting health through bioactivity in the gastrointestinal tract, where they may be in high concentration after ingestion (70–72). In addition, PACs have high affinity for proteins and strongly adhere to cell surfaces and plasma lipoproteins. Therefore, the preparation, extraction, and analysis of tissues for PACs are difficult with currently available methods. Intake of PACs at levels above 2% of diet dry matter is often associated with decreased growth rate and feed efficiency and low true digestibility of protein and essential amino acids in domestic livestock (73). These effects are most likely explained by complex formation between endogenous and food proteins with PACs in the lumen and epithelium of the digestive tract. However, effects of PACs on lipid oxidation, inflammation, immunity, and bacterial adhesion in the gut may have beneficial effects on health. Antioxidant effects in the gut are potentially beneficial to health because oxidized lipids are absorbed and incorporated into lipoproteins, increasing their atherogenic properties (74). Antiadhesion and anti-inflammatory effects are potentially beneficial because the interaction between the gut microflora and the gut-associated lymphoid tissue affects immunity at other mucosal surfaces such as the lungs and urogenital tract (75–78). The limited data from animal studies on bioavailability indicate that molecular weight influences metabolism and absorption of PACs (79). Early research on the oligomeric PACs in grapes and grape seeds indicated extensive absorption and metabolism (79). However, results of this earlier research were questioned because the preparation of the oligomers may have also contained monomeric catechins and other flavonoids (80). Transport of catechin and PAC dimer (B3) and trimer (C2) across the Caco-2 cell monolayer was similar, but the transport of PACs of a higher degree of polymerization was much lower (81). Feeding experiments with rats that received radiolabeled PACs in their diet indicated that no intact PACs could be detected in the plasma or urine (82). However, hawthorn (*Crataegus* spp.) PACs labeled with ^{14}C and of different molecular weights were administered orally to mice and were extensively absorbed (83). In the first hour following administration, 65% of the trimers and 3% of the higher-molecular-weight oligomers were found in the blood. After seven hours, 81% of the trimers and 42% of the oligomers reached the organs, and 1.8% of both the trimers and oligomers were excreted in the urine. Tsang et al. observed PAC dimers (B1, B2, B3, and B4) and trimers in urine from rats after ingestion of grape seed extract (84), whereas PAC oligomers that are not absorbed may be metabolized by colonic microflora to simpler phenolic acids that are absorbed from the colon (85). Urine of mice given isolated cranberry PACs in their drinking water exhibited in vitro bacterial antiadhesion activity (34). This indicates that a certain level of absorption occurred and that bioactive PAC metabolites were present in the urine or that properties of the urine were altered by the PACs such that adhesion was inhibited. The absorption of the unique A-type PAC oligomers in cranberries has not been determined. However, absorption and metabolism of these compounds are critical components of their effects on health.

CONCLUSION

Research indicates that cranberry has a broad range of health benefits that may be attributed, to a large extent, to the PACs. The complexity of this group of phytochemicals has presented many challenges for researchers, especially in the areas of structural elucidation, metabolism and absorption, and interaction with other molecules. The unusual structural features and presence of the A-type linkage make the cranberry PACs intriguing from a medicinal perspective, especially when investigating structure-activity relationships. Additional research is needed to determine pharmacokinetic parameters and dose response associated with ingestion of cranberry PACs or foods containing these PACs. However, a strong link between PACs and biological activity has been presented herein and may support the direction of clinical outcomes discussed in the next chapter.

REFERENCES

[1]Leahy MP, Roderick RMS, Brilliant KMS. The cranberry-promising health benefits, old and new. *Nutr Today*. 36:254–265.

[2]Reed J. Cranberry flavonoids, atherosclerosis and cardiovascular health. *Crit Rev Food Sci Nutr*. 2002; 42:301–316.

[3]Neto CC, Krueger CG, Lamoureaux TL, Kondo M, Vaisberg AJ, Hurta RAR, Curtis S, Matchett MD, Yeung H, Sweeney MI, Reed JD. MALDI-TOF MS characterization of proanthocyanidins from cranberry fruit (Vaccinium macrocarpon) that inhibit tumor cell growth and matrix metalloproteinase expression in vitro. *J Sci Food Agric*. 2006;86:18–25.

[4]Murphy BT, MacKinnon SL, Yan XJ, Hammond GB, Vaisberg AJ, Neto CC. Identification of triterpene hydroxycinnamates with in vitro antitumor activity from whole cranberry fruit (Vaccinium macrocarpon) *J Agric Food Chem.* 2003;51:3541–3545.

[5]Reed JD, Krueger CG, Vestling MM. MALDI-TOF mass spectrometry of oligomeric food polyphenols. *Phytochemistry.* 2005;66:2248–2263.

[6]Haslam E, Cai Y. Plant polyphenols (vegetable tannins): gallic acid metabolism. *Nat Prod Rep.* 1994;11: 41–66.

[7]Krueger CG, Vestling MM, Reed JD. Matrix-assisted laser desorption/ionization time-of-flight mass spectrometry of heteropolyflavan-3-ols and glucosylated heteropolyflavans in sorghum [Sorghum bicolor (L.) Moench]. *J Agric Food Chem.* 2003;51:538–543.

[8]Krueger CG, Dopke NC, Treichel PM, Folts J, Reed JD. Matrix-assisted laser desorption/ionization time-of-flight mass spectrometry of polygalloyl polyflavan-3-ols in grape seed extract. *J Agric Food Chem.* 2000;48: 1663–1667.

[9]Jacques D, Haslam E, Bedford GR, Greatbanks D. Plant proanthocyanidins. 2. proanthocyanidin-A2 and its derivatives. *Journal of the Chemical Society-Perkin Transactions 1.* 1974;2663–2671.

[10]Foo LY, Lu Y, Howell AB, Vorsa N. A-Type proanthocyanidin trimers from cranberry that inhibit adherence of uropathogenic P-fimbriated Escherichia coli. *J Nat Prod.* 2000;63:1225–1228.

[11]Foo LY, Lu Y, Howell AB, Vorsa N. The structure of cranberry proanthocyanidins which inhibit adherence of uropathogenic P-fimbriated Escherichia coli in vitro. *Phytochemistry.* 2000;54:173–181.

[12]Porter ML, Krueger CG, Wiebe DA, Cunningham DG, Reed JD. Cranberry proanthocyanidins associate with low-density lipoprotein and inhibit in vitro Cu2+-induced oxidation. *J Sci Food Agric.* 2001;81: 1306–1313.

[13]Kennedy JA, Matthews MA, Waterhouse AL. Effect of maturity and vine water status on grape skin and wine flavonoids. *Am J Enol Vitic.* 2002;53:268–274.

[14]Wildenradt HL, Singleton VL. Production of aldehydes as a result of oxidation of polyphenolic compounds and its relation to wine aging. *Am J Enol Vitic.* 1974;25:119–126.

[15]Timberlake CF, Bridle P. Interactions between anthocyanins, phenolic compounds, and acetaldehyde and their significance in red wines. *Am J Enol Vitic.* 1976;27:97–105.

[16]Remy S, Fulcrand H, Labarbe B, Cheynier V, Moutounet M. First confirmation in red wine of products resulting from direct anthocyanin-tannin reactions. *J Sci Food Agric.* 2000;80:745–751.

[17]Shoji T, Goda Y, Toyoda M, Yanagida A, Kanda T. Characterization and structures of anthocyanin pigments generated in rose cider during vinification. *Phytochemistry.* 2002;59:183–189.

[18]Krueger CG, Vestling MM. Matrix-assisted laser desorption-ionization time-of-flight mass spectrometry of anthocyanin-polyflavan-3-ol oligomers in cranberry fruit (Vaccinium macrocarpon, Ait.) and spray-dried cranberry juice. *ACS Symposium Series.* 2004;886:232–246.

[19]Hagerman AE, Riedl KM, Jones GA, Sovik KN, Ritchard NT, Hartzfeld PW, Riechel TL. High molecular weight plant polyphenolics (tannins) as biological antioxidants. *J Agric Food Chem.* 1998;46:1887–1892.

[20]Packer L, Rimbach G, Virgili F. Antioxidant activity and biologic properties of a procyanidin-rich extract from pine (Pinus maritima) bark, pycnogenol. *Free Radic Biol Med.* 1999;27:704–724.

[21]Wilson T, Porcari JP, Harbin D. Cranberry extract inhibits low density lipoprotein oxidation. *Life Sci.* 1998;62:PL381–PL386.

[22]Beachey EH. Bacterial adherence: adhesion-receptor interactions mediating the attachment of bacteria to mucosal surfaces. *J Infect Dis.* 1981;143:325–345.

[23]Ronald A. The etiology of urinary tract infection: traditional and emerging pathogens. *Dm Disease-a-Month.* 2003;49:71–82.

[24]Ofek I, Beachey EH. Mannose binding and epithelial-cell adherence of Escherichia-coli. *Infect Immun.* 1978;22:247–254.

[25]Kallenius G, Mollby R, Svenson SB, Winberg J, Lundblad A, Svensson S, Cedergren B. The Pk antigen as receptor for the hemagglutinin of pyelonephritic Escherichia-coli. *FEMS Microbiol Lett.* 1980;7:297–302.

[26]Dowling KJ, Roberts JA, Kaack MB. P-fimbriated Escherichia-coli urinary-tract infection: a clinical correlation. *South Med J.* 1987;80:1533–1536.

[27]Ofek I, Hasty DL, Sharon N. Anti-adhesion therapy of bacterial diseases: prospects and problems. *FEMS Immunol Med Microbiol.* 2003;38:181–191.

[28]Howell AB, Foxman B. Cranberry juice and adhesion of antibiotic-resistant uropathogens. *JAMA.* 2002;287: 3082–3083.

[29]Gupta K, Hooton TM, Stamm WE. Increasing antimicrobial resistance and the management of uncomplicated community-acquired urinary tract infections. *Ann Intern Med.* 2001;135:41–50.

[30]Zafriri D, Ofek I, Adar R, Pocino M, Sharon N. Inhibitory activity of cranberry juice on adherence of type 1 and type P fimbriated Escherichia coli to eucaryotic cells. *Antimicrob Agents Chemother.* 1989;33: 92–98.

[31]Howell AB, Vorsa N, Marderosian AD, Foo LY. Inhibition of the adherence of P-fimbriated Escherichia coli to uro-epithelial-cell surfaces by proanthocyanidin extracts from cranberries (vol 339, pp 1085, 1998). *N Engl J Med.* 1998;339:1408.

[32]Gupta K, Chou MY, Howell A, Wobbe C, Grady R, Stapleton AE. Cranberry products inhibit adherence of p-fimbriated Escherichia coli to primary cultured bladder and vaginal epithelial cells. *J Urol.* 2007;177: 2357–2360.

[33]Howell AB, Leahy M, Kurowska E, Guthrie N. In vivo evidence that cranberry proanthocyanidins inhibit adherence of P-fimbriated E-coli bacteria to uroepithelial cells. *FASEB J.* 2001;15:A284.

[34]Howell AB, Reed JD, Krueger CG, Winterbottom R, Cunningham DG, Leahy M. A-type cranberry proanthocyanidins and uropathogenic bacterial anti-adhesion activity. *Phytochemistry.* 2005;66:2281–2291.

[35]Hagerman AE, Butler LG. Specificity of proanthocyanidin-protein interactions. *J Biol Chem.* 1981;256: 4494–4497.

[36]Jones GW, Richardson LA, Uhlman D. The invasion of hela-cells by salmonella-typhimurium: reversible and irreversible bacterial attachment and the role of bacterial motility. *J Gen Microbiol.* 1981;127: 351–360.

[37]Magnusson KE. Hydrophobic interaction: a mechanism of bacterial binding. *Scand J Infect Dis.* 1982; 32–36.

[38]Liu YT, Black MA, Caron L, Camesano TA. Role of cranberry juice on molecular-scale surface characteristics and adhesion behavior of Escherichia coli. *Biotechnol Bioeng.* 2006;93:297–305.

[39]Mole S, Waterman PG. A critical analysis of techniques for measuring tannins in ecological studies: I. techniques for chemically defining tannins. *Oecologia.* 1987;72:137–147.

[40]Avorn J, Monane M, Gurwitz JH, Glynn RJ, Choodnovskiy I, Lipsitz LA. Reduction of bacteriuria and pyuria after ingestion of cranberry juice. *JAMA.* 1994;271:751–754.

[41]Walker EB, Barney DP, Mickelsen JN, Walton RJ, Mickelsen RA Jr. Cranberry concentrate: UTI prophylaxis. *J Fam Pract.* 1997;45:167–168.

[42]Kontiokari T, Salo J, Eerola E, Uhari M. Cranberry juice and bacterial colonization in children: a placebo-controlled randomized trial. *Clin Nutr.* (Edinburgh, Lothian) 2005;24:1065–1072.

[43]Jepson RG, Craig JC. Cranberries for preventing urinary tract infections. *Cochrane Database of Systematic Reviews.* 2008;26.

[44]Stothers L. A randomized trial to evaluate effectiveness and cost effectiveness of naturopathic cranberry products as prophylaxis against urinary tract infection in women. *Can J Urol.* 2002;9:1558–1562.

[45]Howell AB. Cranberry capsule ingestion and bacterial anti-adhesion activity of urine. *FASEB J.* Late-Breaking Abstracts 2006;20:454.

[46]Greenberg JA, Newmann SJ, Howell AB. Consumption of sweetened dried cranberries versus unsweetened raisins for inhibition of uropathogenic Escherichia coli adhesion in human urine: a pilot study. *J Altern Complement Med.* 2005;11:875–878.

[47]Howell AB. Bioactive compounds in cranberries and their role in prevention of urinary tract infections. *Mol Nutr Food Res.* 2007;51:732–737.

[48]Burger O, Ofek I, Tabak M, Weiss EI, Sharon N, Neeman I. A high molecular mass constituent of cranberry juice inhibits Helicobacter pylori adhesion to human gastric mucus. *FEMS Immunol Med Microbiol.* 2000;29:295–301.

[49]Shmuely H, Burger O, Neeman I, Yahav J, Samra ZI, Niv Y, Sharon N, Weiss E, Athamna A, Tabak M, Ofek I. Susceptibility of Helicobacter pylori isolates to the antiadhesion activity of a high-molecular-weight constituent of cranberry. *Diagn Microbiol Infect Dis.* 2004;50:231–235.

[50]Shmuely H, Yahav J, Samra Z, Chodick G, Koren R, Niv Y, Ofek I. Effect of cranberry juice on eradication of Helicobacter pylori in patients treated with antibiotics and a proton pump inhibitor. *Mol Nutr Food Res.* 2007;51:746–751.

[51]Zhang L, Ma JL, Pan KF, Go VLW, Chen JS, You WC. Efficacy of cranberry juice on Helicobacter pylori infection: a double-blind, randomized placebo-controlled trial. *Helicobacter.* 2005;10:139–145.

[52]Gotteland M, Andrews M, Toledo M, Munoz L, Caceres P, Anziani A, Wittig E, Speisky H, Salazar G. Modulation of Helicobacter pylori colonization with cranberry juice and Lactobacillus johnsonii La1 in children. *Nutrition.* 2008;24:421–426.

[53]Weiss EI, Lev-Dor R, Sharon N, Ofek I. Inhibitory effect of a high-molecular-weight constituent of cranberry on adhesion of oral bacteria. *Crit Rev Food Sci Nutr.* 2002;42:285–292.

[54]Koo H, de Guzman PN, Schobel BD, Smith AVV, Bowen WH. Influence of cranberry juice on glucan-mediated processes involved in Streptococcus mutans biofilm development. *Caries Res.* 2006;40:20–27.

[55]Steinberg D, Feldman M, Ofek I, Weiss EI. Effect of a high-molecular-weight component of cranberry on constituents of dental biofilm. *J Antimicrob Chemother.* 2004;54:86–89.

[56]Steinberg D, Feldman M, Ofek I, Weiss EI. Cranberry high molecular weight constituents promote Streptococcus sobrinus desorption from artificial biofilm. *Int J Antimicrob Agents.* 2005;25:247–251.

[57]Labrecque J, Bodet C, Chandad F, Grenier D. Effects of a high-molecular-weight cranberry fraction on growth, biofilm formation and adherence of Porphyromonas gingivalis. *J Antimicrob Chemother.* 2006;58: 439–443.

[58]Bodet C, Chandad F, Grenier D. Anti-inflammatory activity of a high-molecular-weight cranberry fraction on macrophages stimulated by lipopolysaccharides from periodontopathogens. *J Dent Res.* 2006;85: 235–239.

[59]Bodet C, Piche M, Chandad F, Grenier D. Inhibition of periodontopathogen-derived proteolytic enzymes by a high-molecular-weight fraction isolated from cranberry. *J Antimicrob Chemother.* 2006;

[60]McKay DL, Blumberg JB. Cranberries (Vaccinium macrocarpon) and cardiovascular disease risk factors. *Nutr Rev.* 2007;65:490–502.

[61]Reed JD, Krueger CG, Porter ML. Cranberry juice powder decreases low density lipoprotein cholesterol in hypercholesterolemic swine. *FASEB J.* Late-Breaking Abstracts 2001;15:54.

[62]Maher MA, Mataczynski H, Stefaniak HM, Wilson T. Cranberry juice induces nitric oxide dependent vasodilation and transiently reduces blood pressure. *FASEB J.* 1999;13:A884.

[63]Wilson TEF, Weise C, Porcari J, Backes RJ, White-Kube R. Effect of cranberry juice consumption on blood flow in the arm. *FASEB J.* 2002;16:A239.

[64]Corder R, Warburton RC, Khan NQ, Brown RE, Wood EG, Lees DM. The procyanidin-induced pseudo laminar shear stress response: a new concept for the reversal of endothelial dysfunction. *Clin Sci (Lond).* 2004;107:513–517.

[65]Ndiaye M, Chataigneau M, Lobysheva I, Chataigneau T, Schini-Kerth VB. Red wine polyphenols-induced, endothelium-dependent NO-mediated relaxation is due to the redox-sensitive PI3-kinase/Akt-dependent phosphorylation of endothelial NO-synthase in the isolated porcine coronary artery. *FASEB J.* 2004;18: 455–475.

[66]Neto CC. Cranberry and its phytochemicals: a review of in vitro anticancer studies. *J Nutr.* 2007;137:186S–193S.

[67]Ferguson PJ, Kurowska E, Freeman DJ, Chambers AF, Koropatnick DJ. A flavonoid fraction from cranberry extract inhibits proliferation of human tumor cell lines. *J Nutr.* 2004;134:1529–1535.

[68]Ferguson PJ, Kurowska EM, Freeman DJ, Chambers AF, Koropatnick J. In vivo inhibition of growth of human tumor lines by flavonoid fractions from cranberry extract. *Nutr Cancer.* 2006;56:86–94.

[69]Beecher GR. Proanthocyanidins: biological activities associated with human health. *Pharm Biol.* 2004; 42:2–20.

[70]Jimenez-Ramsey LM, Rogler JC, Housley TL, Butler LG, Elkin RG. Absorption and distribution of C-14-labeled condensed tannins and related sorghum phenolics in chickens. *J Agric Food Chem.* 1994;42:963–967.

[71]Natella F, Belelli F, Gentili V, Ursini F, Scaccini C. Grape seed proanthocyanidins prevent plasma post-prandial oxidative stress in humans. *J Agric Food Chem.* 2002;50:7720–7725.

[72]Terrill TH, Waghorn GC, Woolley DJ, McNabb WC, Barry TN. Assay and digestion of 14C-labelled condensed tannins in the gastrointestinal tract of sheep. *Br J Nutr.* 1994;72:467–477.

[73]Reed JD. Nutritional toxicology of tannins and related polyphenols in forage legumes. *J Anim Sci.* 1995;73:1516–1528.

[74]Staprans I, Pan XM, Rapp JH, Feingold KR. The role of dietary oxidized cholesterol and oxidized fatty acids in the development of atherosclerosis. *Mol Nutr Food Res.* 2005;49:1075–1082.

[75]Azzali G. Structure, lymphatic vascularization and lymphocyte migration in mucosa-associated lymphoid tissue. *Immunol. Rev.* 2003;195:178–189.

[76]Nagler-Anderson C. Man the barrier! strategic defences in the intestinal mucosa. *Nat Rev Immunol.* 2001; 1:59–67.

[77]Renegar KB, Johnson CD, Dewitt RC, King BK, Li J, Fukatsu K, Kudsk KA. Impairment of mucosal immunity by total parenteral nutrition: requirement for IgA in murine nasotracheal anti-influenza immunity. *J Immunol.* (Baltimore, MD: 1950) 2001;166:819–825.

[78]Renegar KB, Kudsk KA, Dewitt RC, Wu Y, King BK. Impairment of mucosal immunity by parenteral nutrition: depressed nasotracheal influenza-specific secretory IgA levels and transport in parenterally fed mice. *Ann Surg.* 2001;233:134–138.

[79]Harmond MF, Blanquet P. The fate of total flavanolic oligomers (OFT) extracted from "vitis vinifera" in the rat. *Eur J Drug Metab Pharmacokinet.* 1978;1:15–30.

[80]Santos-Buelga C, Scalbert A. Proanthocyanidins and tannin-like compounds: nature, occurrence, dietary intake and effects on nutrition and health. *J Sci Food Agric.* 2000;80:1094–1117.

[81]Scalbert A, Deprez S, Mila I, Albrecht AM, Huneau JF, Rabot S. Proanthocyanidins and human health: systemic effects and local effects in the gut. *Biofactors.* 2000;13:115–120.

[82]Donovan JL, Manach C, Rios L, Morand C, Scalbert A, Remesy C. Procyanidins are not bioavailable in rats fed a single meal containing a grapeseed extract or the procyanidin dimer B-3. *Br J Nutr.* 2002;87: 299–306.

[83]Laparra J, Michaud J, and Masquelier J. Etude pharmacocinetiques des oligomeres flavanoliques. *Plant Med Phytother.* 1977;11:133–142.

[84]Tsang C, Auger C, Mullen W, Bornet A, Rouanet JM, Crozier A, Teissedre PL. The absorption, metabolism and excretion of flavan-3-ols and procyanidins following the ingestion of a grape seed extract by rats. *Br J Nutr.* 2005;94:170–181.

[85]Deprez S, Brezillon C, Rabot S, Philippe C, Mila I, Lapierre C, Scalbert A. Polymeric proanthocyanidins are catabolized by human colonic microflora into low-molecular-weight phenolic acids. *J Nutr.* 2000;130: 2733–2738.

Botanical Medicine: From Bench to Bedside
Edited by R. Cooper and F. Kronenberg
© Mary Ann Liebert, Inc.

Chapter 11

Cranberry Products Prevent Urinary Tract Infections in Women: Clinical Evidence

Michael Tempesta and Marilyn Barrett

Cranberries have a history of use for their benefits in preventing urinary tract infections (UTIs). The cranberry is a traditional food, with reports of use dating to the indigenous Americans. American cranberry is a dark red fruit that grows on an evergreen shrub, *Vaccinium macrocarpon* Aiton [Ericaceae], native to bogs, swamps, and wetlands in eastern North America, from Newfoundland in the north to North Carolina in the south and west to central Minnesota (1).

Currently cranberries are sold in a range of food products including fresh fruit, dried sweetened fruit, frozen fruit, juice, juice concentrate, juice powder or concentrate powder, and fruit extracts. Cranberry products are also sold as dietary supplements in forms ranging from dried, ground berries to juice concentrate powders (dehydrated juice) and standardized extracts.

The active constituents in cranberry that are responsible for preventing UTIs are thought to be phenolic compounds known as proanthocyanidins (PACs).

Clinical studies conducted on women with recurrent UTIs have been positive, while the results of those conducted on other populations have been less certain. Although cranberries contain large amounts of organic acids, it is generally agreed that the PACs are responsible for the biological activity, as discussed in Chapter 10.

In this chapter, we present details of an open-label clinical study conducted on women with recurrent UTIs given a cranberry extract standardized to 30% total phenolics. Herein, we also review other clinical studies on cranberry against UTIs using a variety of cranberry products and dosing regimens. Although the results are encouraging, further research will be required to establish the optimal chemical profile and optimal dose of cranberry products in the prevention of UTIs.

[1] Phenolics LLC, El Granada, California 94018-2439; natprod@aol.com
[2] Pharmacognosy Consulting, Mill Valley, California 94941; marilyn@pharmacognosy.com

CHEMISTRY

As discussed in Chapter 10, cranberries contain a number of different chemical constituents, including anthocyanins, PACs, flavonols, organic acids, phenolic acids, volatile oil, and sugars. The most common constituents are sugars and organic acids, which constitute over 90% of all organic compounds in the juice. However, the compounds that are most important therapeutically are thought to be the PACs. These are reported to be present at 418.8 mg/100g whole berries fresh weight and 85.5 mg/L (54.7 mg/8 oz serving) in cranberry juice cocktail (2). PACs are condensed tannins that contain linked flavanol units, mostly epicatechin with smaller amounts of epigallocatechin. The links between flavanol units are either double (both carbon-oxygen-carbon and carbon-carbon; A-type linkage) or single (carbon-carbon; B-type linkage) (see Figure 10.1 in previous chapter). PACs with B-type linkage are found in numerous fruits and berries as well as chocolate (2, 3). PACs with A-type linkage are present in cranberries, blueberries, plums, peanuts, curry, and cinnamon (4) and generally are less common in nature than the B-type PACs (1).

PACs are compounds that belong to a more general chemical class of compounds called polyphenolics or phenolics. One method of characterizing cranberry products is to measure the content of total phenolics. This can be accomplished using UV/VIS spectrometry (Folin-Ciocalteu method). The disadvantage of this method is that it is not specific for PACs, and so unless the sample is purified previous to testing, the results cannot be directly linked to PACs. More specific methods that can separate and quantify the PACs include high-performance liquid chromatography (HPLC), gel-permation chromatography (GPC), and capillary electrophoresis (CE) (4, 5). These methods work well for the more homogeneous B-linked PACs but do not give very accurate levels for the A-type PACs.

MECHANISM OF ACTION

In vitro mode of action studies indicate that cranberry products prevent UTIs by preventing adhesion of pathogenic bacteria to the cells of the bladder and urethra. As the first step in developing infections, bacteria must bind to the host cell and tissues. The *E. coli* strains that cause UTIs have proteinaceous macromolecules (fimbriae) that facilitate the adhesion of bacteria to uroepithelial cells in the urinary tract. Cranberry PACs have been shown to inhibit adhesion of *E. coli* with P-type fimbriae (6). More recent studies have determined that cranberry PACs with A-type linkage are more effective than those with B-type linkage in inhibiting the adhesion of bacteria to cell surfaces (7). Other compounds in cranberry identified in the antiadhesion activity–containing fractions are 1-O-methylgalactose, prunin, and phlorizin (8). The antiadhesion activity is not influenced by the acidity of cranberry juice (neutralization of cranberry juice to pH 7 did not affect the antiadhesion activity) (9). Biochemical studies have demonstrated that cranberry PACs cause the fimbriae on the surface of the bacteria to become compressed, reducing their ability to adhere to cells in the body. Further studies reveal that these compounds may change the shape of the bacteria from rods to spheres and cause chemical changes to bacterial surface membranes (10). Further details of these specific mechanisms are presented by Reed and Howell in Chapter 10.

COMMERCIAL PRODUCTS

There are multiple forms of cranberry available, including juice, cocktail juice, cranberry powders derived from ground berries, cranberry powders derived from dried juice, and extracts. Each of these cranberry products contains significantly different amounts of total phenolics and PACs.

Approximately 1500 g of fresh fruit produces one liter of juice. Thus cranberry juice would be expected to contain approximately 75 mg of PACs per 100 ml. The most commonly available commercial cranberry product may be cranberry juice cocktail, which ranges from 28% to 33% pure juice (11). Cranberry juice cocktail has been reported to contain from 54.7 to 90 mg PACs per 8 oz serving (2, 12).

Dried, ground berries, which are commonly available as cranberry powders, contain 0.2% to 0.5% total phenolic compounds, mostly PACs. The native ratio of PACs to anthocyanins in cranberries or cranberry juices is approximately 10:1. Dried juice concentrates commonly contain 3% to 5% total phenolics, which are mainly PACs (13).

A more concentrated standardized extract containing 30% phenolics has recently become available commercially. It is a unique preparation in that the organic acids and sugars have been removed during the extraction process. The extract, which is trademarked as CranEx, is available in the United States and Europe by Phenolics, LLC. CranEx is an ingredient in numerous commercial preparations, including Cranbiotic@ by Futurebiotics and GNC's Herbal Plus Standardized Cranberry Herbal Supplement.

A CLINICAL STUDY USING A STANDARDIZED CRANBERRY EXTRACT

An open-label pilot study of four months' duration was conducted at Helios Health Center in Boulder, Colorado, using CranEx (14). Included in the study, described by Bailey and colleagues, were 12 women with ages ranging from 25 to 70 years old. The women all had a history of a minimum of six UTIs in the preceding year, and several had had this number of infections or more per year for the past several years. Women who were pregnant, were currently using antibiotics, or had a major illness or diseases other than UTIs were excluded.

Several of the women had been trying cranberry juice on a regular basis or were taking cranberry capsule products from the health food store with varying results. During this study, they did not take any other berry products. All the women were screened prior to administration of the test product and were found to be free of any UTIs. The test product was manufactured using a patented extraction process that results in a cranberry preparation standardized to contain 30% total phenols and a minimum of 25% PACs (15, 16, 17). During the trial, each woman took one capsule containing 200 mg cranberry extract twice daily for 12 weeks. The daily cranberry PAC intake during the study was approximately 100 mg.

A questionnaire was used initially to determine patients' medical histories, and the patients were asked at monthly intervals if any of the information had changed. All of the women in the study had urinalysis within 24 hours before starting on the study preparation and once a month after that for four months. The urinalysis included a dipstick and microscopy exam on a clean voided midstream first morning urine sample. The dipstick test examined the specimen for red blood cells, nitrates, lymphocytes, protein, and glucose as well as measured specific gravity. The microscopic exam looked for red blood cells and white blood cells as well as bacteria and casts. Any samples with positive results were to be cultured and sensitivity toward antibiotics determined. A follow-up of these same patients was conducted approximately two years after the study, and the same questionnaire that had been used initially was reviewed with each patient and any changes noted.

All patients were followed for a period of 12 weeks. The study began in May 2004 and concluded in September 2004. There were no dropouts or withdrawals from the study. None of the women developed a UTI during the study, on the basis of symptoms or laboratory results. Based on the past history of this patient group, 24 to 48 UTI occurrences would have been expected over the course of the study. No patients reported any adverse effects due to the supplement.

A follow-up on the subjects continued for two years after the study. Eight of the subjects did not have any changes in their health since the study began. They did not have access to the specific cranberry product used in the study but took various other cranberry products on the market, that had lower PAC content. The doses of these products ranged from 150 to 300 mg (cranberry powders) per day. If the patients missed taking the cranberry supplements for one to three days, they did not notice any symptoms. Several commented that they took extra capsules for one to two days following more sexual activity than usual, and if they did not do this they could have some UTI symptoms. However, these symptoms did not ever develop into a true UTI and resolved with extra cranberry capsules and an increase in water intake.

Four patients stopped taking cranberry supplements for various unrelated medical reasons. One patient remained free of UTIs, and three developed symptoms that resolved upon resumption of cranberry. Two patients developed UTIs, confirmed by urinalysis, and were treated with antibiotics. They resumed treatment with cranberry and did not have any further symptoms.

In summary, this study indicates that women with a history of recurrent UTIs can prevent those infections with daily use of a cranberry extract high in PACs. Those women who continued to take cranberry supplements even with lower amounts of total phenolics continued to be free from infections two years later.

A REVIEW OF OTHER CLINICAL STUDIES

Other clinical studies also indicate that cranberry may be effective in preventing UTIs in women subject to recurrent infections. A Cochrane review of randomized controlled studies published before January 2007 found ten studies on the use of cranberry products for the prevention of UTIs (18). A meta-analysis performed on four of those studies found that cranberry products significantly reduced the incidence of UTIs after 12 months compared with placebo/control (relative risks [RR] 0.65, 95% confidence interval [CI] 0.46–0.90). Among the ten studies, the evidence was stronger for cranberry products being effective at reducing the incidence of UTIs in women with recurrent UTIs than for elderly men and elderly women or people requiring catheterization (although no direct comparison was made). The authors reported that the optimum dosage and method of administration (e.g., juice, tablets, and capsules) have not been determined. This conclusion most likely resulted from the variation in the preparation, dose, and degree of chemical characterization of the cranberry products tested in the studies.

Besides the Bailey study (14), mentioned in detail above, three other clinical studies were designed to investigate the use of cranberry products for women with a history of recurrent

UTIs. The first was a small crossover study that used a concentrated cranberry preparation. The next two were larger, parallel-group studies that used juice or concentrated juice. All of these studies reported positive results.

The small crossover trial, described by Walker and colleagues (19), studied ten sexually active women who had a history of UTIs (four UTIs during the previous year or at least one UTI within the previous three months). The subjects were given either 400 mg cranberry extract or placebo daily for three months before switching treatments. As a result, cranberry concentrate was found to be more effective than placebo in reducing the occurrence of UTI (p<0.005). Nineteen women entered the study, while ten completed the study and were included in the analysis. While taking cranberry, seven of the ten subjects exhibited fewer UTIs, two subjects exhibited the same number, and one subject experienced one more UTI. From the total of 21 incidents of UTIs recorded among the participants during the six months, 6 UTIs occurred during the time they were taking cranberry (2.6 per subject year). In contrast, a total of 15 UTIs occurred while on placebo (6.0 per subject year).

A parallel-group, placebo-controlled study, authored by Kontiokari and coworkers (20), used a cranberry-lingonberry juice concentrate, described as 7.5 g cranberry concentrate and 1.7 g lingonberry concentrate in 50 ml water. The preparation was compared to a drink containing *lactobacillus* and no treatment. The study included 150 women (mean age approximately 30 years) from the student health services who currently had a UTI (105 cfu *E. coli* per ml). The subjects were given cranberry juice for 6 months or *lactobacillus* for 12 months. The outcome measure was the first recurrence of symptomatic UTI. After 6 months, 16% (8 women) in the cranberry group, 39% (19 women) in the *lactobacillus* group, and 36% (18 women) in the control group presented with at least one infection. Thus cranberry reduced the risk of infection by 20% (95% CI, P=0.023).

Another parallel-group, placebo-controlled study, described by Stothers and colleagues (21), included 150 sexually active women aged 21 through 72 years. They had presented with at least two symptomatic, single-organism, culture-positive UTIs in the previous year but at the time of study were free of infection. The subjects were given cranberry juice (250 ml three times daily), cranberry tablets (1:30 juice concentrate twice daily), or placebo using a double dummy method. In the year of treatment, 32% (16 women) of the placebo group, 20% (10 women) in the juice group, and 18% (9 women) in the tablet group had presented with at least one infection. The mean number of UTIs was 0.72 in the placebo group, 0.30 in the juice group, and 0.39 in the tablet group.

Three clinical studies have explored the effect of cranberry on elderly women and men (mean age approximately 80 years) (22, 23, 24). The largest study was a randomized, placebo-controlled study in which 376 men and women in the hospital consumed either 300 mg per day cranberry juice or placebo drink (22). A total of 21 out of 376 developed a UTI: 7 in the cranberry group and 14 in the placebo group. The differences between groups were not significant, and the study was determined to be underpowered. In another study, 153 elderly women were randomly assigned to consume 300 mg per day cranberry juice or placebo drink (23). The chance that the women drinking cranberry juice would have bacteriuria (≥ 10(5)/mL) in their urine with pyuria was 42% of that for the control group. The chance of remaining in that state in the following month was 27% of that of the control group. In a small crossover study that initially included 38 hospitalized men and women, the participants were given 30 mL cranberry juice or water (24). Only 17 completed treatment, and only 7 were included in the final analysis. Of these remaining 7, those who took cranberry had fewer occurrences of UTI, but the results were only marginally significant.

Two clinical studies were conducted with children with neuropathic bladder requiring intermittent catheterization (25, 26). Daily treatment was either 15 ml cranberry cocktail per kg or 300 ml cranberry juice cocktail. Neither study demonstrated clinical or statistical differences in the number of symptomatic UTIs.

Three clinical studies were conducted on adults with spinal cord injuries and resultant neurogenic bladder (27, 28, 29). A pilot study with 15 subjects reported that a glass of cranberry juice three times daily caused a reduction in bacterial biofilm (27). The two other studies reported no benefit in urinary bacteriuria or UTI. In one study, the participants ingested 2 g concentrated juice for six months (28), and in another study the participants were given 400 mg standardized tablets three times daily for four weeks (29).

The above clinical studies indicate that multiple cranberry products have a range of effectiveness in preventing recurrent UTIs in women. Three of the studies (19, 20, 21) reported a reduction in the incidents of UTIs compared to placebo but not a complete inhibition. In contrast, the study by Bailey and coworkers (14) reported a complete prevention of UTIs during the study. There are several variables that could account for this difference. One variable is the amount of active ingredients, A-type PACs, in the products tested.

The crossover study (19) used a dose of 400 mg daily of a cranberry concentrate (CranActin@) for three months. We estimate that this product may have delivered from 4 to 20 mg of total phenols per day; 15 mg PACs per day. In this study, 6 UTIs occurred while taking cranberry and 15 occurred while taking placebo. This is a 60% reduction compared to placebo. This amount is approximately one-sixth the 100 mg of PACs provided in the preparation used in the Bailey study.

The second study (20) used a cranberry-lingonberry juice concentrate, described as 7.5 g cranberry concentrate and 1.7 g lingonberrry concentrate in 50 ml water taken for six months. We estimate that the cranberry concentrate delivered approximately 250 mg total phenols (35 to 40 mg PACs) per day. In this study, 8 UTIs occurred in the cranberry group, while 18 occurred in the group taking placebo. This is a 55% reduction in symptomatic infections compared to placebo. If our estimates are correct, this product delivered a little over one-third the 100 mg of PACs provided in the preparation used in the Bailey study.

The third study (21) compared 250 ml juice three times daily to cranberry tablets (1:30 juice concentrate) twice daily taken over a year. The two treatments were equally beneficial, reducing the incidence of infection by about 40% compared to placebo. Using data obtained for cranberry juice cocktail, the juice in this study may have delivered 64 to 105 mg PACs.

The Bailey study (14) conducted with a 30% total phenols extract that delivered 100 mg PACs per day for three months reported no incidents of UTIs, whereas 24 to 48 incidents were expected. Although this study lacked a placebo control group, it appears that this preparation was more potent than the other products tested.

In vitro studies indicate that inhibition of adhesion of *E. coli* by PACs to cultured bladder and vaginal epithelial cells occurs in a linear, dose-dependent manner (30). However, comparisons of the estimated amounts of PACs with the results of the three placebo-controlled studies do not indicate a clear dose-response. For example, the amount of daily PACs in the Stothers study (21) may have been close to that used on the Bailey study (14), but the effects on UTI prevention were much weaker, suggesting other factors may play a significant role.

One possible factor is the bioavailability of the PACs in the various preparations may not be similar. Direct comparisons of the bioavailability of various formulations of cranberry have not been undertaken, with the exception of the comparison of juice to tablets in the Stothers study. Another possibility is that there may be other constituents in cranberry that influence the activity of the preparation and/or the PACs. A study published in 1989 reported that cranberry juice contained two inhibitors of the adhesion of uropathogenic *E. coli* (31). One inhibitor was dialyzable and identified as fructose. The other inhibitor was nondialyzable and later identified as A-type PACs. It is possible that the presence of high levels of fructose in cranberry preparations may adversely influence the activity of the preparations. This might explain the potency of the CranEx preparation. Another possibility is that other phenolic compounds in cranberry also have activity. Studies on the virulence of *Streptococcus mutans* indicate that flavonols in cranberry inhibit glucan synthesis on the surface of this bacterium (32). This group proposed that the activity of cranberry against the oral bacterium *S. mutans* may be a combined effect from flavonols and PACs. There have also been reports that cranberry PACs have anti-inflammatory activity (10), which may also play a role in modulation of UTI symptoms.

BIOAVAILABILITY

Bioavailability studies indicate that cranberry PACs are absorbed into the body. A human study found 5% of consumed anthocyanins secreted in the urine over 24 hours following consumption of 200 ml of cranberry juice, with no data on the PACs provided (33). Another human study reported that the urine of those who ingested 250 or 750 ml cranberry juice demonstrated antiadhesion properties when tested ex vivo (34). Urine was taken from volunteers who ingested one or two doses of cranberry juice or placebo. Strains of uropathogenic *E. coli* were incubated in the urine and then tested for adhesion to bladder cells in an in vitro assay. The urine from those who drank cranberry juice prevented the bacteria from adhering in a dose-related manner. A third study reported that eight-week consumption of 1200 mg of dried cranberry juice per day (but not 400 mg per day) by healthy young women produced urine samples that had an inhibitory effect on the adhesion of uropathogenic *E. coli* strains (35). Further commentary on bioavailability is given in Chapter 10.

SAFETY

Cranberry is a food product that has been used for centuries and thereby considered safe for consumption. It is now known that some foods, while safely consumed, can alter the metabolism of certain drugs and thus alter their effectiveness. An example is the effect of grapefruit juice on statin drugs taken to lower cholesterol. However, the studies summarized below do not indicate that such a concern is warranted with cranberry juice.

In this context, several case reports indicated that there might be an interaction between cranberry juice and the anticoagulant warfarin (36). This is a concern because a tight control of warfarin blood levels is necessary to achieve therapeutic benefit and to avoid bleeding complications. The United Kingdom's Committee on the Safety of Medicines has alerted physicians of this possible interaction, publishing 12 possible case reports in a news bulletin in June 2005. However, a randomized, placebo-controlled, double-blind crossover study that explored the possible effect of cranberry on prothrombin time as measured using the International Normalized Ratio (INR) found no such effect (37). The study included seven subjects with atrial fibrillation and stabilized on warfarin who consumed either

250 ml juice or placebo for seven days. After a seven-day washout, the treatment was switched. There was no significant change to INRs. The authors concluded that daily cranberry juice in an amount of 250 ml did not interact with warfarin. A pharmacokinetic study with ten volunteers who took 200 ml cranberry juice three times a day for five days before and five days after ingesting 10 mg racemic warfarin also found that the juice did not alter the anticoagulant effect of warfarin (38).

It has been proposed that the flavonoids in cranberry might influence the activity of P450 enzymes and thus affect the blood levels of certain drugs (36). However, two clinical studies do not indicate this to be the case. A single-dose pharmacokinetic study with 12 healthy volunteers failed to show any interaction between 240 ml cranberry juice and a single dose of 200 mg cyclosporine (a CYP3A and P-glycoprotein substrate) (39). Also, a crossover study did not show any interaction with flurbiprofen (an index of CYP2C9 activity) with 8 oz of cranberry juice (40). A pharmacokinetic study that explored the effects of 200 ml cranberry juice three times a day on probes of CYP2C9, CYP1A2, and CYP3A4 (racemic warfarin, tizanidine, and midazolam, respectively) reported no effect on the activities of these enzymes (38).

CONCLUSION

Further studies are required to establish optimal daily dosing of the cranberry-derived total phenols/PACs for efficient prevention of recurrent UTIs. In vitro and ex vivo studies indicate that these compounds prevent adhesion of *E. coli* to the epithelium of the urinary tract and thus prevent infection. Although in vitro studies indicate a clear dose-response effect with PACs, the clinical picture may be more complicated. There may be interference by high- and low-molecular-weight sugars naturally present in cranberry, reducing the effect of the PACs in prevention of UTIs via this mechanism. Other phenolics, including the anthocyanins, may also play a role in the clinical benefits observed. CranEx@ is a novel extract that is standardized to 30% total phenols, with the majority of sugars and organic acids removed. CranEx@ appears in this pilot study to be much more effective in preventing UTIs than other cranberry products tested clinically. It is clear that all future evaluations using cranberry clinical materials should require a carefully standardized and well-characterized product, to better understand optimal characterization and dosing for the prevention of UTIs.

It is entirely possible that other non-cranberry-based extracts containing concentrates of A-type PACs from blueberry, cinnamon, peanut, plum, avocado, and other food sources may become as useful in prevention of UTIs as concentrated cranberry extracts.

REFERENCES

[1]Upton R, ed. Cranberry fruit, Vaccinium macrocarpon Aiton: standards of analysis, quality control and therapeutics. In: *American Herbal Pharmacopoeia™ and Therapeutic Compendium*. Santa Cruz, CA: American Herbal Pharmacopoeia, booklet.

[2]Gu L, Kelm MA, Hammerstone JF, Beecher G, Holden J, Haytowitz D, Gebhardt S, Prior RL. Concentrations of proanthocyanidins in common foods and estimations of normal consumption. *J Nutr*. 2004;134(3): 613–618.

[3]Gu L, Kelm MA, Hammerstone JF, Beecher G, Holden J, Haytowitz D, Prior RL. Screening of foods containing proanthocyanidins and their structural characterization using LC-MS/MS and thiolytic degradation. *J Agric Food Chem*. 2003;51:7513–7521.

[4]Gu L, Kelm MA, Hammerstone JF, Beecher G, Cunningham D, Vannozzi S, Prior RL. Fractionation of polymeric proanthocyanidins from lowbush blueberry and quantification of procyanidins in selected foods with an optimized normal-phase HPLC-MS fluorescent detection method. *J Agric Food Chem.* 2002;50: 4852–4860.

[5]Prior RL, Lazarus SA, Cao G, Muccitelli H, Hammerstone JF. Identification of procyanidins and anthocyanins in blueberries and cranberries (Vaccinium spp.) using high-performance liquid chromatography/mass spectrometry. *J Agric Food Chem.* 2001;49(3):1270–1276.

[6]Howell AB, Vorsa N, Der Marderosian A, Foo LY. Inhibition of the adherence of P-fimbriated Eschericheria coli to uroepithelial-cell surfaces by proanthocyanidin extracts from cranberries. *N Engl J Med.* 1998;339(15): 1085–1086.

[7]Howell AB, Reed JD, Krueger CG, Winterbottom R, Cunningham DG, Leahy M. A-type cranberry proanthocyanidins and uropathogenic bacterial anti-adhesion activity. *Phytochemistry.* 2005;66(18):2281–2291.

[8]Turner A, Chen SN, Joike MK, Pendland SL, Pauli GF, Farnsworth NR. Inhibition of uropathogenic Escherichia coli by cranberry juice: a new antiadherence assay. *J Agric Food Chem.* 2005;53(23):8940–8947.

[9]Liu Y, Black MA, Caron L, Camesano TA. Role of cranberry juice on molecular-scale surface characteristics and adhesion behavior of Escherichia coli. *Biotechnol Bioeng.* 2006;93(2):297–305.

[10]Liu Y, Gallardo-Moreno AM, Pinzon-Arango PA, Reynolds Y, Rodriguez G, Camerano TA. Cranberry changes the physicochemical surface properties of E. coli and adhesion with uroepithelial cells. *Colloids Surf B Biointerfaces.* 2008;65(1):35–42.

[11]Leung AY, Foster S. *Encyclopedia of Common Natural Ingredients Used in Food, Drugs and Cosmetics.* 2nd ed. New York, NY: John Wiley and Sons; 1996.

[12]McKay DL, Blumberg JB. Cranberries (Vaccinium macrocarpon) and cardiovascular disease risk factors. *Nutr Rev.* 2007:65(11):490–502.

[13]Dietz R, Eurofins Scientific data, private communication, 2006.

[14]Bailey DT, Dalton C, Daugherty FJ, Tempesta MS. Can a concentrated cranberry extract prevent urinary tract infections in women? a pilot study. *Phytomedicine.* 2007;14:237–241.

[15]Bailey DT, Freeberg DR, Gertenbach DG, Gourdin GT, Richheimer SL, Daugherty FJ, Tempesta MS. *Efficient Method for Producing Compositions Enriched in Anthocyanins.* U.S. Patent no. 6,780,442, August 24, 2004.

[16]Gourdin GT, Richheimer SL, Tempesta MS, Bailey DT, Nichols RL, Daugherty FJ, Freeberg DR. *Efficient Method for Producing Compositions Enriched in Total Phenols.* U.S. Patent no. 6,960,360, November 1, 2005.

[17]Gourdin GT, Richheimer SL, Tempesta MS, Bailey DT, Nichols RL, Daugherty FJ, Freeberg DR. *Compositions Enriched in Total Phenols and Methods for Producing Same.* U.S. Patent no. 7,306,815, December 11, 2007.

[18]Jepson RG, Craig JC. Cranberries for preventing urinary tract infections. *Cochrane Database Syst Rev.* 2008;(1):CD001321.

[19]Walker EB, Barney DP, Mickelsen JN, Walton RJ, Mickelsen RA. Cranberry concentrate: UTI prophylaxis. *J Fam Pract.* 1997;45(2):167–168.

[20]Kontiokari T, Sundqvist K, Nuutinen M, Pokka T, Koskela M, Uhari M. Randomized trial of cranberrylingonberry juice and lactobacillus GG drink for the prevention of urinary tract infections in women. *BMJ.* 2001;322(7302):1571–1573.

[21]Stothers L. A randomized trial to evaluate effectiveness and cost effectiveness of naturopathic cranberry products as prophylaxis against urinary tract infection in women. *Can J Urol.* 2002;9(3):1558–1562.

[22]McMurdo ME, Bissett LY, Price RJ, Phillips G, Crombie IK. Does ingestion of cranberry juice reduce symptomatic urinary tract infections in older people in hospital? A double-blind, placebo-controlled trial. *Age Ageing.* 2005;34(3):256–261.

[23]Avorn J, Monane M, Gurwitz JH, Glynn RJ, Choodnovskiy, Lipsitz LA. Reduction of bacteriuria and pyuria after ingestion of cranberry juice. *JAMA.* 1994:271(10):751–774.

[24]Haverkorn MJ, Mandigers J. Reduction of bacteriuria and pyuria using cranberry juice. *JAMA.* 1994;272(8):590.

[25]Foda MM, Middlebrook PF, Garfield CT, Porvin G, Wells G, Schillinger JF. Efficacy of cranberry in prevention of urinary tract infection in a susceptible pediatric population. *Can J Urol.* 1995;2(1):98–102.

[26]Schlager TA, Anderson S, Trudell J, Hendley JO. Effect of cranberry juice on bacteriuria in children with neurogenic bladder receiving intermittent catheterization. *J Pediatr.* 1999;135(6):698–702.

[27]Reid G, Hsiehl J, Potter P, Mighton J, Lam D, Warren D, Stephenson J. Cranberry juice consumption may reduce biofilms on uroepithelial cells: pilot study in spinal cord injured patients. *Spinal Cord.* 2001;39(1): 26–30.

[28]Waites KB, Canupp KC, Armstrong S, DeVivo MJ. Effect of cranberry extract on bacteriuria and pyuria in persons with neurogenic bladder secondary to spinal cord injury. *J Spinal Cord Med.* 2004;27(1): 35–40.

[29]Linsenmeyer TA, Harrison B, Oakley A, Kirshblum S, Stock JA, Millis SR. Evaluation of cranberry supplement for reduction of urinary tract infections in individuals with neurogenic bladders secondary to spinal cord injury. A prospective, double-blinded, placebo-controlled, crossover study. *J Spinal Cord Med.* 2004;27(1):29–34.

[30]Gupta K, Chou MY, Howell A, Wobbe C, Grady R, Stapleton AE. Cranberry products inhibit adherence of p-fimbriated Escherichia coli to primary cultured bladder and vaginal epithelial cells. *J Urol.* 2007;177(6): 2357–2360.

[31]Zafriri D, Ofek I, Adar R, Pocino M, Sharon N. Inhibitory activity of cranberry juice on adherence of type 1 and type P-fimbriated *Escherichia coli* to eukaryotic cells. *Antimicrob Agents Chemother.* 1989;33(1): 92–98.

[32]Gregoire S, Singh AP, Vorsa N, Koo H. Influence of cranberry phenolics on glucan synthesis by glucosyltransferases and Streptococcus metans acidogenicity. *J Appl Microbiol.* 2007;103(5):1960–1968.

[33]Ohnishi R, Ito H, Kasajima N, Kaneda M, Kariyama R, Kumon H, Hatano T, Yoshida T. Urinary excretion of anthocyanins in humans after cranberry juice ingestion. *Biosci Biotechnol Biochem.* 2006;70(7): 1681–1687.

[34]Di Martino P, Agniel R, David K, Templer C, Gaillard JL, Denys P, Botto H. Reduction of Escherichia coli adherence to uroepithelial bladder cells after consumption of cranberry juice: a double-blind randomized placebo-controlled cross-over trial. *World J Urol.* 2006;24(1):21–27.

[35]Valentova K, Stejskal D, Bednar P, Vostalova J, Cihalik C, Vecerova R, Koukalova D, Kolar M, Reichenbach R, Sknouril L, Ulrichova J, Simanek V. Biosafety, antioxidant status and metabolites in urine after consumption of dried cranberry juice in healthy women: a pilot double-blind placebo-controlled trial. *J Agric Food Chem.* 2007;55(8):3217–3224.

[36]Aston JL, Lodolce AE, Shapiro NL. Interaction between warfarin and cranberry juice. *Pharmacotherapy.* 2006 Sep;26(9):1314–1319.

[37]Li Z, Seeram NP, Carpenter CL, Thames G, Minutti C, Bowerman S. Cranberry does not affect prothrombin time in male subjects on warfarin. *J Am Diet Assoc.* 2006;106(12):2057–2061.

[38]Lilja JJ, Backman JT, Neuvonen PJ. Effects of daily ingestion of cranberry juice on the pharmacokinetics of warfarin, tizanidine and midazolam-probes of CYP2C9, CYP1A2, CYP3A4. *Clin Pharmacol Ther.* 2007;81(6):833–839.

[39]Grenier J, Fradette C, Morelli G, Merritt GJ, Vranderick M, Ducharme MP. Pomelo juice, but not cranberry juice, affects the pharmacokinetics of cyclosporine in humans. *Clin Pharmacol Ther.* 2006;79(3): 255–262. Epub 2006 Feb 7.

[40]Greenblatt DJ, von Moltke LL, Perloff ES, Luo Y, Harmatz JS, Zinny MA. Interaction of flurbiprofen with cranberry juice, grape juice, tea, and fluconazole: in vitro and clinical studies. *Clin Pharmacol Ther.* 2006;79(1):125–133.

PART III

Botanical Preparations: A Practitioner's View

Botanical Medicine: From Bench to Bedside
Edited by R. Cooper and F. Kronenberg
© Mary Ann Liebert, Inc.

Chapter 12

Chaste Tree Extract in Women's Health: A Critical Review

Tieraona Low Dog

The history of botanical medicine is universal, having been used by all cultures and all peoples across the span of time. Fossil records date the human use of medicinal plants to at least the Middle Paleolithic Age some 60,000 years ago, demonstrating the resourceful nature of our ancestors, who used their ingenuity to discover and effectively use plant medicines. Over the centuries, botanical medicine gave birth to the modern sciences of botany, pharmacy, perfumery, and chemistry. With all of the advancements in modern medicine and science, it would be easy to dismiss herbal medicine as quaint: a discipline spoken of only in the past tense. However, in many parts of the world, including modern China, India, and many countries in South America and Africa, it remains a primary source of medicine. And in the West, botanical medicine is a growing part of a movement known as "complementary and alternative medicine (CAM)," which loosely translates as a collection of practices and approaches that fall principally outside those taught in conventional medical training centers.

Women are the largest consumers of health care, and this extends to their utilization of CAM. The 2002 National Health Interview Survey, which included more than 17,000 women, found that women utilized CAM more than men; 69% reported using CAM within the previous 12 months. Higher levels of CAM use were associated with increased education, higher income, and a lower health status. In general, women between 50 and 59 years of age composed the subgroup with the highest rates of use (1). Researchers have attempted to uncover the reasons why women turn to CAM in general and to botanical medicine in particular. A recent study in the United Kingdom found that the desire to have personal control over their health was the strongest motive for women to use herbal medicine. Secondarily was their dissatisfaction with conventional treatment and its disregard for a holistic approach, as well as concerns about the side effects of medications (2).

As a health practitioner for more than 25 years, this author has gained significant knowledge in the use of botanical medicines in women's health. There are significant challenges facing the clinician when attempting to recommend botanical medicines, particularly when it comes to the research and the marketplace. This chapter is not intended to be an

Arizona Center for Integrative Medicine, University of Arizona Health Sciences Center, Tucson, Arizona 85701; tlowdog@ahsc.arizona.edu

exhaustive summary of herbal medicine in women's health; there are entire books written on the subject. Instead, this chapter is intended to be a discussion of opportunities and challenges facing clinicians.

I have chosen to focus on only one herb, chaste tree berry (*Vitex agnus castus*), of which I am intimately familiar, having used it extensively in practice for almost three decades. This herb is popular for addressing the symptoms of premenstrual syndrome (PMS) and can also be found in a variety of products addressing infertility and the irregular menses that often occurs around menopause.

By examining the science behind this plant, this chapter is intended to illustrate more broadly the shortcomings of research and the marketplace while highlighting the challenges facing medical practitioners who wish to help guide and educate the patient on its proper use.

THE MENSTRUAL YEARS

There are several conditions that can be problematic for women during their menstrual years. PMS is estimated to affect up to 90% of menstruating women, with the most severe cases occurring in 2% to 5% of women between the ages of 26 and 35 years (3). It is characterized by the presence of physical and behavioral symptoms that occur repetitively in the latter half of the menstrual cycle. For milder forms of PMS, the primary conventional interventions consist of dietary changes (i.e., reducing caffeine and salt consumption), exercise, nonsteroidal anti-inflammatory medications, and possibly oral contraceptives. A growing number of the female population is also experiencing problems with infertility, which is defined as the inability to become pregnant after 12 months of regular unprotected intercourse. Ovulatory disorders are the primary cause for female infertility, and while fertility treatments are more widely available, they are expensive and not without adverse effects. As there is a rather limited range of treatment options for these conditions, it should come as little surprise that many women are curious about exploring other approaches.

CHASTE TREE BERRY (*VITEX AGNUS CASTUS*)

Perhaps the most popular of the herbal remedies for PMS and anovulatory disorders is chaste tree berry (*Vitex agnus castus*). The Latin name *agnus castus* means "chaste lamb," in reference to the early belief that the fruit reduced sexual desire, which is also the basis for its other common name, monk's pepper.

An important source reference for herbal remedies is the German Commission E, a panel of experts charged with evaluating the safety and effectiveness of herbal medicines sold in pharmacies. The Commission E has approved the use of chaste tree extract for the treatment of PMS, cyclical mastalgia, and menstrual irregularity (4).

MECHANISM OF ACTION

Several mechanisms have been proposed to explain the beneficial effects of a chaste tree extract on PMS, cyclical mastalgia, irregular menses, and infertility. It is known that a chaste tree preparation acts, in part, by reducing prolactin, increasing progesterone, and binding opioid receptors (5). This binding of opioid receptors (6) may be the primary mechanism involved in PMS. Women with severe PMS show symptoms of transient impairment of central opioid tone during the luteal phase of their menstrual cycle (7). Symptoms such as anxiety, food cravings, and physical discomfort are directly and inversely proportional to the decline of β-endorphin levels (8). This rapid decline in β-endorphin levels may cause a mild opioid-withdrawal syndrome, leading women to experience an increase in pain, headache, mood swings, and water retention (9). Compounds in chaste tree berry also bind dopamine (D2) receptors in the hypothalamus and anterior pituitary, inhibiting the release of prolactin (10). Prolactin plays a role in breast stimulation and may result in cyclical mastalgia. Nonlactating women with elevated levels of prolactin often present with ovulatory disorders, infertility, and/or galactorrhea. Elevation of prolactin can cause corpus luteum insufficiency, defined as an abnormally low level of progesterone three weeks after the onset of menstruation, through suppression of luteinizing hormone (LH). Women with corpus luteum insufficiency typically have a shortened second half of their menstrual cycle and may have difficulty conceiving and maintaining pregnancy.

CLINICAL EVIDENCE

PMS

The most rigorous study to date of chaste tree for PMS was a three-month, double-blind, placebo-controlled trial by Schellenberg that randomized 170 women diagnosed with PMS to receive 20 mg fruit extract (ZE 440: 60% ethanol m/m, extract ratio 6–12:1; standardized for casticin) or placebo (11). Five of the six self-assessment items indicated significant superiority for chaste tree (irritability, mood alteration, anger, headache, and breast fullness). Other symptoms, including bloating, were unaffected by treatment. Overall, the reduction in symptoms was 52% for the active versus 24% for placebo (P < 0.001). The authors of the trial concluded, "*Agnus castus* is a well tolerated and effective treatment for premenstrual syndrome, the effects being confirmed by physicians and patients alike."

A study comparing 20–40 mg per day of chaste tree extract to 20–40 mg per day of fluoxetine for women (ages 25–45) diagnosed with premenstrual dysphoric disorder (PMDD) and having regular menstrual cycles failed to note any significant difference between the two groups with respect to the Hamilton Depression Rating Scale (HAM-D), Clinical Global Impression Scale-Severity of Illness (CGI-SI), or Clinical Global Impression-Improvement (CGI-I) (12). Unfortunately, the authors did not provide any details regarding the chaste tree product (e.g., extraction method, extract strength, etc.).

An older, randomized, double-blind, placebo-controlled study of 600 women with PMS taking chaste tree (600 mg capsules three times a day) for three months showed improvement only in restlessness (13). The study suffers from a significant dropout rate; only 217 participants were included in the final evaluation. This dose is also much higher than typically used. One comparative trial found chaste tree to be as equally effective as pyridoxine for relieving PMS symptoms; however, the efficacy of pyridoxine in PMS remains inconclusive (14).

Safety

A drug-monitoring study conducted on a proprietary chaste tree product, Agnolyt (Agnolyt contains 9 grams of a 1:5 tincture for each 100 grams of aqueous-alcoholic solution; Dr. Madaus GmbH and Co., Cologne, Germany), reported that 32 of 1,542 (2.1%) women treated with an average of 42 drops daily of Agnolyt solution for over five months experienced side effects. Most common were gastrointestinal complaints, acne, and nausea (15). The relative lack of significant adverse events, however, is reassuring.

Based upon this evidence and the rather benign, though admittedly troublesome, nature of mild PMS, it seems reasonable for clinicians to recommend chaste tree for women who choose not to use oral contraceptives or have only minor benefit from lifestyle changes. However, as many of these women may be of an age where pregnancy could be likely to occur, it would be useful to have safety information that specifically addresses this issue. Indeed, it is rather surprising that there is a paucity of information regarding safety during pregnancy, since chaste tree has been studied for female infertility and is recommended for this purpose by some herbalists and midwives.

Infertility

There is some scientific basis for its use in infertility. Chaste tree extracts have been shown to restore progesterone levels and prolong the hyperthermic phase in the basal body temperature curve when used daily for at least three months (16). Increasing progesterone levels and enhancing the function of the corpus luteum can improve female fertility. Two small evaluations in women with infertility not related to endocrine disorders (i.e., hyperprolactinemia, androgen, or thyroid) have been published. The first included 18 women with corpus luteum insufficiency, as evidenced by low progesterone levels three weeks after onset of menstruation. Progesterone levels increased in nine women, returning to normal ranges in seven participants. Fourteen of the 18 women achieved a sustained hyperthermic basal body temperature during the luteal phase. Two women became pregnant during the three-month trial using 40 drops per day of Agnolyt (9 grams of 1:5 extract per 100 g solution; 58% ethanol; Madaus). The authors of the second study (n=48 women with corpus luteum insufficiency) reportedly used chaste tree initially to correct the luteal phase abnormality and then, if needed, implemented hormone therapy to increase fertility (17).

In addition to these small studies using chaste tree as a monotherapy, in 1998, a double-blind, placebo-controlled trial included 96 women with menstrual irregularities (secondary amenorrhea n=38, luteal insufficiency n=31, and idiopathic infertility n=27) who were randomized to receive placebo or Mastodynon solution (30 drops BID) for three months (Mastodynon: 10 g tincture contains 2 g crude drug 53% ethanol; *Vitex agnus castus*, *Caulophyllum thalictroides*, Cyclamen, Ignatia, Iris, and *Lilium tigrinum*: manufactured by Bionorica). Only 66 women were available for evaluation. The authors reported that pregnancy occurred more than twice as often in the treatment group (n=8; 15%) than in the placebo group (n=3; 7%) (18). Of course, there were more than twice the number of women desiring pregnancy in the treatment group, and the trial suffered from a significant number of dropouts. It is also difficult to ascertain if it was chaste tree or the combination of ingredients that was responsible for the purported effect. It is unclear how much blue cohosh (*Caulophyllum thalictroides*) is present in the product; however, there are significant concerns regarding its safety in early pregnancy, given that compounds in blue cohosh are teratogenic in rat embryo cultures (19).

Menstrual irregularity, anovulation, and infertility can also result from hyperprolactinemia. A randomized, double-blind, placebo-controlled study of 52 women with latent hyperprolactinemia and luteal phase defect was conducted using 20 mg per day of chaste tree fruit aqueous alcohol dry extract (Strotan Capsules: 3 mg dry extract per capsule [10–16:1 extract 60% ethanol]; Strathmann AG) or placebo (20). Blood was drawn on days 5 through 8 and on day 20 of the menstrual cycle, before and after three months of therapy for hormonal analysis. Thirty-seven women were available for statistical evaluation (placebo: n = 20, treatment: n = 17). Chaste tree lowered prolactin release in response to thyroid releasing hormone (TRH) stimulation compared to placebo (p < 0.001), lengthened the luteal phase by five days, and restored low progesterone levels to the normal range after three months of use. Beta-estradiol levels were increased during the luteal phase in those receiving chaste tree; all other hormone levels remained unchanged. No side effects were noted within the study.

In a small, open clinical trial using a combination product, Vitex Mastodynon, the authors reported a reduction in prolactin levels and normalization of menstrual cycles in 13 women with hyperprolactinemia when used daily for three consecutive menstrual cycles (21). Two of the women taking the product during the study became pregnant without any adverse effects to the fetus. The same comments mentioned previously with this product hold true here as well.

Interestingly, given the aforementioned data, it might be hard to reconcile the occasional recommendation by herbalists for using chaste tree to promote breast milk production. However, the effect on prolactin might be dose related. A study in men found that treatment with 120 mg of chaste tree (BNO 1095 by Bionorica) increased prolactin levels by 16% compared to placebo (p < 0.03), the 240 mg dose resulted in no change in prolactin, and only the 480 mg dose caused a reduction in prolactin compared to placebo (22).

MY OWN CLINICAL EXPERIENCE

Taken as a whole, this research is highly intriguing to me, given my own clinical experience. Chaste tree has always been one of my favorite and most versatile herbs in clinical practice. It is hard to imagine a PMS treatment plan that did not include this herb or a formulation for the perimenopausal woman experiencing irregular menstruation. I have worked with dozens of women over the years who successfully used chaste tree to regulate their menstrual cycles and then went on to become pregnant after many months or years of trying. I have also found chaste tree beneficial for maintaining pregnancy in women with repeated first-trimester miscarriages when taken for the first 12 to 14 weeks.

CASE REPORT

While working at the Indian Health Service in Albuquerque, New Mexico, I cared for a patient in her twenties who was diagnosed with hyperprolactinemia secondary to a pituitary microadenoma. After the appropriate work-up and referrals, I prescribed bromocriptine, which she discontinued approximately four weeks later because of nausea, vomiting, and headaches. I recommended chaste tree (500 mg/d crude dried fruit), and her prolactin levels fell and her menses returned, though there was little change on MRI. She stayed on the chaste tree for the year I was her physician, with her prolactin remaining in the high normal range.

THE MARKETPLACE CONUNDRUM

Given the dramatic increase in the use of botanical remedies and the sheer number of products, it is understandable that consumers and health care professionals alike have difficulty navigating the supplement marketplace as well as translating the research into clinical guidance. Questions such as "Which product should I take?" "At what dose?" "Will it interact with my medication?" "Is it safe?" and "Will it work?" plague anyone who has ever looked down a supplement aisle. Herein lies one of the key problems with translating the research into clinical practice. In the event that a woman and her clinician decide that a trial of chaste tree would be a good idea for addressing her PMS, invariably the conversation will turn to the questions of "which product" at "what dose." The practitioner will most likely tell her to buy a "good-quality product" and take what it "says on the label." Or the astute practitioner might recommend that she use the product that was studied in a clinical trial (at a dose of 20 mg per day). However, the product used in the best clinical trial, ZE440, is not available in the United States at the time of this writing. And what consumer or practitioner would know how to interpret "60% ethanol m/m, extract ratio 6–12:1, standardized for casticin" to find an equivalent product?

DECIPHERING THE PRODUCT LABEL

A quick perusal of the product aisle at a local health food shop in Tucson, Arizona, yielded no fewer than 22 products containing chaste tree, either alone or in combination with other herbs such as black cohosh, black haw, blue cohosh, cramp bark, dong quai, evening primrose oil, ginseng, hops, nettles, raspberry leaf, partridge berry, schisandra, valerian, wild yam, and a host of others—each product promising to "balance your female hormones"—whatever that precisely means! We can look at three products containing only chaste tree to illustrate some of the difficulties clinicians face when recommending herbal products. Figure 12.1 shows the supplement fact boxes on labels from three of them.

The first label indicates a similar dose to the one used in a clinical trial (40 mg vs. 20 mg). But how does one interpret the label? Is this material an extract? If so, at what strength? Or does each capsule contain 40 mg of ground-up crude chaste tree fruit? Not likely, as 40 mg of chaste tree would not fill a capsule of any size. The second label indicates that the product contains 215 mg of chaste tree berry and 25 mg of *Vitex agnus castus*. What exactly does this mean? Chaste tree berry is the same as *Vitex agnus castus*. Therefore, does this mean 215 mg of crude chaste tree and 25 mg of extract? And if so, what is the strength of the extract?

The third label is from a product providing a relatively higher dose of chaste tree than used in the clinical trial, but since the label does not provide the strength of extract, there is no way to know what "225 mg" means. Unlike the other products, it claims that it is standardized to a compound in chaste tree. In this case, it is agnusides, not casticin. Does that matter?

Supplement Facts

Serving Size: 1 Capsule
Servings per Container: 90

	Amount Per Serving	% Daily Value
Vitex Agnus Castus (Chastetree berry)	40 mg	*

*Daily value not established.

Figure 12.1. First Label

Supplement Facts

Serving Size: 1 Capsule
Servings per Container: 60

	Amount Per Serving	% Daily Value*
Chaste Tree Berry	215 mg	**
Vitex Agnus Castus	25 mg	**

* Based on a 2,000 calorie diet
**Daily value not established.

Figure 12.2. Second Label

Supplement Facts

Serving Size: 1 Capsule
Servings per Container: 240

	Amount Per Serving	% Daily Value
Chasteberry Extract (standardized to 0.5% agnusides)(Vitex agnus-castus)	225 mg	*

*Daily value not established.

Figure 12.3. Third Label

Figures 12.1–12.3. Examples of Three Supplement Fact Boxes for Chaste Tree Products

It is difficult, and often impossible, for the average clinician, even the most open minded and interested, to translate the information from clinical studies to the products found in the marketplace. And perhaps, even beyond this confusion, concerns about the quality of dietary supplements in general, and botanical remedies in particular, make recommending products challenging. There are numerous reports in the popular media and professional literature regarding adulteration and contamination of products, as well as variation between what is printed on the label and what is actually present in the bottle. While many manufacturers produce high-quality botanical products, the unscrupulous and incompetent have, unfortunately, tarnished the industry, making it difficult for consumers and clinicians to separate the good from the bad. While it is hoped that the new CGMPs (Current Good Manufacturing Practices) will improve quality throughout the industry, realistically, this uncertainty in quality is a very real barrier for many clinicians, who do not want to recommend a product that may turn out to harm their patient because of poor quality.

CHALLENGES WITH THE RESEARCH

Clinicians and consumers often believe that one brand of a particular herbal product is interchangeable with another: the belief that if you hear about one study, you can generalize the results to any product containing that herb. But this is not true. The herbal preparations used often vary considerably from trial to trial, making comparison difficult, as products may not be biologically or pharmacologically equivalent. Because of the complex nature of botanicals and variation in constituents between species, plant part, and preparation, it is essential that researchers clearly provide an adequate description of the product used in their clinical trial. Descriptions should include identification (Latin binomial and authority), plant part (root, leaf, seed, etc.), and type of preparation (tea, tincture, extract, oil, etc.). Tincture and extract description should include the identity of the solvent and the ratio of solvent to plant material. The botanical should be well characterized, and if standardized to a particular constituent, then that information should also be included. If the research product bears little resemblance to crude plant material or simple extracts found in the marketplace, then that should also be clearly stated. Precise and clear dose and dosage form should be provided. The study that used chaste tree for the treatment of PMDD had no description of the product in the paper, making it impossible for other researchers to replicate the study or for a clinician to adequately counsel a patient about product choice. Peer-reviewed journals must mandate that this information be part of any paper accepted for publication.

CRITICAL COMMENTARY

As was seen in the local health food store in Tucson, herbal products generally contain a mixture of plants. This is often because herbalists generally prescribe herbal mixtures instead of single-herb preparations, based upon the premise that when properly prepared, herbal mixtures offer greater efficacy. An example would be the perimenopausal woman who is complaining of irregular menses, moodiness, and occasional hot flashes. One approach might be to consider a formulation that included chaste tree and black cohosh. Chaste tree would be included to help with the irregular menstruation and black cohosh to address the moodiness and hot flashes. However, clinical trials are generally not conducted on herbal formulations, and when they are, the formulations are not constructed using any scientifically founded, rigorous process. The marketplace is no better. Products often have up to a dozen herbs thrown together in haphazard fashion, with no basis for the combination in tradition or modern research. Unfortunately, given the number of traditional medical systems that utilize herbal formulations, the focus on botanical monotherapies may be a critical shortcoming in botanical research.

While most herbal practitioners consider the "whole herb" to be active, there may be times when the basic science demonstrates that a primary activity is the result of a particular compound or compounds. For instance, casticin appears to be the compound most responsible for reducing prolactin levels (23). This might be critically important in a clinical trial for hyperprolactinemia or infertility. It would be important for this information to be clearly conveyed so that clinicians treating patients could appropriately recommend the right type of product. Along this same line of reasoning, the compound, agnuside, but not casticin, has been shown to exert estrogen-like activity in vitro (24). Would guaranteeing a minimum level of agnuside in chaste tree extracts yield a superior product for the irregular menses seen in perimenopause (a very common use of chaste tree)?

When reviewing the doses used in research and the "serving sizes" recommended for products in the marketplace, there is little consistency to be found. One could look back at the doses recommended in the historic literature, but the waters get murky quite quickly, especially in the United States. In addition to the folk traditions of the past 200 years, the influence of both the eclectic and physiomedicalist practices of the nineteenth century can still be felt in American herbalism. Eclectic practitioners tended to use large, or "heroic," doses of botanicals, including many that would be considered toxic. The physiomedicalist approach abhorred this heroic approach and tended to use smaller doses, or "drop" dosing. Clearly, there is a need for evidence-based, modern research to include dose-ranging studies prior to conducting any large clinical trial. Scientifically based dose ranges for particular dosage forms would also give clinicians and consumers greater confidence in the use of herbal remedies.

DOSE LEVELS

In the case of chaste tree, the dose may have a great deal to do with the clinical effect, as seen in the study in men showing an inhibition of prolactin only at a higher dose. Without proper dose-ranging studies, one could easily imagine a negative result using the very low dosages of chaste tree seen in some of the previous research, in a clinical trial assessing its efficacy for latent hyperprolactinemia. This would be an important study, given that the drugs currently approved for hyperprolactinemia, namely, cabergoline and bromocriptine, have side effects that many women find intolerable, including nausea, headache, fatigue, insomnia, vertigo, and much more rarely psychiatric manifestations such as depression or hallucinations.

SAFETY PROFILES

Most clinicians are willing to recommend, and certainly many women are willing to try, a remedy that might relieve PMS symptoms if deemed to have a relatively good safety profile. But it is rare to find a clinician who would recommend a product such as chaste tree berry for enhancing fertility without detailed reproductive safety data readily available. Thus, one of the most important research questions for chaste tree, and for any other herb being marketed to women during their reproductive years, should be "Is it safe during pregnancy?" Women are taking chaste tree for PMS, irregular menstruation, and infertility. There are some basic science and clinical trial data that support these uses, but there is little research adequately addressing its safety, particularly during the first trimester. And while no significant adverse events have been reported, there remains a tremendous need for safety studies. This question must be answered before any research could be conducted assessing the possible role of chaste tree in female infertility.

CONCLUSIONS

The challenges presented in this chapter are very real and complicated by a chaotic marketplace and often disorganized research agenda. As revealed throughout history and confirmed through contemporary research, plants have played an important role in women's health. However, there remains much work to be done "from bench to bedside." It is important to identify which botanicals are most efficacious for a given condition as well as how they compare with conventional treatments in terms of safety, effectiveness, and cost. Pharmacokinetic and pharmacodynamic studies are essential as well as research on safety during pregnancy and lactation.

Chaste tree appears to be a viable and safe approach for PMS, especially for women who choose not to take oral contraceptives and for whom lifestyle changes are not enough. Chaste tree may have the potential to address certain types of female infertility, which could be very cost effective if proven clinically effective. For PMS and infertility, the herb will be taken by women of reproductive age—so the question of safety in pregnancy is an extremely important one. If chaste tree can correct latent hyperprolactinemia, this would mean a safer and more tolerable treatment for many women. But before this can be studied, dose-ranging studies in women specifically looking at prolactin levels are imperative. And basic science is needed to determine what constituent(s), if any, should be considered for standardization based upon the condition being treated.

There is definitely a need for more rigorous and creative research in the area of botanicals and women's health. The researcher studies the efficacy and mechanism of a given therapy so that broad numbers of patients may potentially benefit from the treatment. Clinicians working in the field of women's health are keenly aware that treatments must often be tailored to meet the individual needs of the woman and that there is often not one simple answer. Clinicians and researchers could benefit greatly from more extensive dialogue with each other—so that each can share their unique experiences and worldviews, learning from each other to improve both research and clinical care. For in spite of the lack of rigorous research for many botanicals, it is highly likely that many women will continue to seek out these therapies as a means of self-treatment and self-care.

REFERENCES

[1]Upchurch DM, Chyu L, Greendale GA, Utts J, Bair YA, Zhang G, Gold EB. Complementary and alternative medicine use among American women: findings from the National Health Interview Survey, 2002. *J Womens Health* (Larchmt). 2007;16:102–113.

[2]Vickers K, Jolly KB, Greenfield SM. Herbal medicine: women's views, knowledge and interaction with doctors: a qualitative study. *BMC Complement Altern Med*. 2006;6:40.

[3]American College of Obstetrics and Gynecology: Committee opinion. *Int J Gynecol Obstet*. 1995:50:80.

[4]Blumenthal M, Goldberg A, Brinckmann J, eds. *Herbal Medicine. Expanded Commission E Monographs. Integrative Medicine, Communications*. 1st ed. Newton, MA: Integrative Medicine Communications; 2000.

[5]Webster DE, Lu J, Chen SN, Farnsworth NR, Wang ZJ. Activation of the mu-opiate receptor by *Vitex agnus-castus* methanol extracts: implication for its use in PMS. *J Ethnopharmacol*. 2006 Jun 30;106(2):216–221.

[6]Meier B, et al. Pharmacological activities of *Vitex agnus castus* extracts *in vitro*. *Phytomedicine*. 2000;7: 373–381.

[7]Rapkin AJ, Shoupe D, Reading A, Daneshgar KK, Goldman L, Bohn Y, Brann DW, Mahesh VB. Decreased central opioid activity in premenstrual syndrome: luteinizing hormone response to naloxone. *J Soc Gynecol Investig*. 1996;3: 93–98.

[8]Giannini AJ, Melemis SM, Martin DM, Folts DJ. Symptoms of premenstrual syndrome as a function of beta-endorphin: two subtypes. *Prog Neuropsychopharmacol Biol Psychiatry*. 1994;18:321–327.

[9]Mortola JF. Premenstrual syndrome. *Trends Endocrinol Metab*. 1996;7:184–189.

[10]Wuttke W, Jarry H, Christoffel V, Spengler B, Seidlová-Wuttke D. Chaste tree (*Vitex agnus-castus*): pharmacology and clinical indications. *Phytomedicine*. 2003 May;10(4):348–357.

[11]Schellenberg R. Treatment for the premenstrual syndrome with *agnus castus* fruit extract: prospective, randomised, placebo controlled study. *BMJ*. 2001;322:134–137.

[12]Atmaca M, Kumru S, Tezcan E. Fluoxetine versus *Vitex agnus castus* extract in the treatment of premenstrual dysphoric disorder. *Hum Psychopharmacol*. 2003;18:191–195.

[13]Turner S, Mills S. A double-blind clinical trial on a herbal remedy for premenstrual syndrome: a case study. *Complement Ther Med*. 1993:1:73–77.

[14]Lauritzen CH, Reuter HD, Repges R, et al. Treatment of premenstrual tension syndrome with *Vitex agnus-castus*: controlled, double-blind study versus pyridoxine. *Phytomedicine*. 1997;4:183–189.

[15]Dittmar FW, Bohnert KJ, Peeters M, et al. Premenstrual syndrome treatment with a phytopharmaceutical. *TW Gynakologie*. 1992;5:60–68. (Original paper in German.)

[16]Newall CA, et al. *Herbal Medicines: A Guide for Health-Care Professionals*. London: Pharmaceutical Press; 1996:19–20.

[17]Propping D, Katzorke T, Belkien L. Diagnosis and therapy of corpus luteum deficiency in general practice. *Therapiewoche*. 1988;38:2992–3001.

[18]Original work by Gerhard et al. 1998. Presented at the Oklahoma City Women's Health Conference Sept 27, 2000.

[19]Kennelly EJ, Flynn TJ, Mazzola EP, et al. Detecting potential teratogenic alkaloids from blue cohosh rhizomes using an *in vitro* rat embryo culture. *J Nat Prod*. 1999;62(10): 1385–1389.

[20]Milewicz A, et al. Vitex agnus castus extract in the treatment of luteal phase defects due to latent hyperprolactinemia: results of a randomized placebo-controlled double-blind study. *Arzneimittelforschung*. 1993;43: 752–756.

[21]Roeder DA. Therapy of cyclic disorders with *Vitex agnus-castus*. Zeitschrift fur *Phytotherapie*. 1994;14: 155–159.

[22]Merz PG, Gorkow C, Schrodter A, et al. The effects of a special *Agnus castus* extract (BP1095E1) on prolactin secretion in healthy male subjects. *Exp Clin Endocrinol Diabetes*. 1996;104:447–453.

[23]Hu Y, Xin HL, Zhang QY, Zheng HC, Rahman K, Qin LP. Anti-nociceptive and antihyperprolactinemia activities of *Fructus Viticis* and its effective fractions and chemical constituents. *Phytomedicine*. 2007 Oct;14(10):668–674.

[24]Hu Y, Hou TT, Zhang QY, Xin HL, Zheng HC, Rahman K, Qin LP. Evaluation of the estrogenic activity of the constituents in the fruits of *Vitex rotundifolia* L. for the potential treatment of premenstrual syndrome. *J Pharm Pharmacol*. 2007 Sep;59(9):1307–1312.

INDEX